C0-BWL-307

# WILSON'S DISEASE

*Editor*
Daniel Bergsma, M.D.

*Associate Editors*
I. Herbert Scheinberg, M.D.
Irmin Sternlieb, M.D.

*Assistant Editor*
Camille Jackson

*Art and Production Director*
Hal L. Childs

*Birth Defects Original Article Series, Vol. IV, No. 2; April, 1968*

Received for publication November 2, 1967.



Library of Congress Catalog Card Number: 68-22582.

Printed in U.S.A.

To enhance medical communication in the birth defects field, The National Foundation publishes an *Original Article Series,* a *Reprint Series,* monthly *Abstracts of Selected Articles* and provides a series of films and related brochures.

Further information can be obtained from:

Daniel Bergsma, M.D.
Director-Medical Department
The National Foundation-March of Dimes
800 Second Avenue
New York, New York 10017

# FOREWORD

In September, 1960, an International Symposium on Wilson's Disease was held in London under the direction of Drs. John M. Walshe and John N. Cumings. The results of that Symposium were published (Wilson's Disease, Some Current Concepts, edited by John M. Walshe and John N. Cumings, Blackwell Scientific Publications, Oxford 1961) as a summary of the knowledge of the disorder. This proved to be of considerable value to those physicians and biochemists investigating Wilson's disease.

Early in 1964 Dr. Masataka Arima, a pediatrician who has studied the genetics of Wilson's disease, introduced me, via correspondence, to Professor Yawara Yoshitoshi. Over the course of the next few months we formulated plans for a Second International Symposium devoted to Wilson's disease to be held at the time of, though independently from, the meetings in Japan of the 1966 World Congress of Gastroenterology and the International Association for the Study of Liver Diseases. The views of other researchers were sought and there was general agreement that the work that had been done since the 1960 meeting merited another intensive exchange of information.

The present volume consists of papers presented at these meetings which were held on September 20th-21st, 1966 at the International House of Japan in Tokyo. Although taped recordings of the discussions were made, it proved impractical to incorporate either transcripts or summaries of them in the volume. However, each author was asked to edit the manuscript which he had presented at the meeting and was urged to feel free to include material, or modify his paper, in the light of the vigorous discussions at the Symposium.

It is obvious that this volume is the product of many minds and hands. Without the work of the Japanese members of the Organizing Committee there would, of course, have been no Symposium at all. Each of the authors responded cheerfully – and in almost all cases reasonably promptly! – to our urgings to complete preparation and revision of their manuscripts.

Finally, I should like to thank expressly those individuals of The National Foundation-March of Dimes who helped so greatly in preparing this volume in final form, and to the Foundation itself for assuring its publication.

I. Herbert Scheinberg

*March 4, 1968*

# Contents

# Introductory Remarks

I. Herbert Scheinberg, M.D.

All of us who came from overseas would like to thank Professors Yoshitoshi, Miyake, Nakao and Takatsu for the extraordinarily delightful arrangements they made for us. For many of us this was our first visit to Japan and all of us were made to feel at home.

Over half a century ago Wilson[1] and Garrod[2] independently and almost simultaneously laid the dual cornerstones of our present understanding of hepatolenticular degeneration: Wilson extracted the syndrome from a group of heterogeneous neurologic diseases, and Garrod first defined inborn errors of metabolism, although no one at that time knew that Wilson's disease would prove to be one. No one knew . . . but Wilson, in his earliest monograph, was aware of the familial nature of the disease, and by 1921 Hall[3] first clearly suggested that Wilson's disease was in fact inherited in autosomal recessive fashion.

Within a year of Wilson's monograph a hint appeared in the literature, in a paper by Rumpel,[4] that abnormalities in metal metabolism might have something to do with Wilson's disease, and in the succeeding two decades Lüthy, Haurowitz and Glazebrook[5-7] incriminated copper as the probable villain. Even before Wilson's work, Kayser[8] and Fleischer[9] had observed the rings, which Wilson finally accepted as an almost universal sign of his disease, and which contain copper.

The breakthrough which led to the greatest diagnostic and therapeutic advances was made by Mandelbrote, Stanier, Thompson and Thruston[10] when they showed that only the urine of a patient with Wilson's disease, among specimens from a number of individuals with various neurologic disorders, contained a large concentration of copper. Soon thereafter, Cumings[11] demonstrated an excessive amount of copper in the tissues of the nervous system of patients with this illness and, even more importantly, suggested that removal of copper by British anti-Lewisite might arrest the progression of the disease. Denny-Brown and Porter[12] administered BAL, around 1950, to five patients with Wilson's disease and found marked improvement in three of these.

In the next year the clinical significance of deficiency of ceruloplasmin in the serum of patients with Wilson's disease was demonstrated and it became possible, for the first time, to diagnose this illness while the patient was still free of signs or symptoms of the disorder (Scheinberg and Gitlin[13]).

Finally, in 1956, Walshe[14] discovered that penicillamine, or $\beta$, $\beta$-dimethylcysteine, administered orally to patients with Wilson's disease, greatly promoted the excretion of copper in the urine. Thereby it became feasible to produce, and maintain for a long period, a negative balance of copper in patients with this illness.

The disease discussed in this symposium is a striking example of the interaction of heredity and environment. Its pathogenesis is understood to a degree which is true of very few diseases. It may be diagnosed, with certainty, in individuals who are apparently in the best of health. Its treatment is often followed by dramatic therapeutic results. And, with sufficiently early diagnosis and prophylaxis, the appearance of clinical manifestations may, perhaps, be completely prevented.

## *REFERENCES*


1. Wilson, S.A.K.: Progressive lenticular degeneration. A familial nervous disease associated with cirrhosis of the liver. *Brain,* **34:**295-509, 1912.
2. Garrod, A. E.: Inborn errors of metabolism (Croonian Lectures). *Lancet,* **ii:**1, 73, 142, 214, 1908.
3. Hall, H. C.: La Dégénérescence Hépato-Lenticulaire. Maladie de Wilson — Pseudo-Sclérose. Masson et Cie, Paris, 1921.
4. Rumpel, A.: Über das Wesen und die Bedeutung der Leberveränderungen und der Pigmentierungen bei den damit verbundenen Fällen von Pseudosklerose, zugleich ein Beitrag zur Lehre von der Pseudosklerose (Westphal-Strümpell). *Dtsch. Z. Nervenheilk.,* **49:**54-73, 1913.
5. Lüthy, F.: Über die hepato-lentikuläre Degeneration (Wilson-Westphal-Strümpell). *Dtsch. Z. Nervenheilk.,* **123:**101-181, 1931-1932.
6. Haurowitz, F.: Über eine Anomalie des Kupfestoff Wechsels. *Hoppe-Seylers Z. physiol. Chem.,* **190:**72-74, 1930.
7. Glazebrook, A. J.: Wilson's disease. *Edinb. med. J.,* **52:**83-87, 1945.
8. Kayser, B.: Über einen Fall von angeborener grünlicher Verfärbung der Kornea. *Klin. Mbl. Augenheilk.,* **40:**22-25, 1902.
9. Fleischer, B.: Die periphere braun-grünliche Hornhautverfärbung als Symptom einer eigenartigen Allgemeinerkrankung. *Münch. Med. Wschr.,* **56:**1120-1123, 1909.
10. Mandelbrote, B. M.; Stanier, M. W.; Thompson, R. H. S. and Thruston, M. N.: Studies on copper metabolism in demyelinating diseases of the central nervous system. *Brain,* **17:**212-228, 1948.
11. Cumings, J. N.: The copper and iron content of brain and liver in the normal and in hepatolenticular degeneration. *Brain,* **71:**410-415, 1948.
12. Denny-Brown, D. and Porter, H.: The effect of BAL (2, 3-dimercaptopropanol) on hepatolenticular degeneration (Wilson's disease). *New Engl. J. Med.,* **254:**917-925, 1951.
13. Scheinberg, I. H. and Gitlin, D.: Deficiency of ceruloplasmin in patients with hepatolenticular degeneration (Wilson's disease). *Science,* **116:**484-485, 1952.
14. Walshe, J.M.: Wilson's disease. New oral therapy. *Lancet,* **i:**25-26, 1956.

## Organizing Committee

**Masashi Miyake, M.D.,** University of Tokyo Faculty of Medicine, Tokyo, Japan

**Kiku Nakao, M.D.,** University of Tokyo Faculty of Medicine, Tokyo, Japan

**I. Herbert Scheinberg, M.D.,** Albert Einstein College of Medicine, Bronx, New York

**Tadao Takatsu, M.D.,** University of Tokyo Faculty of Medicine, Tokyo, Japan

**Yawara Yoshitoshi, M.D.,** University of Tokyo Faculty of Medicine, Tokyo, Japan

## Participants

**Masataka Arima, M.D.,** Toho University School of Medicine, Tokyo, Japan

**Iwao Arioka, M.D.,** Nara Medical University, Kashihara, Nara, Japan

**R. Quentin Blackwell, Ph.D.,** U.S. Naval Medical Research Unit No. 2, Taipei, Taiwan

**Georges Boudin, M.D.,** Hôpital Saint-Antoine, Paris, France

**Paul A. Farrer, M.B., B.S.,** University of Rochester School of Medicine and Dentistry, Rochester, New York

**James W. Fresh, M.D. CDR, MC,** U.S. Naval Medical Research Unit No. 2, Taipei, Taiwan

**Norman P. Goldstein, M.D.,** Mayo Graduate School of Medicine, Rochester, Minnesota

**Tadashi Inose, M.D.,** Yokohama University School of Medicine, Yokohama, Japan

**Shibanosuke Katsuki, M.D.,** Faculty of Medicine, Kyushu University, Fukuoka, Japan

**Venard R. Kinney, M.D.,** Mayo Graduate School of Medicine, Rochester, Minnesota

**Joachim Lange, M.D.,** University of Bonn and Municipal Hospital, Gummersbach, West Germany

**John T. McCall, Ph.D.,** Mayo Graduate School of Medicine, Rochester, Minnesota

**Kazuo Mori, M.D.,** University of Tokyo Faculty of Medicine, Tokyo, Japan

**Toshiji Mozai, M.D.,** University of Tokyo Faculty of Medicine, Tokyo, Japan

**Mitsumasa Nagase, M.D.,** University of Tokyo Faculty of Medicine, Tokyo, Japan

**Toshitsugu Oda, M.D.,** University of Tokyo Faculty of Medicine, Tokyo, Japan

**Kazuteru Ogihara, M.D.,** University of Tokyo Faculty of Medicine, Tokyo, Japan

**Makoto Okumura, M.D.,** Faculty of Medicine, Kyushu University, Fukuoka, Japan

**Chales A. Owen, Jr., M.D.,** Mayo Graduate School of Medicine, Rochester, Minnesota

**Bernard Pépin, M.D.,** Hôpital Saint-Antoine, Paris, France

**Hans Popper, M.D.,** Mount Sinai Medical School, New York, New York

**Huntington Porter, M.D.,** New England Medical Center Hospitals, Boston, Massachusetts

**Isamu Sano, M.D.,** University of Osaka, Osaka, Japan

**I. Herbert Scheinberg, M.D.,** Albert Einstein College of Medicine, Bronx, New York

**Sheila Sherlock, M.D.,** Royal Free Hospital, London, England

**Toshio Shikata, M.D.,** University of Tokyo Faculty of Medicine, Tokyo, Japan

**Mitiyuki Shimizu, M.D.,** Showa University Medical School, Tokyo, Japan

**Hirotsugu Shiraki, M.D.,** University of Tokyo Faculty of Medicine, Tokyo, Japan

**Mervin Silverberg, M.D.,** Bronx-Lebanon Hospital Center, Bronx, New York

**Irmin Sternlieb, M.D.,** Albert Einstein College of Medicine, Bronx, New York

**W. Newlon Tauxe, M.D.,** Mayo Graduate School of Medicine, Rochester, Minnesota

**Toshio Terao, M.D.,** University of Tokyo Faculty of Medicine, Tokyo, Japan

**Jun-bi Tu, M.D.,** Kingston General Hospital, Kingston, Ontario, Canada

**John M. Walshe, Sc.D., F.R.C.P.,** University of Cambridge, Cambridge, England

**Raymond H. Watten, Capt. MC USN,** U.S. Naval Medical Research Unit No. 2, Taipei, Taiwan

**Yoshiji Yamane, M.D.,** University of Tokyo Faculty of Medicine, Tokyo, Japan

**Yawara Yoshitoshi, M.D.,** University of Tokyo Faculty of Medicine, Tokyo, Japan

# Copper Metabolism in the Rat*

CHARLES A. OWEN, JR., M.D., Ph.D.** and JANE B. HAZELRIG, M.S.†

Copper metabolism was studied in rats with intravenous tracer doses of $^{64}Cu$. The $^{64}Cu$ concentrated rapidly in the liver and thence was excreted into the bile or returned to the blood as ceruloplasmin. The concentration of $^{64}Cu$ rose in several organs only after the $^{64}Cu$-ceruloplasmin had emerged, as if the ceruloplasmin were donating copper to the tissues. In copper-toxic rats, Wilson's disease was partially simulated; exaggerated hepatic uptake of $^{64}Cu$, reduced $^{64}Cu$-ceruloplasmin, and elevated hepatic and urinary copper.

During the past few years we have been studying the metabolism of copper in the rat by using $^{64}Cu$-labeled cupric acetate.[1] In general, when injected, radiocopper concentrates primarily in the liver, whether the liver is in an intact rat or is isolated in a perfusion system. Part of the hepatic copper is promptly excreted in the bile and the remainder is slowly returned to the bloodstream. This difference in time-concentration patterns suggests that the liver must be functioning as at least two separate subunits or compartments with regard to copper metabolism. Evidence for a third compartment will be presented. Once the radiocopper, now incorporated into ceruloplasmin, has returned to the blood of intact rats, the concentration of $^{64}Cu$ begins to increase in certain tissues. Therefore, it appears that ceruloplasmin functions as a copper donor for such tissues.

## Methods

*Animals.* – Male Sprague-Dawley rats were used; most of them weighed 250 to 300 gm.

*Perfusion of isolated rat livers.* – The technic was essentially that of Brauer and associates.[2] The freshly removed rat liver was perfused, via its portal vein, with 100 to 120 ml of fresh, pooled, heparinized rat blood. The perfusion apparatus was housed in a cabinet at 37°C and relative humidity greater than 50%. The perfusing blood was exposed to a 95% $O_2$-5% $CO_2$ gas mixture, prewarmed and humidified. The blood flowed through the liver under a hydrostatic pressure of 12 cm of blood, which, in the normal liver, is sufficient to maintain a hepatic blood flow rate well above the 1 ml/gram/minute considered minimally adequate. (Such livers make bile and excrete sulfobromophthalein normally for at least five hours.) Most perfusions were carried out for five hours. Bile was collected half-hourly and blood hourly, and the radioactivity in the liver was assayed at the end of the perfusion. During the perfusion, the radioactivity in the perfusing blood and in the liver was recorded continuously from two heavily shielded sodium iodide crystal-counter units.

*Tissue $^{64}Cu$.* – Small organs were assayed in their entirety in a well-counter (sodium iodide, thallium-activated crystal) against an aliquot of the dose of cupric-$^{64}Cu$ acetate injected into the rat or perfusion system. Aliquots of large organs (skin, muscle) were assayed and the weight of the whole organ was assumed to be 45.5% of body weight for muscle,[3] 18.5% for skin,[4] or 5.0% for blood.[5]

*Blood $^{64}Cu$.* – Whole blood and plasma were assayed in the well-counter against aliquots of the dose. In the liver perfusions, the exact blood volume was known and the plasma volumes were calculated from the hematocrit value (Wintrobe).

Ceruloplasmin-$^{64}Cu$ was estimated by complexing the free copper in the plasma with diethyldithiocarbamate and removing the complex with activated charcoal. The unadsorbed $^{64}Cu$ was assumed to be in ceruloplasmin.[6]

*Plasmatic ceruloplasmin.* – Ceruloplasmin was measured in "units" as 1,000 times the average change per minute in optical density at 435 m$\mu$ when 0.5 ml of plasma was added to an optimal concentration of buffered *p*-phenylenediamine (PPD). The readings were

---

*This investigation was supported in part by Research Grant AM-3932 from the National Institutes of Health, Public Health Service.

**Consultant, Section of Clinical Pathology and Section of Biochemistry, Mayo Clinic; Professor of Medicine (Medical Research), Mayo Graduate School of Medicine (University of Minnesota); Rochester, Minnesota.

†Consultant, Section of Biophysics, Mayo Clinic; Rochester, Minnesota.

taken each minute between the fifth and 15th minutes after the plasma was mixed with substrate (method described in personal communication from Dr. G. A. Fleisher, Section of Biochemistry, Mayo Clinic).

## ABOUT THE SENIOR AUTHOR

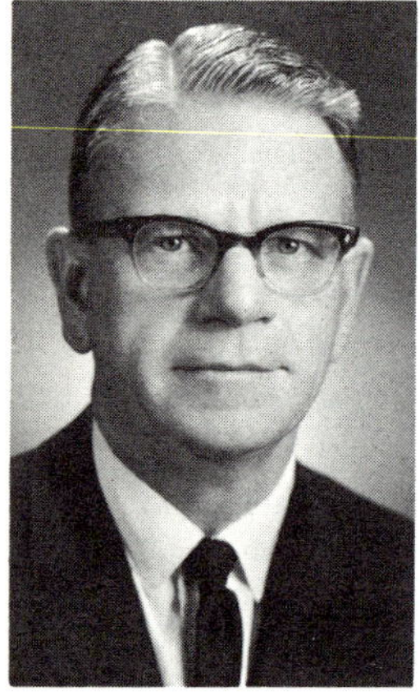

Dr. Charles Archibald Owen, Jr., head of the Section of Clinical Pathology and of a section of biochemistry in the Mayo Clinic, and professor of medicine (medical research) in the Mayo Graduate School of Medicine, University of Minnesota, Rochester, was born in Assiut, Egypt in 1915.

He received the degree of bachelor of arts in 1936 from Monmouth College and received the degree of doctor of medicine in 1941 from the State University of Iowa. In 1950 he received the degree of doctor of philosophy in medicine from the University of Minnesota. He was a research fellow in the State University of Iowa in 1938 and 1939.

Dr. Owen was certified as a specialist in pathology in 1954 by the American Board of Pathology, Inc. He is a fellow of the College of American Pathologists and a member of the American Association for the Advancement of Science, the American Association of Clinical Chemists, the American Chemical Society, the American Thyroid Association, the American Gastroenterological Association, the American Medical Association, the Society of Nuclear Medicine, the American Physiological Society, the American Society of Clinical Pathologists, the American Society for Experimental Pathology, the American Society of Hematology, the Central Society for Clinical Research, the International Society for Hematology, the New York Academy of Sciences, the Minnesota Society of Clinical Pathologists (president 1963-64), the Society for Experimental Biology and Medicine, the Zumbro Valley Medical Society, the Minnesota State Medical Association, the Society of the Sigma Xi, the Alumni Association of the Mayo Graduate School of Medicine, the Alpha Omega Alpha medical honor society and the Phi Rho Sigma professional medical fraternity.

Doctor Owen has contributed extensively to the literature on hematology, clinical pathology and biochemistry and in 1959 his book, *Diagnostic Radioisotopes*, was published by Charles C. Thomas. He is also the author of a chapter, with Dr. Eunice V. Flock, "Synthesis Transport and Degradation of Thyroid Hormones," in the volume, *The Thyroid*, published in 1964 by the International Academy of Pathology.

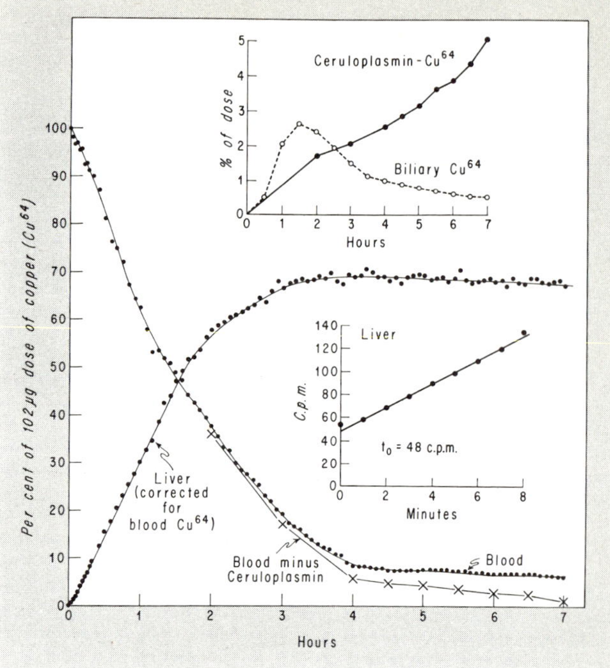


Fig. 1. Representative results of perfusion of a normal rat liver with 102 μg of copper labeled with $^{64}$Cu as cupric acetate. (Reproduced from Owen, C. A., Jr. and Hazelrig, J. B.: Metabolism of Cu$^{64}$-Labeled Copper by the Isolated Rat Liver. *Amer. J. Physiol.* **210**:1059-1064, 1966. By permission of the publisher.)

### Results

*Synthesis of ceruloplasmin by isolated rat liver.* — One hour after the liver had been perfused with blood containing $^{64}$Cu, almost half the dose was in the liver but only a small amount had returned to the blood as ceruloplasmin-$^{64}$Cu. The ceruloplasmin-$^{64}$Cu emerged in increasingly larger amounts during the next four hours. The patterns of hepatic uptake of $^{64}$Cu and release of the labeled ceruloplasmin closely resembled those found in the intact rat. A typical perfusion pattern is shown in Figure 1.

*Excretion of biliary $^{64}$Cu.* — Unlike ceruloplasmin-$^{64}$Cu which was just beginning to be secreted into the blood by the end of the first hour, biliary $^{64}$Cu was excreted rapidly and reached its peak between the first and second hours. Then, as ceruloplasmin-$^{64}$Cu was being released into the blood in steadily greater amounts, the biliary $^{64}$Cu excretion began to diminish (Fig. 1).

*Storage compartment in liver.* — From Table I it is clear that, as the dose of copper was increased, an increasingly large fraction of the dose accumulated in the isolated liver in five hours. This increased uptake was not accompanied by an increment in the biliary excretion of copper (Table II); the excretion was found, by linear regression analysis, to be essentially constant in doses up to 100 μg. Further, the cumulative percent of dose of copper which was returned to the plasma as ceruloplasmin actually decreased as the dose increased (Table III). Since the increased hepatic uptake of copper was accompanied by a constant excretion in the bile (in doses up to 100 μg) and a reduced secretion of ceruloplasmin, there was a net accumulation, or storage, in the liver with the progressively larger doses.

*Three-compartment hepatic system.* — A number of variations can be created about a basic model in which the central compartment (plasma) has free copper interchange with three hepatic compartments: one leading to storage, one to biliary excretion, and one to the synthesis of ceruloplasmin.[7] One compartmental system which satisfactorily conforms to our data is illustrated in Figure 2. Here the central compartment (plasma) is shown to contain copper in exchange with erythrocytes (and thus is the only significant nonhepatic tissue in the isolated liver system) and with three compartments of the liver. Figure 3 compares experimental data from perfusion experiments at four different doses of labeled copper with predictions based on the model.

TABLE I

**Hepatic Uptake of $^{64}$Cu-Labeled Copper (in Five Hours) by Isolated, Perfused Rat Liver**

| Dose (μg of Cu) | No. of experiments | Hepatic uptake of Cu: μg | Hepatic uptake of Cu: % of dose |
|---|---|---|---|
| 1 | 2 | 0.33 | 33 |
| 5 | 15 | 2.1 | 42 |
| 10 | 1 | 5.5 | 55 |
| 25 | 2 | 13.5 | 54 |
| 50 | 2 | 22.7 | 45 |
| 100 | 9 | 63.3 | 63 |
| 300 | 1 | 261 | 87 |
| 500 | 2 | 451 | 90 |
| 1,000 | 2 | 778 | 78 |

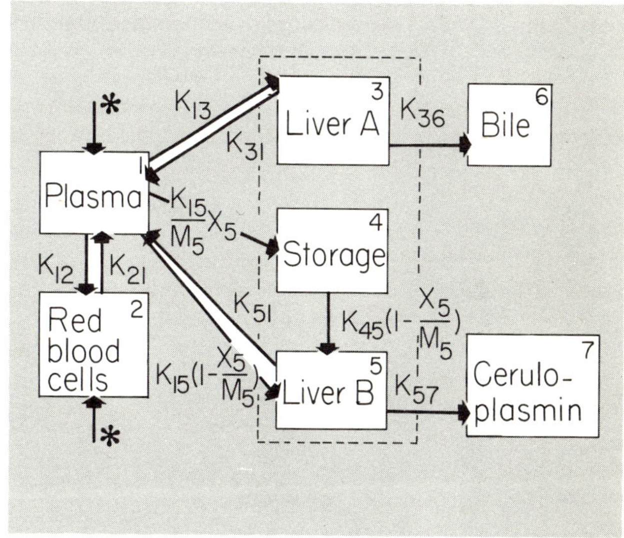


Fig. 2. Proposed model for handling of copper by isolated, perfused rat liver. Notations: $X_i$ = percent of administered dose in compartment *i* at time *t*; $K_{ij}$ = fraction of dose in compartment *i* being transferred to compartment *j* per unit time; M = maximal capacity of liver compartment, *B* expressed as percent of dose.

TABLE II

**Biliary Excretion of $^{64}$Cu by Isolated, Perfused Rat Liver**

| Dose (μg of Cu) | No. of experi-ments | % of dose,* hourly and total: 1 | 2 | 3 | 4 | 5 | Total | Total (μg) |
|---|---|---|---|---|---|---|---|---|
| 1 | 2 | 3.5 | **4.1** | 3.4 | 2.0 | 1.0 | 14.0 | 0.14 |
| 5 | 15 | 3.5 | **6.6** | 5.0 | 3.4 | 2.2 | 20.7 | 1.04 |
| 10 | 3 | 3.2 | **5.3** | 4.5 | 3.0 | 2.0 | 18.0 | 1.80 |
| 25 | 2 | 5.3 | **7.6** | 5.6 | 3.7 | 1.9 | 24.1 | 6.03 |
| 47 | 1 | **8.5** | 5.1 | 3.1 | 1.4 | 0.9 | 19.0 | 8.93 |
| 100 | 9 | 2.7 | **4.2** | 3.0 | 1.8 | 1.7 | 13.4 | 13.4 |
| 300 | 1 | 3.1 | **3.9** | 1.4 | 0.5 | 0.4 | 9.3 | 28.2 |
| 500 | 2 | 2.8 | **4.9** | 2.3 | 1.4 | 0.2 | 11.6 | 58.0 |
| 1,000 | 2 | 1.1 | **2.0** | **2.0** | 0.9 | 0.6 | 6.6 | 66.0 |

*Peak excretion shown in bold face.

TABLE III

**Synthesis and Secretion Into Plasma of Ceruloplasmin-$^{64}$Cu by Isolated, Perfused Rat Liver**

| Dose (μg of Cu) | No. of experi-ments | Ceruloplasmin-$^{64}$Cu in plasma: Produced in fifth hour (% of dose) | Produced in 5 hours: % of dose | Produced in 5 hours: μg |
|---|---|---|---|---|
| 1 | 2 | 2.7 | 9.6 | 0.10 |
| 5 | 15 | 2.4 | 8.1 | 0.40 |
| 10 | 3 | 1.8 | 6.2 | 0.62 |
| 25 | 2 | 2.6 | 6.0 | 1.5 |
| 47 | 1 | 3.0 | 4.9 | 2.3 |
| 100 | 9 | 0.7 | 2.7 | 2.7 |
| 300 | 1 | 0.6 | 1.3 | 3.9 |
| 500 | 2 | 0.6 | 1.6 | 8 |
| 1,000 | 2 | 0.2 | 1.4 | 14 |

The agreement between observed values and predicted ones is sufficiently good that a three-compartment hepatic system of some sort seems likely to have biologic reality. We are currently testing the compartmental model by studying abnormal rat livers—from copper-deficient rats, from rats on a high copper intake, from rats treated acutely with carbon tetrachloride, and from rats treated with drugs of the puromycin class.

*Copper deficiency.* – When 75- to 100-gm rats were placed on a diet of bovine milk powder and copper-free water, they rapidly became copper deficient and anemic. Representative data are shown in Table IV.

When the livers of these severely copper-deficient rats were perfused with normal rat blood, the return of $^{64}Cu$

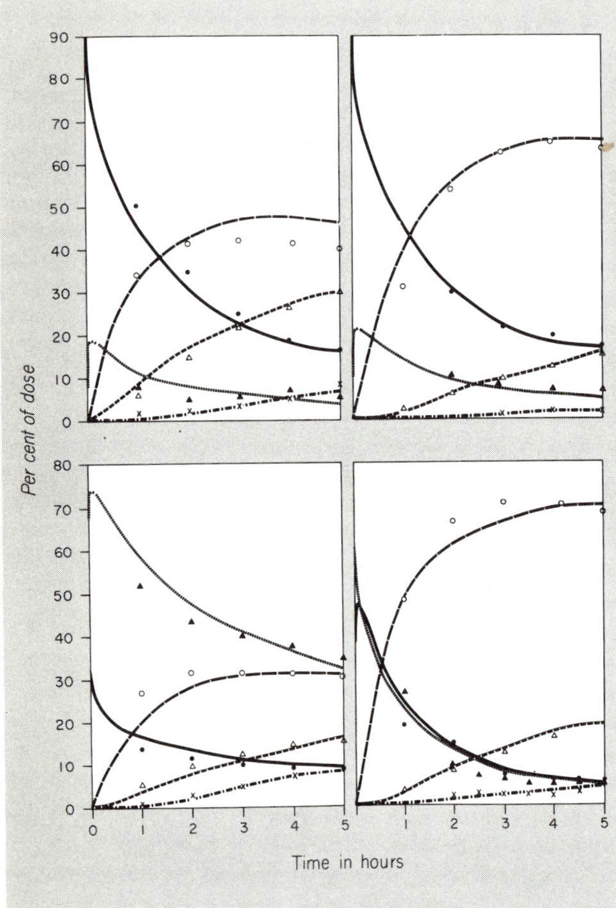


Fig. 3. Actual handling of copper by isolated, perfused, normal rat liver compared with predictions based on proposed model shown in Fig 2. Four dose levels of copper are compared: *Upper Left,* 5 μg; *Upper Right,* 100 μg; *Lower Left,* 1 μg and *Lower Right,* 25 μg. Points are experimental data and lines are theoretical predictions. Symbols: plasma = solid line and solid circles; erythrocytes = dotted line and solid triangles; liver = long-dash line and open circles; cumulative bile = short-dash line and open triangles; cumulative ceruloplasmin = dot-and-dash lines and X's. (Reproduced from Hazelrig, J. B.; Owen, C. A., Jr. and Ackerman, E.: A Mathematical Model for Copper Metabolism and Its Relation to Wilson's Disease. *Amer. J. Physiol.* **211:** 1075-1081, 1966.

**TABLE IV**

## Copper Deficiency in Rats Receiving Only Bovine Powdered Milk and Copper-Free Drinking Water

| Months of treatment | Mean hemoglobin (gm/100 ml blood) | Mean plasma copper (μg/100 ml) | Mean hepatic copper (μg/gm) | Mean PPD* (units/ml plasma) |
|---|---|---|---|---|
| 0 (controls)† | 14.3±1.3 | 123±13 | 4.4±0.5 | 54.1±10.2 |
| 1‡ | 14.7 (6) | 28 (3) | 2.8 (3) | 5.0 (3) |
| 2 | 12.6 (8) | .... | 3.7 (1) | 7.3 (3) |
| 3 | 12.0 (6) | 29 (2) | 3.3 (2) | .... |
| 4 | 10.4 (4) | .... | .... | .... |
| 5 | 9.1 (4) | 3 (1) | .... | .... |
| 6 | 9.0 (4) | 19 (2) | 1.2 (2) | 7.1 (3) |
| 7-8 | 6.0 (6) | 9 (1) | 0.4 (1) | 3.3 (8) |

*PPD: oxidation of *p*-phenylenediamine in optical density units (see text).

†Shown as mean ± SD.

‡For these and subsequent ranks, numbers in parentheses show number of rats studied.

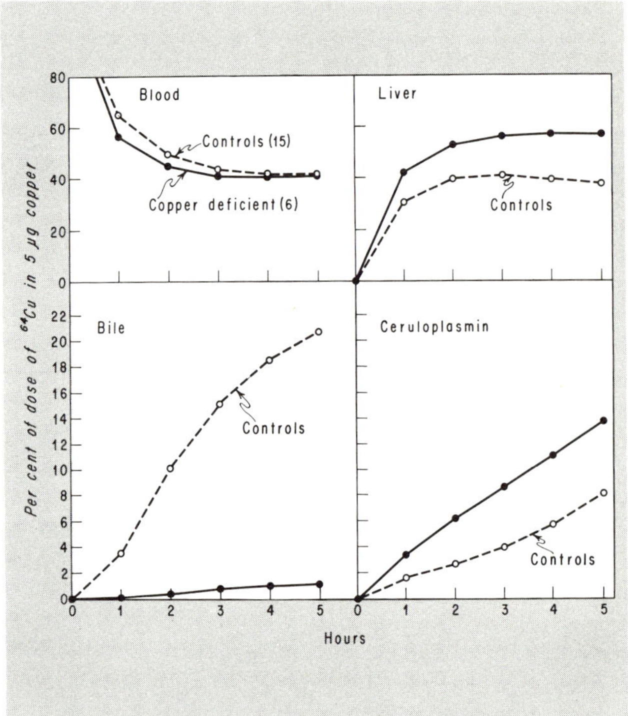


Fig. 4. Results of perfusions of copper-deficient livers. The handling of 5 μg of copper, as cupric-$^{64}Cu$ acetate, by 15 normal and 6 copper-deficient isolated, perfused rat livers is compared. The increased hepatic uptake of copper by the copper-deficient livers, despite a normal rate of clearance of copper from the blood and an exaggerated release of labeled ceruloplasmin, is explained by the almost complete absence of biliary excretion of the $^{64}Cu$.

to the blood, as ceruloplasmin, and the excretion into the bile were remarkably altered (Fig. 4). Practically no $^{64}Cu$ appeared in the bile during the five hours of perfusion. In contrast, ceruloplasmin-$^{64}Cu$ was returned to the blood so rapidly that by the end of one hour as much of the labeled protein had been synthesized and released as the normal liver accomplished in its fifth hour.

### TABLE V

## Copper Toxicity in Rats Receiving Normal (Rockland Pellet) Diet but Water Containing 0.125% Cupric Acetate

| Months of treatment | Mean hemoglobin (gm/100 ml blood) | Mean plasma copper (μg/100 ml) | Mean hepatic copper (μg/gm) | Mean PPD* (units/ml plasma) |
|---|---|---|---|---|
| 0 (controls)† | 14.3±1.3 | 123±13 | 4.4±0.5 | 54.1±10.2 |
| 1‡ | 13.7 (4) | 160 (1) | 85.8 (1) | 56 (5) |
| 2 | 15.3 (6) | 171 (1) | 92.3 (1) | 82 (2) |
| 3 | 15.0 (4) | 160 (1) | 76.3 (1) | .... |
| 4 | 13.4 (4) | 162 (1) | 138.0 (1) | 64 (4) |
| 5 | 14.8 (4) | 146 (1) | 81.0 (1) | 62 (3) |

*PPD: oxidation of *p*-phenylenediamine in optical density units (see text).

†Shown as mean ± SD.

‡For these and subsequent ranks, numbers in parentheses show number of rats studied.

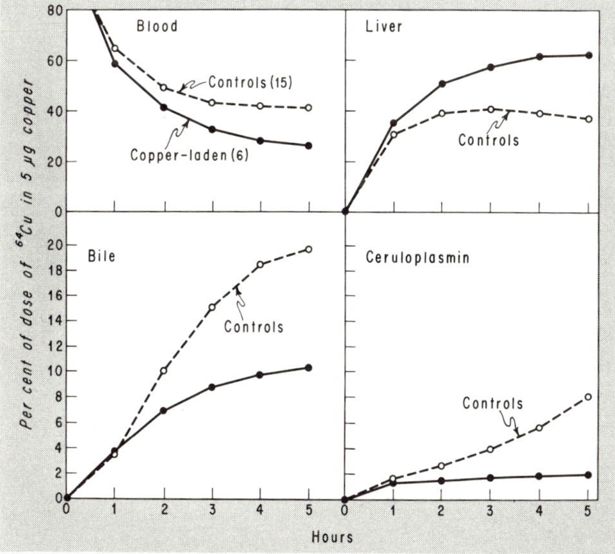


Fig. 5. Results of perfusions of copper-laden livers. The handling of 5 μg of copper, as cupric-$^{64}Cu$ acetate, by 15 normal and 6 copper-laden isolated, perfused rat livers is compared. The increased hepatic uptake of copper by the copper-laden livers, despite a nearly normal rate of clearance of copper from the blood, is explained by reduced secretion of ceruloplasmin-$^{64}Cu$ and excretion of biliary $^{64}Cu$.

In one instance, both the perfused liver and the pooled blood for perfusion were obtained from severely copper-deficient rats. The usual rapid outpouring of ceruloplasmin-$^{64}Cu$ occurred. In addition, there was an actual increase in the oxidative activity of the plasma. In this perfusion, the dose of copper was 100 μg; of this, 11.6 μg emerged from the liver in ceruloplasmin and the PPD activity increased 5.6 units/ml plasma (from 2.4 to 8.0). These two values are in reasonably good agreement because each is about one-tenth of the normal plasma level.

*Copper toxicity.* — When the rats were placed on a normal diet of food, but given water containing 0.125% cupric acetate, the concentration of copper in the liver increased rapidly (Table V). The metabolism of $^{64}Cu$ by these copper-laden livers again differed from normal (Fig. 5); more copper accumulated in the liver while biliary excretion and synthesis of ceruloplasmin were significantly depressed.

*Distribution of $^{64}Cu$ in intact rat.* — Although a 100-μg dose of copper, as cupric-$^{64}Cu$ acetate, is far greater than the amount of free copper in the plasma of an adult rat, this dose was originally required in order to follow the tissue distribution of $^{64}Cu$ for at least three to four days. More recently, availability of $^{64}Cu$ of higher specific activities has permitted repetition of the study with 5-μg doses for up to three days.

Uniform tissue patterns were found. In liver, a peak concentration was reached within the first few hours, followed by a steady, slow decrease which lasted as long as the $^{64}Cu$ could be assayed (Fig. 6). In blood, the $^{64}Cu$ decreased precipitously within the first hour. This was followed by an increase in concentration of $^{64}Cu$ in the plasma, as ceruloplasmin-$^{64}Cu$, which reached its peak at about 12 hours and then by a slow decrease (Fig. 7). In kidney, the highest concentration occurred at the time that urinary excretion of $^{64}Cu$ was greatest—the first few hours. However, considerably more of the $^{64}Cu$ accumulated in the kidneys than appeared in the urine.

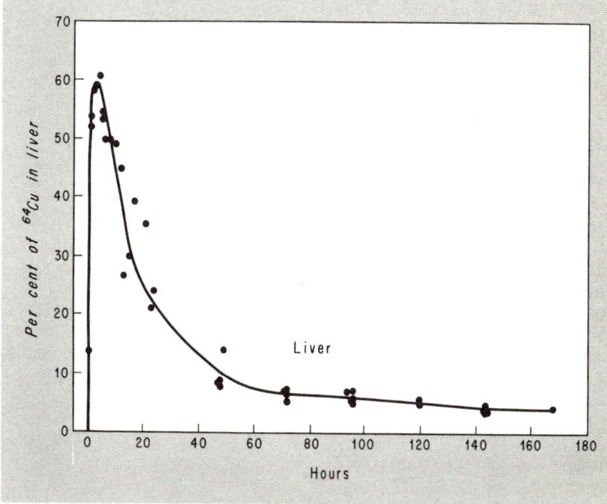


Fig. 6. Hepatic $^{64}Cu$, as percent of a 100-μg dose of labeled copper during one week, in normal rats.

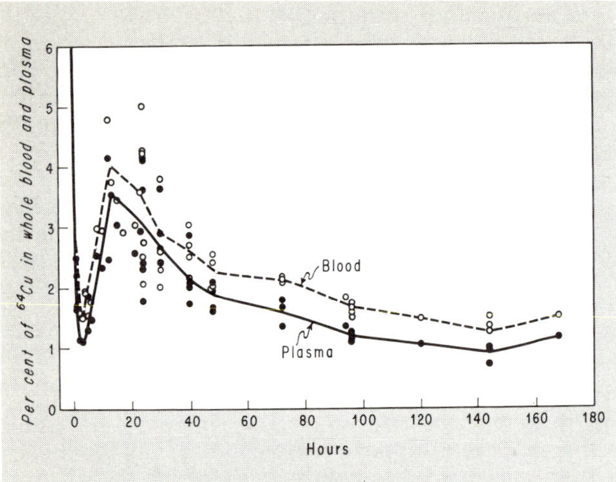


Fig. 7. $^{64}$Cu in whole blood and in plasma, as percent of a 100-μg dose of labeled copper, during one week, in normal rats. A significant fraction of the $^{64}$Cu was in the erythrocytes throughout the interval.

In certain organs, notably testes (Fig. 8), heart, and brain, a different pattern emerged. The $^{64}$Cu was at its peak concentration three to five minutes after it was injected intravenously. There followed a steady decrease during the next few hours. Then, as ceruloplasmin-$^{64}$Cu was emerging from the liver, the $^{64}$Cu in the various tissues began to increase, reaching a secondary peak one to three days later.

## Discussion

From study of the fate of $^{64}$Cu-labeled copper in the normal rat or in the carefully controlled abnormal rat, a certain pattern of copper metabolism seems evident.

Copper is absorbed from the upper part of the small intestine preferentially.[8] Whether given orally or intravenously, there is a rapid accumulation of the copper in the liver. The concentration of new copper, labeled with $^{64}$Cu, rapidly diminished in the blood and most of the tissues; only the liver, kidney, and gastrointestinal wall show an early increase. Since these three organs excrete copper, their aberrant patterns are probably related to this function.

Within a few minutes after $^{64}$Cu reaches the liver, the isotope can be detected in the bile. The biliary excretion is maximal within an hour or two and then decreases as the concentration of $^{64}$Cu in the blood decreases. Proportionately smaller amounts of the $^{64}$Cu label appear to be excreted in the bile as the dose of copper is increased above 100 μg. When placed in the stomach of normal rats, the biliary copper is scarcely absorbed,[8] suggesting that biliary excretion of copper may be a homeostatic regulating mechanism to control excess copper in the body. This homeostatic concept receives support from the observation of decreased $^{64}$Cu excretion in the bile of copper-deficient rats.

The normal rat liver generally secretes little labeled ceruloplasmin into the blood during the first hour but, after that, steadily greater amounts emerge.[9] In the intact rat the peak in the blood is reached within the first 24 hours. The level in the blood is maintained for about the next 24 hours before it begins to decrease.

The rat liver tends to concentrate proportionately more $^{64}$Cu as the dose of copper increases from 1 to 1,000 μg. However, the increased hepatic uptake is not accompanied by proportionately increased biliary excretion or ceruloplasmin synthesis. Therefore it seems reasonable that there is a storage area within the liver for the excess copper. This is the basis for postulating a three-compartment hepatic system: one compartment for the copper destined to become ceruloplasmin, one for excretion in the bile (unless the liver is too severely depleted of copper), and one for storage if the other two compartments are taxed maximally.[7] Since the whole hepatic process is accelerated in copper deficiency and retarded in copper loading, it seems likely that the depleting or filling of the hepatic storage compartment contributes directly to the experimentally observed changes.

If the results with 100-μg doses of copper are representative of the physiologic state, the concentration of $^{64}$Cu in certain tissues begins to increase only after the label returns to the blood in the form of ceruloplasmin. The short half-life of $^{64}$Cu makes it difficult to confirm with truly physiologic doses this concept of ceruloplasmin as the copper donor.

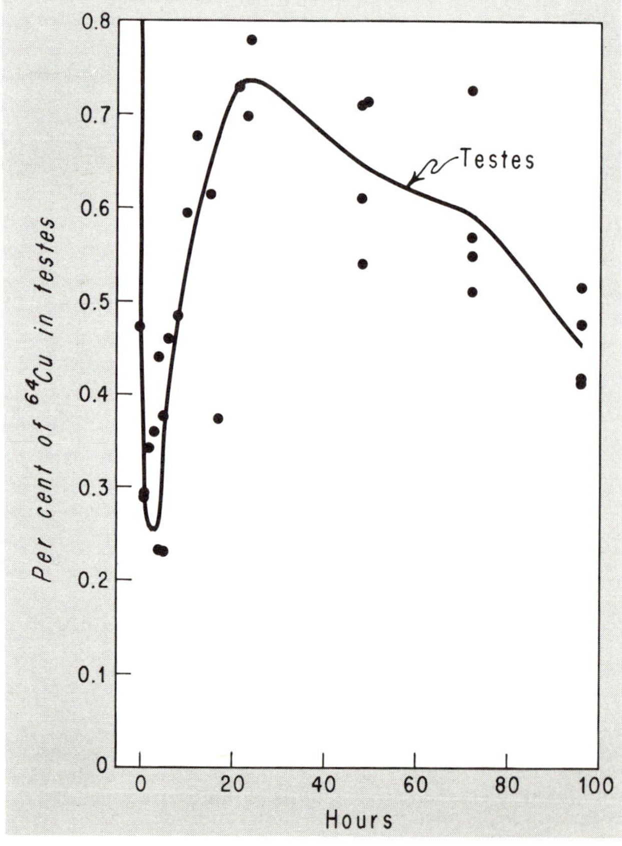


Fig. 8. Testicular $^{64}$Cu, as percent of a 100-μg dose of labeled copper, during four days, in normal rats.

**Summary**

Metabolism of $^{64}$Cu-labeled copper has been studied in the intact rat and in the isolated, perfused rat liver. The hepatic handling of varying doses of copper is practically identical in the two systems.

The rapid excretion of copper in the bile, the delayed emergence of labeled ceruloplasmin in the blood, and the liver's ability to store excess copper suggest that a three-compartment hepatic system is in contact with the blood. Predictions of rates of movement of copper from blood to liver and back to blood, as well as to bile, based on such a compartmental model were in good agreement with experimental data when doses of 1, 5, 25, and 100 $\mu$g of copper were studied in the isolated, perfused rat liver. Changes in the handling of copper by livers from copper-deficient or copper-laden rats were found to be compatible with the mathematical model.

Since secretion of ceruloplasmin-$^{64}$Cu from the liver into the blood preceded the buildup of $^{64}$Cu in the tissues, at least when the dose of copper was 100 $\mu$g, it is suggested that ceruloplasmin may function as the copper donor for the tissues.

## REFERENCES

1. Owen, C. A., Jr.: Copper metabolism and Wilson's disease. In Knisely, R. M.; Tauxe, W. N. and Anderson, Elizabeth B.: Dynamic clinical studies with radioisotopes. Oak Ridge, Tennessee, USAEC Division of Technical Information Extension, pp. 581-604, 1964.
2. Brauer, R. W.; Pessotti, R. L. and Pizzolato, P.: Isolated rat liver preparation: Bile production and other basic properties. *Proc. Soc. exp. Biol.* **78:**174-181, 1951.
3. Caster, W. O.; Poncelet, J.; Simon, A. B. and Armstrong, W. D.: Tissue weights of the rat. I. Normal values determined by dissection and chemical methods. *Proc. Soc. exp. Biol.* **91:**122-126. 1956.
4. Owen, C. A., Jr.: Distribution of copper in the rat. *Amer. J. Physiol.* **207:**446-448, 1964.
5. Owen, C. A., Jr. and Orvis, A. L.: Elution of chromium from rat erythrocytes. *Amer. J. Physiol.* **210:**573-575, 1966.
6. Owen, C. A., Jr.: Metabolism of radiocopper ($Cu^{64}$) in the rat. *Amer. J. Physiol.* **209:**900-904, 1965.
7. Hazelrig, J. B.; Owen, C. A., Jr. and Ackerman, E.: A mathematical model for copper metabolism and its relation to Wilson's disease. *Amer. J. Physiol.* **211:**1075-1081, 1966.
8. Owen, C. A., Jr.: Absorption and excretion of $Cu^{64}$-labeled copper by the rat. *Amer. J. Physiol.* **207:**1203-1206, 1964.
9. Owen, C. A., Jr., and Hazelrig, J. B.: Metabolism of $Cu^{64}$-labeled copper by the isolated rat liver. *Amer. J. Physiol.* **210:**1059-1064, 1966.

# The Role of Amino Acids in Physiologic and Pathologic Copper Transport: *In Vitro* and *in Vivo* Studies

MERVIN SILVERBERG, M.D.*; PETER Z. NEUMANN, M.D.** and A. DANIEL ROTENBERG, Ph.D.***

L-amino acids in physiologic concentrations facilitate the passage of copper-64 ($^{64}Cu$) across cell membranes, and increase the uptake of $^{64}Cu$ by rat and human liver slices, and human erythrocytes. The exact nature of the transport is uncertain. In erythrocytes, labile and stable copper fractions are noted and the former is likely amino acid bound. Untreated Wilson's disease liver slices show a 50% defect in uptake compared to normal and cirrhotic controls. The defect may be primary, or related to saturated intracellular binding sites.

One of the main problems in explaining the basic defect in Wilson's disease has been the inability to definitely outline the kinetics of copper transport through the various body compartments, even in the normal. Up until 1963, copper in the circulation was considered to exist only in two forms: 1) 90-95% was ceruloplasmin bound, a form in which the copper was unavailable for transport across cell membranes at physiological pH's; 2) 5-10% was albumin bound, which was considered to be dissociable and was thought to be the immediate transport form of copper. Neumann and Sass-Kortsak[2] demonstrated a third small but physiologically active form of copper, in serum, bound to amino acids (AA). These copper-AA complexes have been recently isolated by Sass-Kortsak. (Personal communication).

The present paper will attempt to show that amino acids, particularly histidine and its complexes, facilitate the transport of copper across inert cellophane membranes into mammalian tissues and finally may be involved in the basic defect in copper transport in patients with Wilson's disease.

*Director of Adolescent Unit and Chief of the Gastroenterology Research Program, Bronx-Lebanon Hospital Center, Assistant Clinical Professor of Pediatrics, Albert Einstein College of Medicine and Attending Physician, Bronx Municipal Hospital Center, Bronx, New York.

**Research Associate in the Gastrointestinal Unit, and Clinical Assistant at the Montreal Children's Hospital, Montreal, Canada.

***Biophysicist to Department of Radiology at the Montreal General Hospital, Montreal, Canada

In all the experiments, $^{64}$cupric acetate was used, with a specific activity of 10-40 mc/$\mu$g of copper prepared by fast neutron bombardment of $^{64}Zn$.

In our first experiment we set out to answer the question: can amino acids affect the transfer of $^{64}Cu$ through a semipermeable membrane?

A 4 gm% purified human albumin solution in Krebs-Ringer-Bicarbonate (KRB) buffer of pH 7.4 with added unlabeled and $^{64}Cu$ acetate was dialyzed through a semipermeable membrane against the same albumin solution, with no added copper, at 37°C, with constant shaking.

To another aliquot of the same albumin solution, the 20 naturally occurring amino acids were added in physiologic concentration and the same experiment was carried out. The percent of $^{64}Cu$ dialyzed across the semipermeable membrane was determined serially up to 24 hours.

Similar experiments were carried out using fresh serum of normal donors and of the patient with Wilson's disease. An aliquot of this serum was first dialyzed against five changes of five times the volume KRB buffer of pH 7.4 for a period of three hours each in order to dialyze out all diffusible constituents of serum, including amino acids. Following this "predialysis," a mixture of copper and $^{64}$copper acetate was added to the aliquots of the dialyzed serum in amounts to achieve an albumin, copper molar ratio of 1:2, which is an excess of copper, down to physiological ratios of 1:0.0001, and then were dialyzed against either the

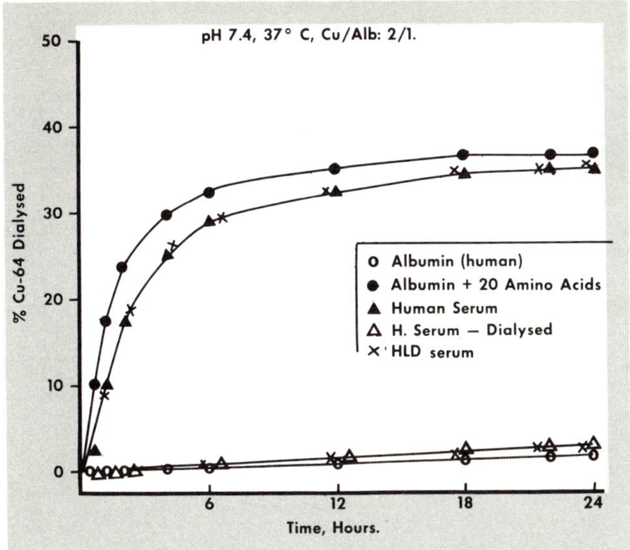


Fig. 1. The Effect of Amino Acids on the *in Vitro* Transfer of $^{64}$Copper via a Semipermeable Membrane.

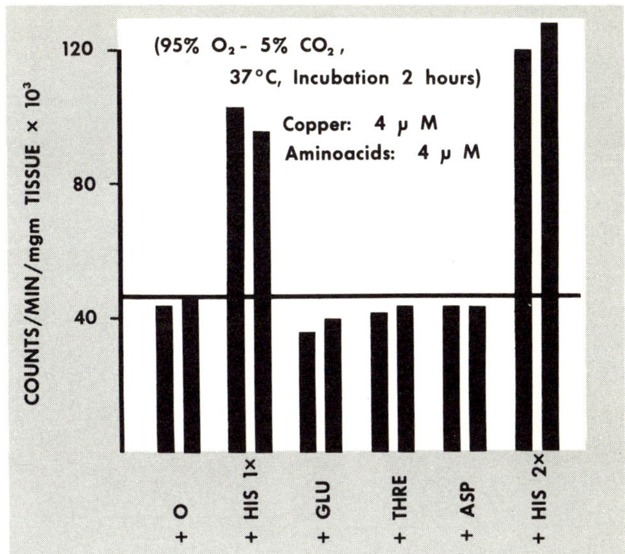


Fig. 3. $^{64}$Copper Transport in Normal Human Liver Slices —2 cases.

"native" or "predialyzed" serum with no added copper (Fig. 1).

Insignificant amounts of $^{64}$Cu transfer were noted up to 24 hours when the albumin (open circles) or predialyzed human sera (open triangles) were used. When native serum (closed triangles) or albumin plus AA (closed circles) were used, a 40% transfer was noted. The sera of patients with Wilson's disease (X's) behaved like normal sera. Therefore we can conclude that AA compete effectively with binding sites on human albumin and facilitate the transfer of Cu across a semipermeable membrane.

The next question was — does this AA facilitated transport operate in metabolically active animal and human cell systems? We studied fresh male Wistar rat liver slices, human liver slices, and human RBC's. Labeled cupric acetate was added to the medium in physiologic concentration, or in excess amounts, together

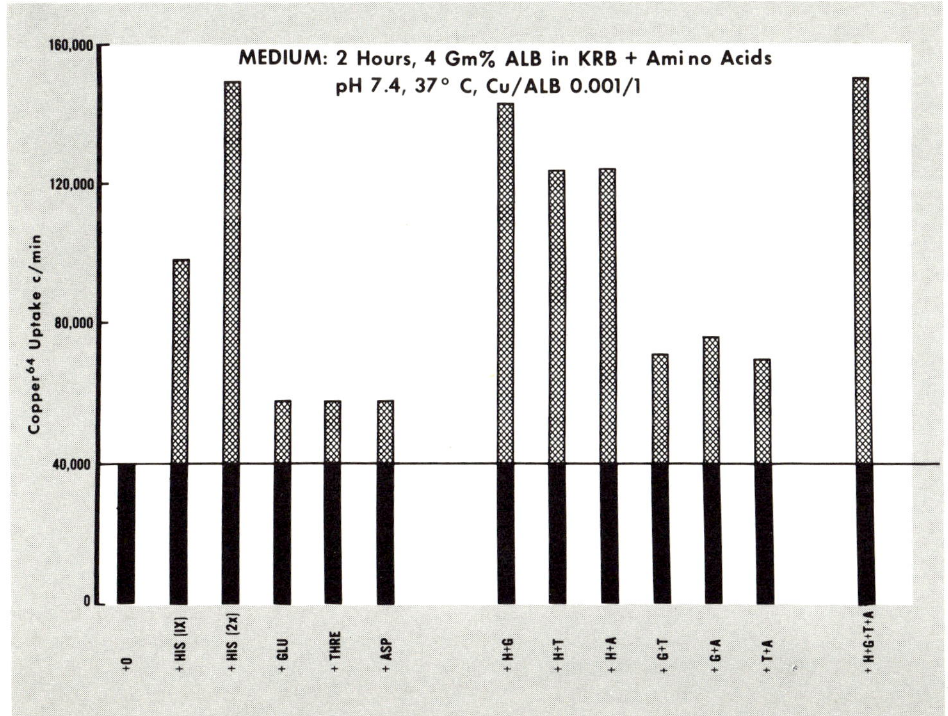


Fig. 2. Effect of Amino Acids on $^{64}$Copper Uptake by Rat Liver Slices.

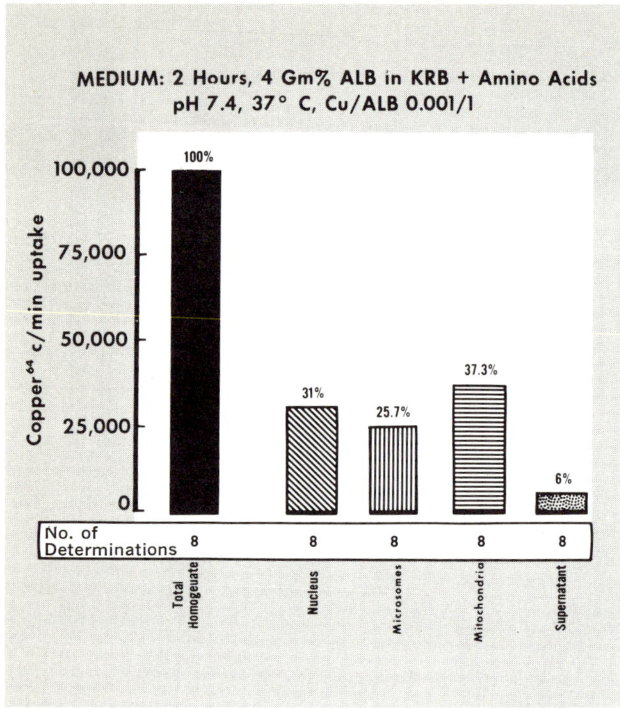


Fig. 4. 64Copper Content of Rat Liver Cell Fractions.

with L-amino acids — the latter individually or in combination, in equimolar concentration. The flasks were incubated in a Dubnoff metabolic shaker at 37°C for three hours in 95% $O_2$-5% $CO_2$ atmospheres. Similar experiments were done at 20°C and with varying concentration of $O_2$. Following incubation, the slices were immediately removed, washed three times with 20 ml of ion-free water, blotted, and counted in a Picker Scintillation counter.

Figure 2 shows the marked enhancing effect on $^{64}$Cu of histidine (his.). Glutamine (glu.), threonine (thre.), and asparagine (asp.), show very little effect. The amino acid complexes containing histidine, particularly histidine and glutamine, resulted in an uptake of $^{64}$Cu greater than the sum of the effects of individual amino acids. Combinations not containing histidine were relatively ineffective. The ratio of c.p.m./mgm tissue to c.p.m./mgm medium is shown at the right. The ratio greater than one excludes the possibility of simple diffusion as the transport mechanism for copper. The system was shown to be dependent on temperature, $O_2$ and operated against a chemical concentration gradient.[3]

Figure 3 shows the results of incubation studies in two sets of human liver slices with normal histology obtained by open biopsy. Again, histidine appears to be the most potent amino acid in facilitating the movement of $^{64}$Cu from the medium into tissue.

Figure 4 shows that the transport $^{64}$Cu was indeed inside the liver cells. The subcellular distribution of $^{64}$Cu of the liver slice homogenates, as determined by the technic of Hogeboom, shows that after two hours incubation 31% of the activity is in the nuclear fraction, 25.7% in the microsomes, 37.3% in mitochondria, and 6% in the supernatant.

We next set out to investigate the kinetics of copper transport in RBC and to assess the role of amino acids in this function. Bush[1] showed that copper existed within RBC's as labile and stable pools in normal humans, and suggested that the stable pool corresponded to erythrocuprein. The dialyzable labile pool has never been described.

The relationship between copper transport in RBC and amino acid facilitation was shown to be similar to

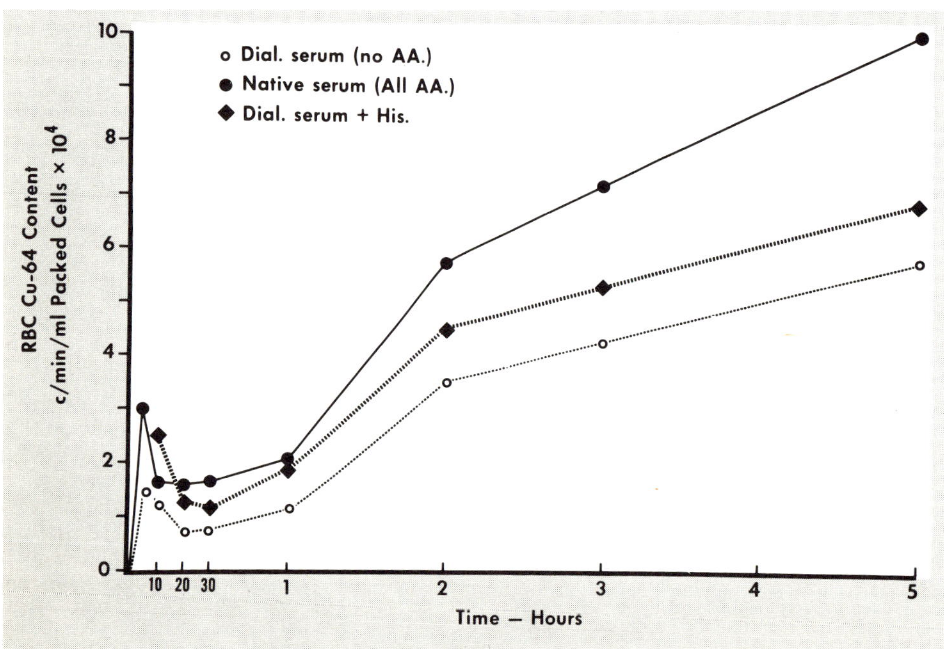


Fig. 5. The Effect of Amino Acids on the Uptake of 64Copper by Erythrocytes *in Vitro*.

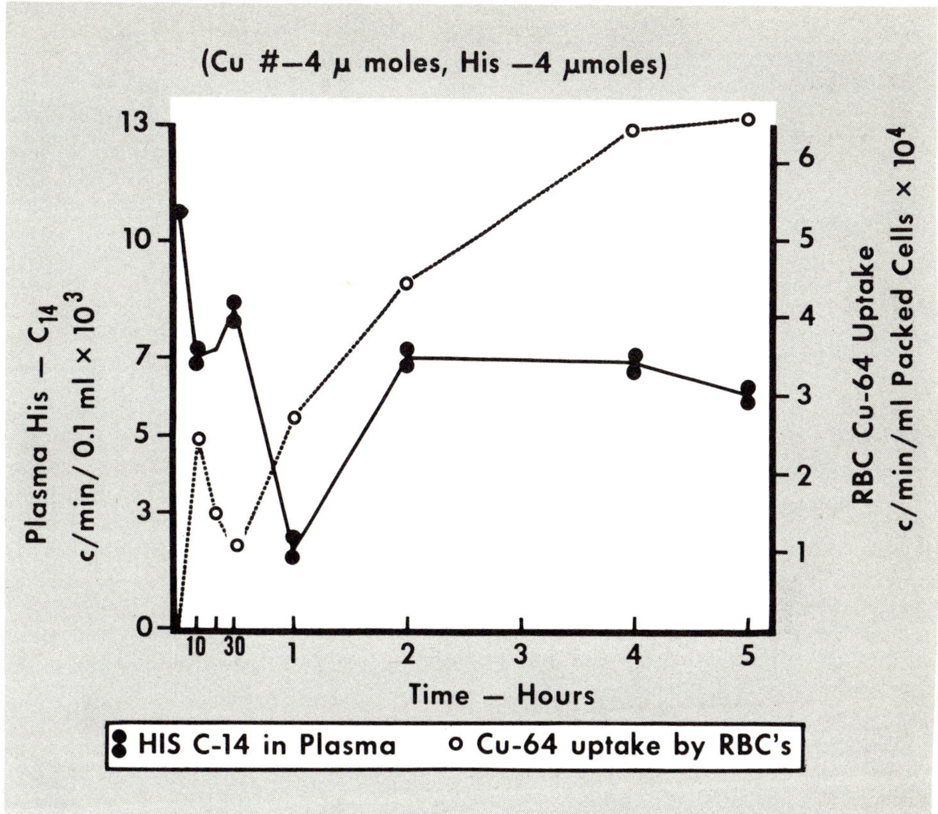


Fig. 6. The *in Vitro* Relationship of Plasma $^{14}C$ Histidine Level to $^{64}$Copper uptake by Erythrocytes.

the previous experiments using liver slices, although potentiation was not as dramatic. There appears to be an initial rapid uptake followed by an efflux of copper from the RBC and then a secondary rise in RBC $^{64}Cu$ activity in one hour (Fig. 5).

In a similar experiment, when both $^{64}Cu$ (open circles) and $^{14}C$ histidine (double closed circles) were added to the incubation medium, we could show a positive correlation between the RBC uptake of $^{64}Cu$ and the disappearance of $^{14}C$ histidine from the medium. The $^{14}C$ histidine does not appear to participate in the secondary rise of $^{64}Cu$ activity in the RBC, hence the corresponding rise in $^{14}C$ histidine activity in the plasma medium (Fig. 6). The participation of $^{14}C$ histidine in the $^{64}Cu$ transport is suggested.[4] Recently, Winter and Christenson have shown a similar phenomenon of transport and countertransport of amino acids in and out of RBC.[6]

At this point we may bring up the question — can a defect in amino acid facilitated copper transport be one of the underlying abnormalities in Wilson's disease? *In vivo* studies were made in four patients with Wilson's disease and four normal controls. Figure 7 shows the significant features of the patients. We should note two things: R.W. was and still is asymptomatic, and M.F. had near normal serum ceruloplasmin levels. Figure 8 (A & B) are contour maps reconstructed from a gamma scanogram of a normal human and a Wilson's disease patient up to one and one-half days following the intravenous injection of 1 mc of $^{64}Cu$. Note the rapid initial uptake over the liver followed by a discharge of activity with 150,000 counts/min. over the normal liver at 35 hours. Also note the widespread distribution of activity in the gut. In contrast, in the typical Wilson's contour map, there is a delay in uptake of copper, no evidence of discharge of activity — and only 85,000 counts/min.

## *ABOUT THE SENIOR AUTHOR*

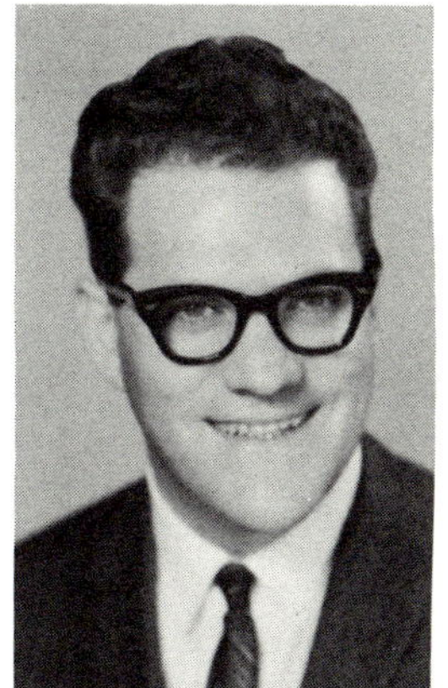

Dr. Mervin Silverberg received his medical degree from McGill University in 1954 followed by residency training in Pediatrics in Montreal and Boston. He was Director of the Gastrointestinal Unit at the Montreal Children's Hospital from 1961 to 1967.

Dr. Silverberg is now Director of Adolescent Unit and Chief of the Gastroenterology Research Program at the Bronx-Lebanon Hospital Center. He is Assistant Clinical Professor of Pediatrics at the Albert Einstein College of Medicine and Attending Physician at the Bronx Municipal Hospital Center.

| | F.B | M.F. | R.W | E.T |
|---|---|---|---|---|
| Age (yrs.) Sex | 12M | 38F | 10M | 13F |
| Symptoms, (mos.) | 3 | 4 | 0 | 3 |
| K-F rings | + | + | 0 | + (slit) |
| Liver (cms.) | 2 | 1 | 0 | 2 |
| Serum uric acid (mgm%) | 0.9 | 2.5 | 4.8 | 2.1 |
| Ceruloplasmin | 7.0 | 21.0 | 2.2 | 1.9 |
| Urine Cu (ugm/24 hrs.) | 210 | 131 | 158 | 572 |
| AA-uria | ++ | + | 0 | ++ |
| Cirrhosis | + | + | + | + |

Fig. 7. Significant Clinical and Laboratory Data of HLD.

over the liver area at 35 hours, – about 50% of the normal. There is also an unusual concentration of $^{64}$Cu in the kidneys and no activity in the gut. The same results were obtained with tracer and loading (0.5 mgm) doses of injected copper.

The question now was, could we reproduce this apparent transport defect on a cellular basis in Wilson's disease?[5]

Experiments were performed comparing the results of $^{64}$Cu facilitated transport by amino acids, using liver slices from human normals, postnecrotic cirrhosis, and Wilson's disease. Duplicate procedures were employed only when sufficient tissue was available (Figs. 9 and 10).

Two things can be concluded from these studies: 1) the potentiating effects of histidine on $^{64}$Cu transport occurs in cirrhotics and Wilson's disease, as well as in normals, and is effective within a wide spectrum of copper concentrations. 2) This potentiating effect is 40-50% less effective when the liver slices in Wilson's disease patients are compared to both other types of patients. It is important to note that despite the fact that all the Wilson's disease livers showed histologic evidence of widespread postnecrotic cirrhosis, one case with asymptomatic disease had normal concentration of copper in the liver slices used, and still showed the transport defect. There is a possibility that the apparent defect could be the expression of copper-saturated binding sites within the liver cells. However, the fact that the defect was unchanged in the asymptomatic patient whose liver slices contained normal amounts of copper makes this alternative less likely.

In conclusion, we have shown that copper transport across inert and metabolically active cell membranes is closely allied to amino acid transport and is facilitated against a concentration gradient.

The presence of a copper transport defect in four patients with Wilson's disease is suggested by: 1) the 40-50% *in vivo* defect in hepatic uptake of $^{64}$Cu using radio scanning technics; 2) the 40-50% *in vitro* defect in $^{64}$Cu uptake by liver slices of Wilson's disease, when compared to controls; and 3) the 6-20 times elevation of nonceruloplasmin-bound circulating copper in patients with Wilson's disease.

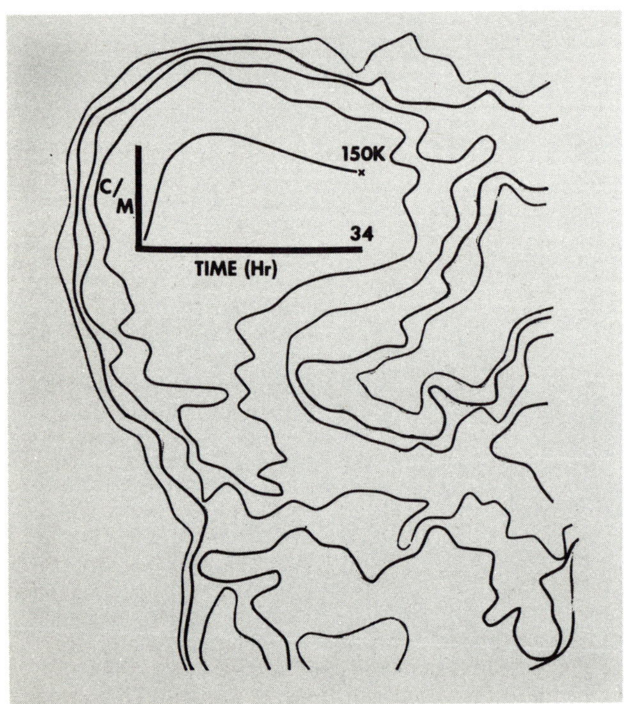


Fig. 8a. Contour Map of $^{64}$Cu Scan of Normal.

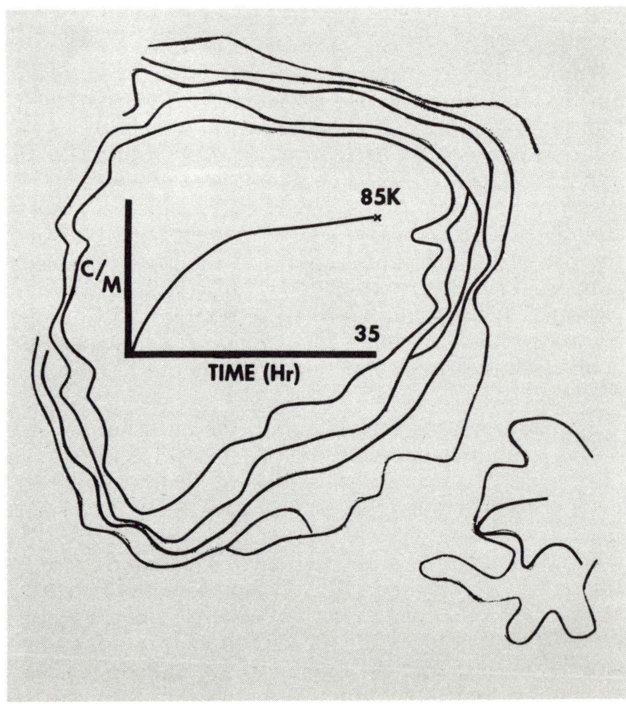


Fig. 8b. Contour Map of $^{64}$Cu Scan of HLD.

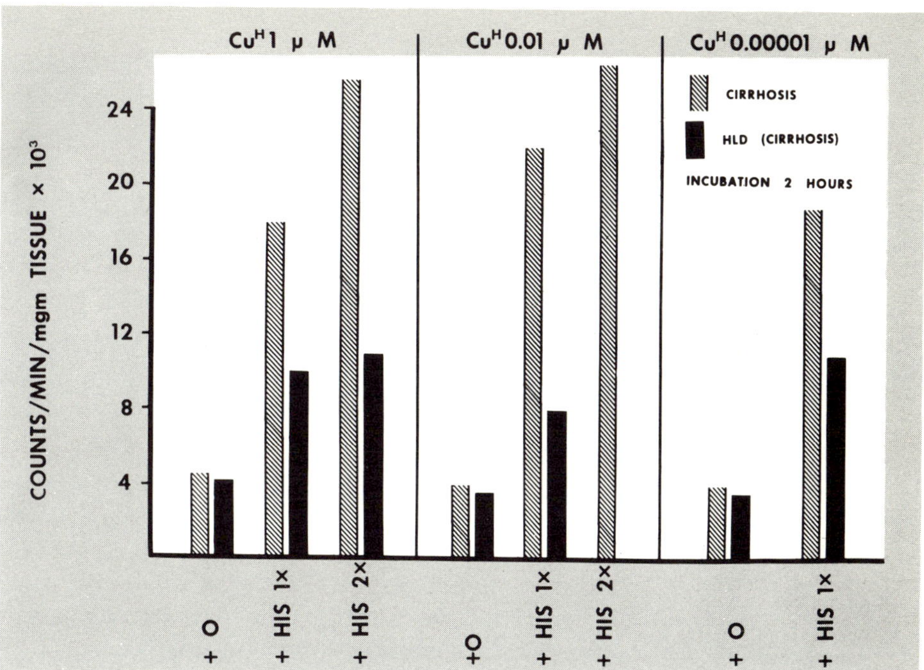


Fig. 9. 64Copper Transport in Human Liver Slices – 2 cases. Normal vs. Wilson's Disease.

## REFERENCES


1. Bush, J. A.; Mahoney, J. P.; Gubiler, C. J.; Cartwright, G. E. and Wintrobe, M. M.: Studies on copper metabolism. XXI. The transfer of radiocopper between erythrocytes and plasma. *J. Lab. clin. Med.* **47**:898, 1956.
2. Neumann, P. Z. and Sass-Kortsak, A.: Binding of copper by serum proteins. *Vox. Sang.* **8**:111, 1963.
3. Neumann, P. Z. and Silverberg, M.: Active copper transport in mammalian tissues; its possible role in Wilson's disease. *Nature,* **210**:414, 1966.
4. Neumann, P. Z. and Silverberg, M.: Metabolic pathways of red blood copper in normal humans and in Wilson's disease. *Proc. Can. Fed. Biol. Soc.* **8**:49, 1965.
5. Neumann, P. Z. and Silverberg, M.: *In vivo* and *in vitro* studies of hepatic copper transport in normal humans and Wilson's disease (hepatolenticular degeneration, HLD). *Gastroenterology,* **50**:3, 1966.
6. Winter, C. G. and Christensen, H. N.: Migration of amino acids across the membrane of the human erythrocyte. *J. biol. Chem.,* **239**:872, 1964.


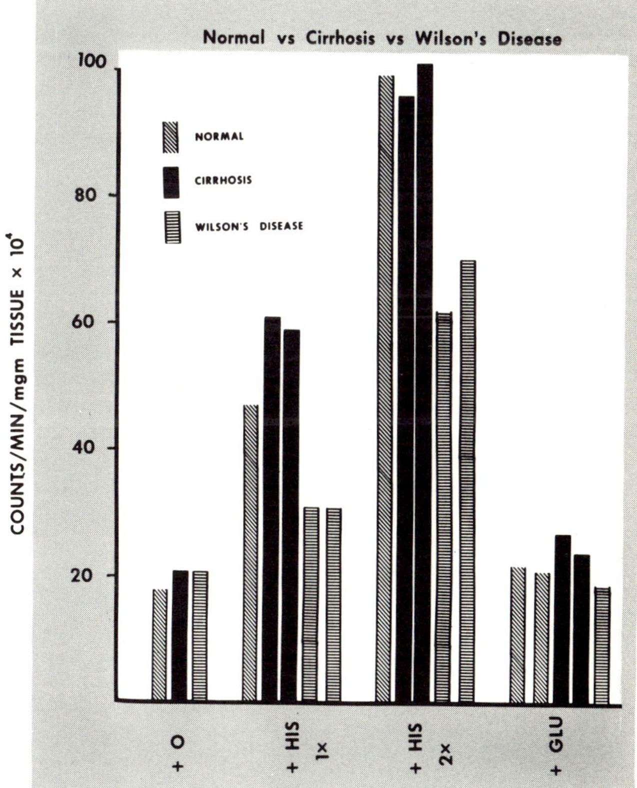


Fig. 10. 64Copper Transport in Human Liver Slices.

# Copper Metabolism in the Rat: Studies of the Biliary Excretion and Intestinal Absorption of $^{64}$Cu-Labeled Copper*†

Paul A. Farrer, M.B., B.S.** and Stephen P. Mistilis, M.B., B.S.***

Copper excretion and absorption and the extent to which bile copper undergoes intestinal reabsorption in the rat were studied using $^{64}$Cu as Cu++-acetate and Cu (II) EDTA. A parallelism was found to exist between the increasing nondialyzability of biliary $^{64}$Cu on the one hand, and its progressively increasing malabsorption on the other with time following intravenous injection of the label. It is thought that normally most of the copper in bile is associated with a specific copper protein (but not ceruloplasmin) and that this precludes the mineral from significant reabsorption in the gut.

Under normal circumstances fecal elimination is the predominant manner in which copper is excreted from the body.[1-4] The normal fecal loss is considered to result from 1) nonabsorption of a relatively large fraction of exogenous copper present in the diet, and 2) biliary and transmural excretion into the intestine of endogenous copper derived from the metabolic "pool" of the element in the body. With respect to copper that has been assimilated into the body, the bile represents the major excretory pathway in man and in a number of other species including the rat.[5-7] The precise chemical nature of endogenous bile copper, its source, and the mechanism of its excretion are still largely unknown. Using the isolated perfused rat-liver preparation, Jeunet *et al*[8] demonstrated the passage of ceruloplasmin into the bile, but the measured concentrations of biliary ceruloplasmin were too low to account for all the copper normally excreted in this manner. Thus the actual chemical form in which the relatively larger fraction of nonceruloplasmin copper is normally excreted in the bile and just how its excretion comes about remain undetermined.

At the same time, the mechanism of absorption of exogenous copper is incompletely understood; and even less is known about the reabsorption of endogenous biliary copper or its enterohepatic circulation. Excessive absorption of the mineral has been thought by some workers to occur in Wilson's disease.[3,9,10] The possibility that increased reabsorption of endogenous bile copper is responsible or contributes toward the net positive balance of the mineral in this disorder has not been explored.

This report describes an investigation of the physiology of copper excretion and absorption in the rat. The study was also designed to define the extent to which bile copper is reabsorbed in the intestinal tract of the rat and to compare the excretion and absorption of copper-64 in two chemically different forms: ionic cupric acetate and chelated Cu (II) EDTA.

## Methods

$^{64}$Cu as cupric acetate and Cu (II) EDTA ($\log K_1 = 18.5$)[11] was obtained from the Australian Atomic Energy Commission Research Establishment, Lucas Heights, N.S.W. Doses were based on the stated specific activity and calculated in terms of micrograms ($\mu$g) copper.

Doses of 0.25 – 100 $\mu$g Cu as cupric acetate and Cu (II) EDTA were given intravenously to adult male Sprague-Dawley rats. Radiocopper in bile was assayed in rats with operative external biliary fistulas; intestinal (transmural) excretion of label was determined by assaying $^{64}$Cu in intestinal contents, feces and intestinal washings at the conclusion of experiments. Bile was collected in three successive fractional collections (0-4 hours, 4-8 hours, and 8-24 hours post *i.v.* injection) and bile aliquots were subjected to repeated dialysis (one

*Supported by a research grant-in-aid (P.A.F.) from The New South Wales State Cancer Council, Sydney, Australia.

**Departments of Radiology and Medicine, University of Rochester School of Medicine, Rochester, N.Y.

***Senior Research Fellow and Assistant Director, The A. W. Morrow Department of Gastroenterology, Royal Prince Alfred Hospital, Camperdown, Sydney, Australia.

†Work carried out in the Department of Medicine, University of Sydney, Sydney, Australia.

vol. bile *vs* 100 vol. normal saline, pH 6.5 – 6.9 at 0°C), and precipitation with trichloroacetic acid (final concentration of 5% at 0°C).

In attempting to further characterize the nature of biliary copper in the rat, a one ml aliquot of bile collected between four and eight hours after intravenous injection of 100 μg copper (as $^{64}$Cu (II) EDTA) was subjected to gel filtration at room temperature using "Sephadex" (Pharmacia) G-25 (exclusion limit: average molecular weight of 5000). Gel filtration was performed using a column (2.0 cm diameter, 25 cm length) that had been previously equilibrated with Tris-phosphate buffer (pH 8.0) containing 0.9% sodium chloride; a ten cm height of saline was maintained above the "Sephadex" surface.

Intestinal absorption of exogenous $^{64}$Cu-acetate and $^{64}$Cu (II) EDTA was determined following doses of 0.50 – 1000 μg Cu injected intrapylorically on the duodenal side of the pylorus. The animals were sacrificed at 24 hours, exsanguinated by cardiac puncture, the entire gastrointestinal tract was resected and the total radioactivity remaining in carcass, liver and blood was used as the index of absorption.

For the absorption of biliary copper, bile was obtained through external biliary fistulas from animals previously given an intravenous dose of 100 μg copper labeled with $^{64}$Cu. Known amounts (0.5 – 10 μg) of copper in the biliary fractions taken at 0-4 hours, 4-8 hours, and 8-24 hours (both undialyzed and dialyzed) were then injected intrapylorically and absorption during 24 hours was determined similarly. In studying the absorption of nondialyzable (indiffusible) biliary radiocopper a constant intrapyloric dose of 2.5 μg of bile copper was used.

The absorption of nondialyzable serum radiocopper was determined in separate experiments. Rats that had received two intravenous doses of 100 μg Cu as $^{64}$Cu-acetate 12 hours apart were sacrificed 24-36 hours after the second dose, exsanguinated, and their serum pooled. On repeated dialysis over 90% of the serum radioactivity was found to be nondialyzable, presumed to be ceruloplasmin-bound.[12] Doses of 1.25 and 2.5 μg of labeled ceruloplasmin-copper were administered intrapylorically and the 24-hour absorption of the label was determined.

Biliary fistulas, intravenous (femoral vein) injections and intrapyloric administrations of labeled material were performed under ether anesthesia. Intrapyloric injections were made under direct visualization through a laparotomy incision. The rats were kept in restraining cages for the duration of the experiment. Radioactive samples were measured in a "Packard" NaI (T1) "autogamma" well-type scintillation spectrometer. Whole-body (carcass) radioactivity was assayed in a "Packard" Armac counter. Appropriate "standards" (known fractions of the given dose) were counted with the samples and corrections were made for physical decay and background.

## Results

*Biliary excretion of intravenously administered copper* (Figs. 1, 2, 3)

Prompt biliary excretion of $^{64}$Cu results, following its intravenous administration. With increasing doses, the fraction of the given dose as well as the absolute amount of copper excreted in the 24-hour bile increases, but significantly more excretion takes place in later time intervals. The larger the dose of copper, the greater the fractional excretion but in steadily diminishing increments so that the increments are not proportional to the dose. The results are quantitatively similar regardless of the chemical form of injected copper. However, the stepwise increment in fractional excretion with increasing dosage is more evident in the case of the $^{64}$Cu (II) EDTA complex.

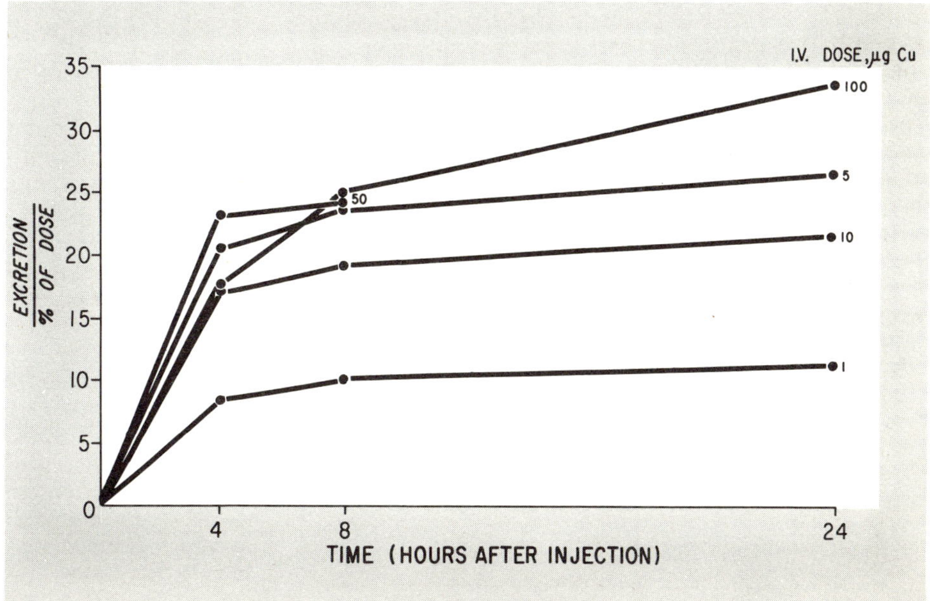


Fig. 1. Cumulative biliary excretion of $^{64}$Cu-acetate after intravenous injection in rats with external biliary fistulas. (Excretion as percentage of the administered dose).

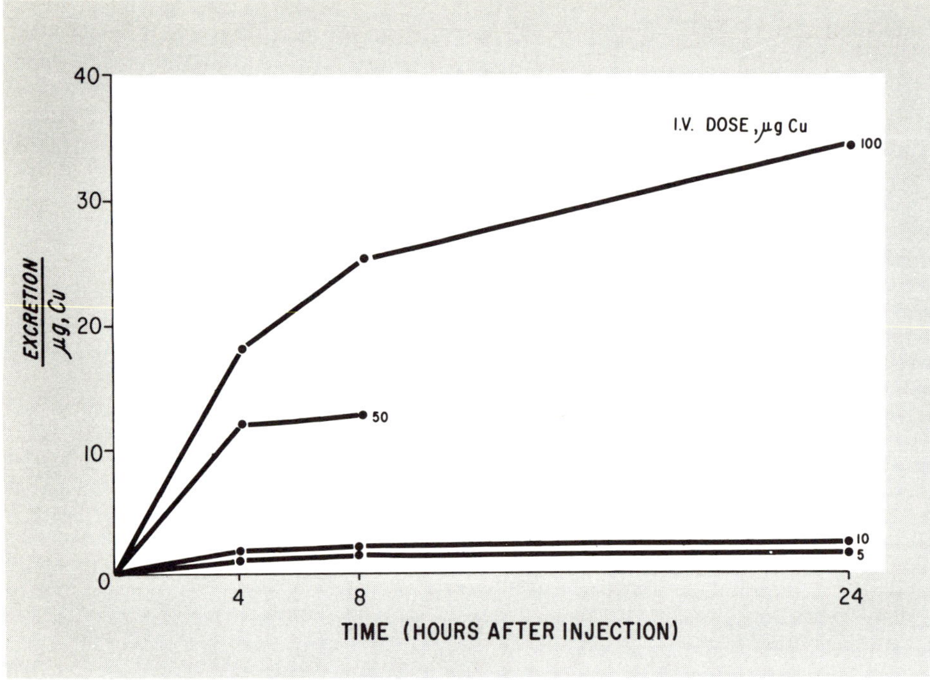


Fig. 2. Cumulative biliary excretion of *i.v.* $^{64}$Cu-acetate in terms of µg copper excreted in 24 hours.

*Hepatic uptake of $^{64}$Cu* (Tables I and II)

Table I summarizes the hepatic uptake of intravenously injected $^{64}$Cu-acetate in doses of 0.25—100 µg Cu. With increasing dosage the hepatic uptake of copper also increases. With smaller doses, peak concentration in the liver is reached earlier and by 24 hours there is considerable reduction in liver copper concentration compared to the four-hour uptake value. On the other hand, the larger the dose of copper the later the peak concentration in the liver and the less the difference between hepatic uptake at four hours and 24 hours (Table II). The hepatic uptake of $^{64}$Cu at 24 hours is also seen to increase with progressively larger doses of intravenously administered $^{64}$Cu (II) EDTA, but at the largest dose level used (100 µg Cu), the hepatic retention of label is considerably less (18.0 µg) than in the case of ionic copper (29.6 µg) (Table I).

## ABOUT THE SENIOR AUTHOR

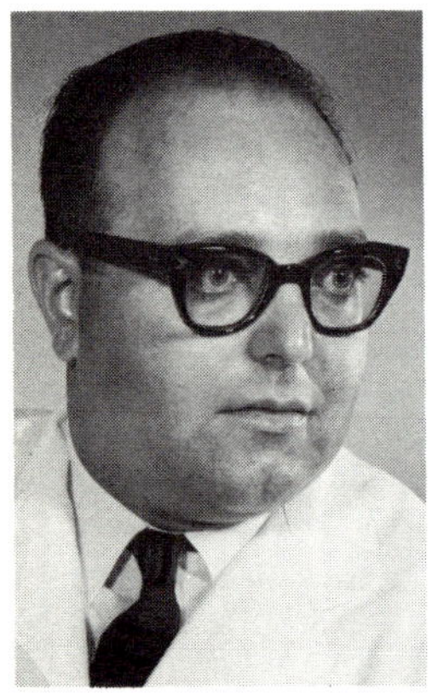

Dr. Paul A. Farrer was born in Budapest, Hungary in 1935, and at present is Senior Instructor in Radiology and Medicine in the School of Medicine, University of Rochester, and Assistant Radiologist (Nuclear Medicine) at Strong Memorial Hospital, Rochester, New York. He earned his medical degree at the University of Sydney, Australia in 1960, and received his clinical training at Royal Prince Alfred Hospital, Sydney. Between 1963 and 1965 he worked in the Radioisotope Unit of the Department of Medicine, University of Sydney as a Medical Research Fellow of The New South Wales State Cancer Council. Dr. Farrer joined the faculty of the University of Rochester in 1966. He was elected Associate Member of The College of Radiologists of Australasia in 1964.

*Transmural excretion of copper into the intestine*

In rats with operative external bile-fistulas (hence with no biliary connection to the gut), a rather constant fraction of the dose (approximately 5%) is recovered in the gastrointestinal tract, luminal content and feces in 24 hours following the intravenous administration of $^{64}$Cu-acetate in doses of 1—100 µg Cu. About half (3% of the dose) is present in the luminal contents and feces, the remainder being "fixed" in the intestinal wall; the former represents direct transmural excretion of copper into the bowel (as well as the gastric and salivary excretion of the element).

*Determination of nondialyzable and 5% TCA—precipitable biliary $^{64}$Cu following intravenous labeled copper* (Tables III, IV) (Fig. 4)

The average proportions of nondialyzable biliary radiocopper present in the three bile-fractions (0-4 hr, 4-8 hr, 8-24 hr) following intravenous doses of 5-100 µg of $^{64}$Cu show a progressive increase with increasing time postinjection. Increasing nondialyzability of biliary $^{64}$Cu is observed regardless of the chemical form in which the copper is injected (i.e. ionic or chelated) in this dose range.

Similarly, the average proportions of biliary radioactivity precipitated by trichloroacetic acid in a final concentration of 5% are also found to increase progressively with time after intravenous administration of $^{64}$Cu. About half to two-thirds of the $^{64}$Cu in the 8-24-hour bile is so precipitated following intravenous copper doses of 5—100 μg cupric acetate and Cu (II) EDTA.

*"Sephadex" G-25 filtration of 4-8 hr. bile collection following $^{64}$Cu (II) EDTA i.v.*

Approximately 30% of the total radioactivity of the bile added to the column was eluted and recovered in a total effluent volume of 16 ml collected after the hold-up volume (17 ml containing no detectable radioactivity) had passed.

*Absorption of $^{64}$Cu in 24 hours following intrapyloric doses of exogenous cupric acetate and Cu (II) EDTA* (Fig. 5)

A relatively constant fraction of the injected copper (about 40%) is retained at 24 hours when cupric acetate is given intrapylorically in the dose range of 0.50—10.0 μg Cu. With larger doses less is absorbed and with doses of 200—1000 μg Cu only 10% is retained. Similar

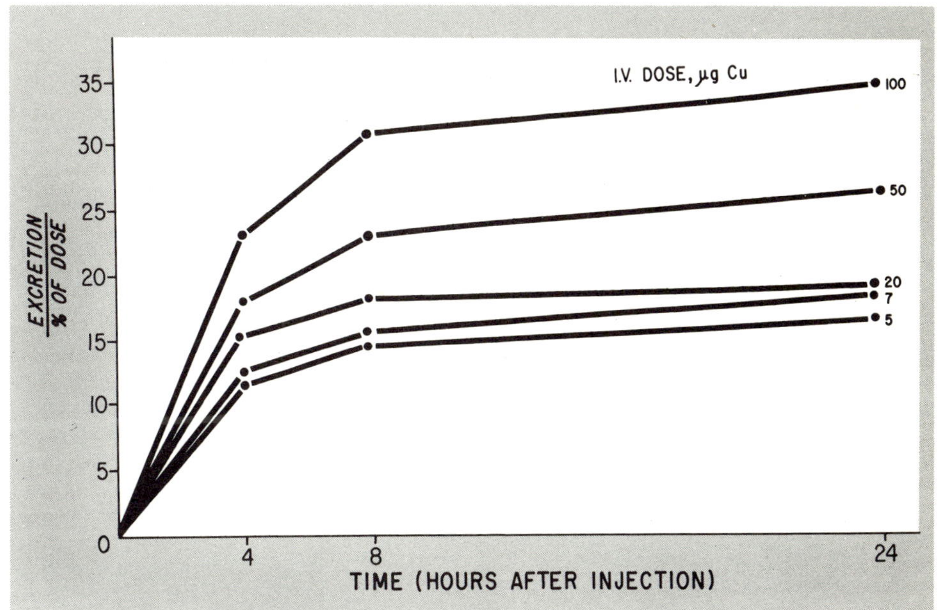


Fig. 3. Cumulative biliary excretion of $^{64}$Cu (II) EDTA after intravenous injection in rats with external biliary fistulas. (Excretion as percentage of the administered dose).

**TABLE I**

**PERCENTAGE AND ABSOLUTE HEPATIC UPTAKE OF $^{64}$Cu AT 24 HOURS FOLLOWING INTRAVENOUS DOSES OF CUPRIC ACETATE AND Cu (II) EDTA**

| Dose, μg Cu | No. of Experiments | Uptake Mean % of Dose (Range) | Mean, μg Cu |
|---|---|---|---|
| **Cupric Acetate** | | | |
| 0.25 μg | 2 | 8.5 ( 7.5-9.5 ) | 0.02 |
| 0.50 μg | 3 | 14.7 (13.4-15.9) | 0.07 |
| 1 μg | 2 | 20.4 (17.8-23.0) | 0.20 |
| 5 μg | 2 | 23.8 (22.6-25.1) | 1.19 |
| 10 μg | 7 | 19.8 (16.9-22.7) | 1.98 |
| 40 μg | 3 | 11.2 ( 9.3-12.8) | 4.48 |
| 100 μg | 8 | 29.6 (16.9-39.1) | 29.6 |
| **Cu (II) EDTA** | | | |
| 0.25 μg | 4 | 12.6 ( 8.3-18.4) | 0.03 |
| 0.50 μg | 2 | 13.7 (13.0-14.3) | 0.07 |
| 1 μg | 2 | 10.7 ( 8.7-12.7) | 0.10 |
| 5 μg | 2 | 18.4 (16.7-20.2) | 0.92 |
| 7 μg | 2 | 13.7 (13.6-13.7) | 0.96 |
| 50 μg | 2 | 12.2 (11.0-13.3) | 6.1 |
| 100 μg | 4 | 18.0 (11.7-24.0) | 18.0 |

TABLE II

## PERCENTAGE AND ABSOLUTE HEPATIC UPTAKE OF $^{64}Cu$ FOLLOWING INTRAVENOUS $^{64}Cu$-ACETATE

| Dose, µg Cu | 4 hours Mean % of Dose (Range) | Mean µg Cu | 8 hours Mean % of Dose (Range) | Mean µg Cu | 24 hours Mean % of Dose (Range) | Mean µg Cu |
|---|---|---|---|---|---|---|
| 100 µg | 32.0 (28.5-35.5) | 32.0 | 42.7 (34.9-50.5) | 42.7 | 29.6 (16.9-39.1) | 29.6 |
| 40 µg | 36.3 (34.8-38.6) | 14.5 | 18.7 (17.5-28.6) | 7.5 | 11.2 ( 9.3-12.8) | 4.5 |

TABLE III

## NONDIALYZABLE BILIARY $^{64}Cu$ AS PERCENTAGE OF TOTAL BILIARY RADIOACTIVITY FOLLOWING INTRAVENOUS CUPRIC ACETATE AND Cu (II) EDTA

| Dose, µg Cu | No. of Experiments | Bile Fraction (Postinjection) | Percent Nondialyzable | | |
|---|---|---|---|---|---|
| | | | Mean | Range | S.D. |
| $^{64}Cu$-acetate | | | | | |
| 10 µg | 3* | 0-4 hrs. | 37.0% | -------- | ------ |
| 100 µg | 9 | 0-4 hrs. | 49.5% | 48.8-58.2 | ± 7.2 |
| 100 µg | 9 | 4-8 hrs. | 71.9% | 63.6-77.4 | ± 6.1 |
| 100 µg | 9 | 8-24 hrs. | 84.3% | 81.7-88.0 | ± 2.8 |
| $^{64}Cu$ (II) EDTA | | | | | |
| 5 µg | 2 | 0-4 hrs. | 51.0% | 48.0-54.0 | ± 4.2 |
| 10 µg | 2 | 0-4 hrs. | 42.0% | 36.0-46.0 | ± 5.7 |
| 100 µg | 3* | 0-4 hrs. | 62.0% | -------- | ------ |
| 10 µg | 1 | 8-24 hrs. | 71.0% | -------- | ------ |
| 100 µg | 3 | 8-24 hrs. | 84.0% | 79.0-88.0 | ± 4.6 |

*Pooled samples.

TABLE IV

## 5% TRICHLOROACETIC ACID—PRECIPITATED BILIARY $^{64}Cu$ AS PERCENTAGE OF TOTAL BILIARY RADIOACTIVITY FOLLOWING INTRAVENOUS CUPRIC ACETATE AND Cu (II) EDTA

| Dose, µg Cu | Precipitated Radioactivity as Per Cent of Total Bile — $^{64}Cu$ | | |
|---|---|---|---|
| | 0-4 hr. Bile | 4-8 hr. Bile | 8-24 hr. Bile |
| Cupric Acetate | | | |
| 1 µg | 37.0 (1)* | ------ | ------ |
| 5 µg | 24.5 (2) | ------ | 49.0 (2) |
| 10 µg | 21.2 (3) | 50.0 (2) | 55.7 (2) |
| 100 µg | 14.5 (2) | 32.1 (2) | 55.0 (2) |
| Cu (II) EDTA | | | |
| 5 µg | 37.5 (1) | ------ | ------ |
| 7 µg | 34.5 (2) | 63.5 (2) | 60.5 (2) |
| 10 µg | 30.0 (2) | 56.0 (2) | 55.5 (2) |
| 20 µg | 34.0 (2) | 57.1 (2) | 66.3 (1) |
| 50 µg | 22.7 (2) | 53.5 (1) | 67.6 (2) |
| 100 µg | 13.6 (3) | 37.0 (2) | 61.8 (2) |

*Numbers in parentheses refer to the number of different determinations. Values tabulated are the means.

results are obtained with $^{64}$Cu (II) EDTA although with a 200 μg dose the 24-hour retention of 16.7% of the dose is twice the value obtained with 200 μg ionic copper (8.7%).

*Absorption of biliary copper labeled with $^{64}$Cu* (Table V) (Fig. 6)

When biliary copper is given intrapylorically in doses of 0.50 to 10.0 μg about 16% of the dose is absorbed or at least retained in the body at 24 hours. At a constant dose of 2.5 μg nondialyzable bile copper, absorption decreases progressively when the fractions of bile collected at later times are injected (15% absorption for the 0-4-hour fraction and 9% absorption for the 8-24-hour fraction). Progressively diminishing fractional absorption of $^{64}$Cu is also observed as later bile-fractions are used from $^{64}$Cu (II) EDTA-injected donors, a constant 2.5 μg Cu dose being used in each instance. There is somewhat greater 24-hour retention of $^{64}$Cu (presumably also better absorption) using the 0-4-hour bile-EDTA fraction (21%) than with the same fraction of bile-acetate (14.8%), the elemental copper dose being identical (2.5 μg) in each instance.

*Absorption of nondialyzable serum $^{64}$Cu*

When 1.25 μg nondialyzable serum radiocopper (presumably ceruloplasmin-bound) is given intrapylorically, 14.6% of the dose is retained in the body at 24 hours. In two animals given intrapyloric doses of 2.5 μg each, the fractions retained at 24 hours were 7.4% and 8.2% respectively.

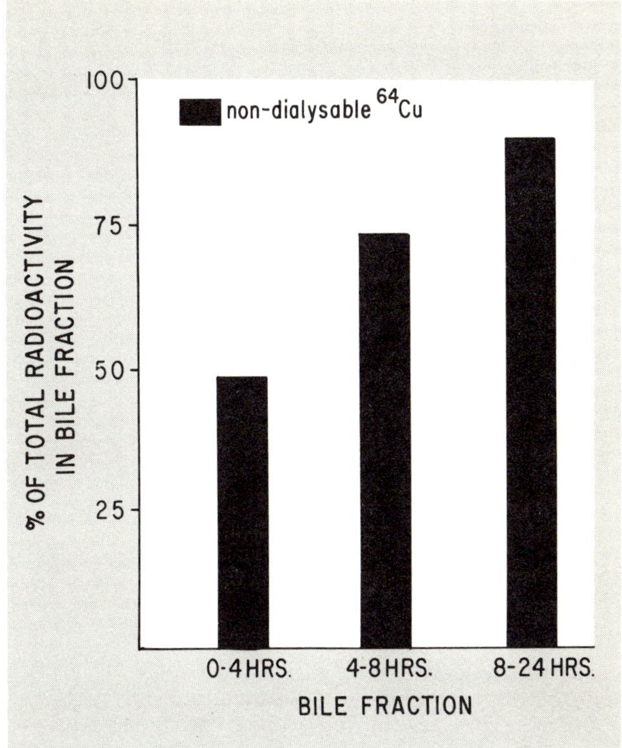


Fig. 4. Dialysis of bile fractions after *i.v.* $^{64}$Cu-acetate (100 μg Cu). The figure shows the increasing proportions of nondialyzable $^{64}$Cu present in successive fractional collections of bile in rats with external biliary fistulas.

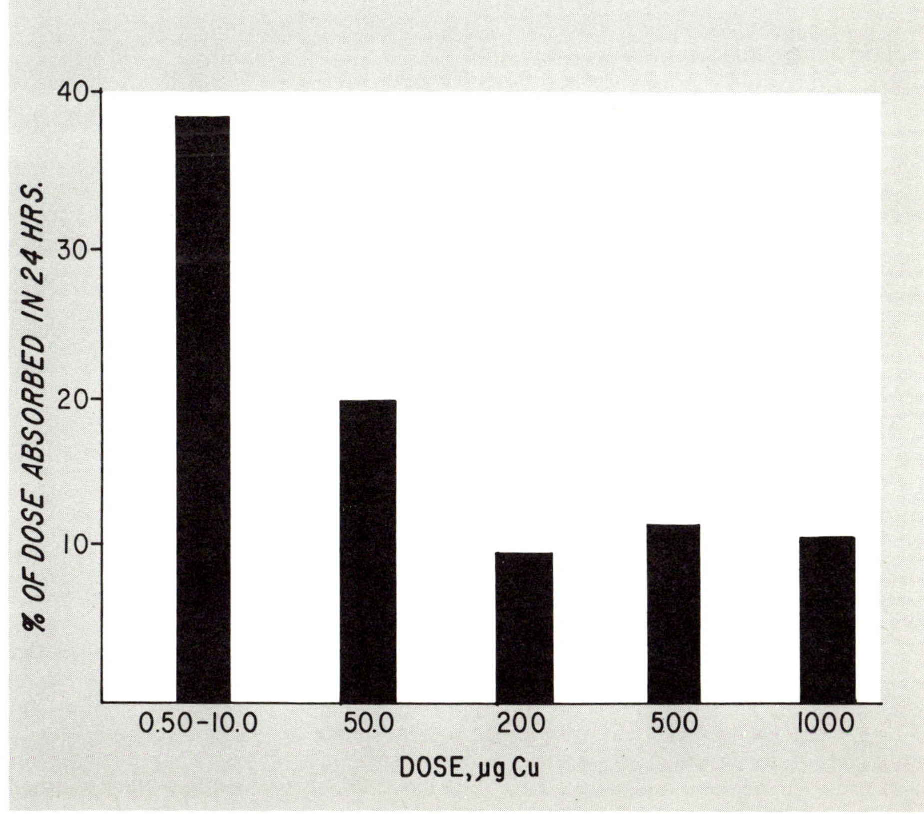


Fig. 5. Absorption of $^{64}$Cu-acetate. The figure depicts the percentage of dose absorbed in 24 hours following 0.50–1000 μg Cu injected into the pylorus.

**TABLE V**

## ABSORPTION OF $^{64}Cu$ IN 24 HOURS FOLLOWING INTRAPYLORIC DOSES OF ENDOGENOUS BILIARY $^{64}Cu$

| Intrapyloric Dose μg Cu | Bile Fraction | No. of Experiments | % of Dose Absorbed (Mean ± S.D.) | Mean μg Cu |
|---|---|---|---|---|
| 2.5 | 0-4 hr.* | 3 | 14.8 ± 1.6 | 0.37 |
| 10.0 | 0-4 hr.* | 2 | 19.5 ± 5.5 | 1.95 |
| 0.5 | 4-8 hr.* | 2 | 13.5 ± 2.3 | 0.07 |
| 2.5 | 4-8 hr.* | 2 | 12.7 ± 1.7 | 0.32 |
| 2.5 | 0-4 hr.+ | 3 | 21.2 ± 4.4 | 0.53 |
| 2.5 | 4-8 hr.+ | 2 | 12.7 ± 0.5 | 0.32 |
| 2.5 | 8-24 hr.+ | 1 | 7.6 | 0.19 |
| 2.5 | 0-4 hr.# | 5 | 15.5 ± 2.8 | 0.39 |
| 2.5 | 4-8 hr.# | 6 | 12.3 ± 4.8 | 0.31 |
| 2.5 | 8-24 hr.# | 3 | 9.5 ± 2.9 | 0.24 |

* Bile from $^{64}Cu$-acetate-injected "donor" rats.
\+ Bile from $^{64}Cu$ (II) EDTA-injected "donor" rats.
\# Dialyzed bile from $^{64}Cu$-acetate-injected "donor" rats.

### Discussion

The results here are in good agreement with Owen's reported observations[13] of the magnitude and patterns of biliary excretion following intravenous doses (up to 100 μg) of cupric acetate in the rat. Prompt biliary excretion of copper occurs following intravenous administration in this dose range and the amount excreted increases with increasing copper loads. The amount of copper excreted in rat bile appears to depend on the amount of bile formed, at least in that a continuous flow of bile at physiologic (even base-line) rates is necessary (approximately 0.5 ml/hour). The excretion of copper in the bile appears to be related most importantly to the amount and concentration of copper present in the liver. A reasonably close parallelism is noted between the delay in reaching peak hepatic concentrations of $^{64}Cu$ and the continuation of significant biliary $^{64}Cu$ excretion for longer periods of time as progressively larger intravenous doses are given. Studies of the perfused, isolated rat liver have shown that the hepatic cell mass has a limited capacity for removing copper from the blood and seems to be a limiting factor for the amount of copper excreted in the bile in brief periods of time.[14]

In mice, the excretion and concentration of copper in the bile increase with the size of the intravenous dose,[15] and even with continued copper administration the larger the copper load the greater the fecal copper excretion. In copper-loaded rats the capacity of the liver to excrete a tracer dose of copper is not impaired, and the excretion of $^{64}Cu$ in the bile is directly related to the concentration of $^{64}Cu$ in the liver.[16] In rabbits maintained on a high inorganic copper diet, in addition to elevated serum ceruloplasmin levels, there is increased $^{64}Cu$ in the liver and the bile.[17]

In contrast, the concentrations of copper in bile in Wilson's disease are in the normal range and not commensurate with the markedly increased hepatic copper pool present.[2,18] Also, radioactive copper is excreted in the stools to a lesser extent in Wilson's disease than in control subjects.[2,3,9] These observations would be consistent with the suggestion of Gitlin and coworkers that the elevated tissue-copper levels in Wilson's disease are probably due to a defect in biliary copper excretion rather than to excessive absorption from the gut.[15]

Progressively larger proportions of the $^{64}Cu$ excreted in the bile are nondialyzable and precipitated in 5% trichloroacetic acid (TCA) with the passage of time following the intravenous injection of labeled copper in the rat. Eventually about 80% of the label is nondialyzable and 60% TCA-precipitated, and this is true for all dose levels in the range of 1-100 μg and regardless of the chemical form of the injected copper. This would be consistent with rat bile containing a specific copper protein in which the copper is bound very tightly. It is unlikely that ceruloplasmin is the protein concerned, since in a separate experiment in which a rat was injected intravenously with serum containing 2.5 μg $^{64}Cu$ (prepared from the exhaustively dialyzed pooled sera of $^{64}Cu$-injected "donor" rats), only 1.8% of the dose was excreted in the bile in 24 hours; the liver at that time had 9.2% of the administered dose. (In contrast, animals receiving 2.5 μg $^{64}Cu$-acetate also by the intravenous route were found to have mean 24-hour bile excretion and hepatic uptake values of 12.0% and 22.1% respectively.) Our findings in the rat concur with those of Aisen and coworkers in the rabbit[19] and support the thesis that little ceruloplasmin is excreted directly into the bile.

The protein composition of bile has been the subject of a number of studies and many serum proteins have also been identified to be present in bile.[20,21,22,23] Two biliary protein components specific for bile were reported by Clausen *et al*[24] and more recently Yoon, Shim and Kil[25] detected three bile-specific protein components in normal human hepatic bile. (Yoon and coworkers also found ceruloplasmin to be present, thereby

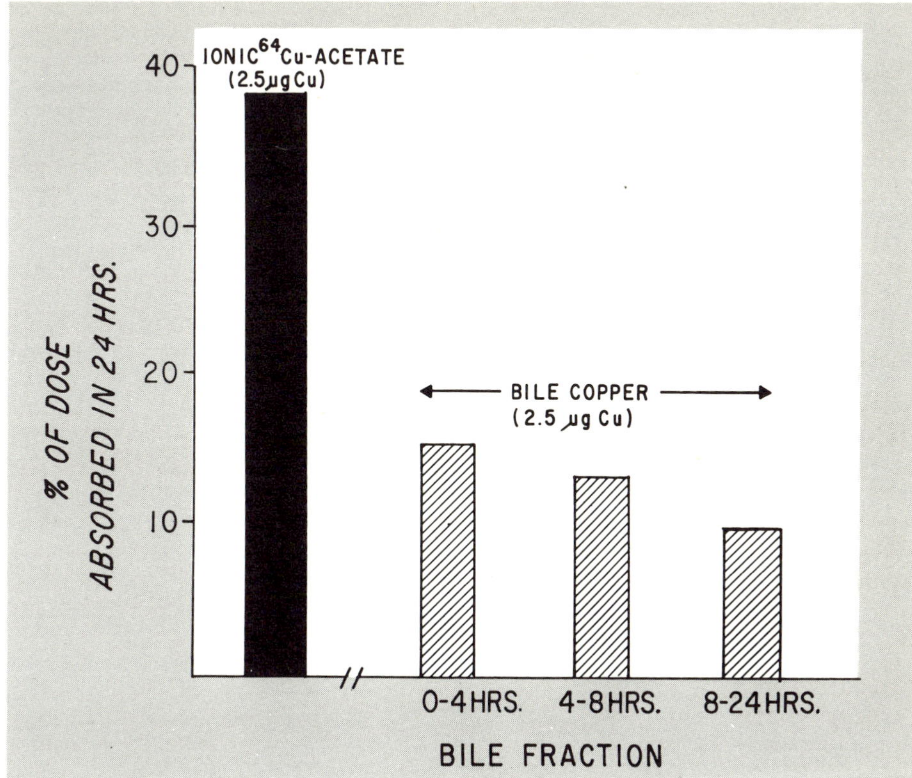


Fig. 6. Absorption of nondialyzable bile copper (2.5 μg $^{64}$Cu). The figure shows the percentage of the dose absorbed in 24 hours when nondialyzable bile $^{64}$Cu from successive bile-collections is injected into the pylorus in a constant dose of 2.5 μg Cu. The absorption of cupric acetate (2.5 μg Cu) is shown by way of comparison.

confirming the observations of Jeunet and associates in the rat.[8]) At present the biosynthetic site and physiologic functions of these bile-specific proteins are not known; however, their existence is relevant to our suggestion that under normal circumstances most of the copper in bile is firmly bound to a specific copper metalloprotein and that the latter is not ceruloplasmin.

Biliary copper is poorly absorbed even in small doses in the rat, in contrast to the relatively greater absorption of comparable doses of exogenous copper. This cannot be ascribed to the endogenous copper content of rat bile (about 0.5 μg/ml[7]) since the doses of bile used in the present study were usually one ml or less and never exceeded two ml. A parallelism seems to exist between the increasing nondialyzability and protein-binding of biliary radiocopper on the one hand, and the increasing malabsorption of the contained $^{64}$Cu on the other, as time goes on following intravenous administration of $^{64}$Cu in rats. This suggests an alteration in the nature of the copper-containing moiety, as a result of which the binding of copper in bile becomes progressively stronger and its availability for reabsorption in the gut lesser and lesser. In this way, the maintenance of normal copper balance is in part related to the excretion of the mineral in a protein-bound form in the bile and its preclusion from significant reabsorption in the intestinal tract. In Wilson's disease the copper in the bile perhaps exists in a form that makes it relatively more available for intestinal reabsorption; if this could be proven, then the abnormal accumulation of copper in the disease would be related to a qualitative as well as a quantitative[15] defect in the biliary excretion of the mineral.

## REFERENCES


1. Mahoney, J. P.; Bush, J. A.; Gubler, C. J.; Moretz, W. H.; Cartwright, G. E. and Wintrobe, M. M.: Studies on copper metabolism. XV. The excretion of copper by animals. *J. Lab. clin. Med.* **46**:702, 1955.
2. Bush, J. A.; Mahoney, J. P.; Markowitz, H.; Gubler, C. J.; Cartwright, G. E. and Wintrobe, M. M.: Studies on copper metabolism. XIV. Radioactive copper studies in normal subjects and in patients with hepatolenticular degeneration. *J. clin. Invest.* **34**:1766, 1955.
3. Bearn, A. G. and Kunkel, H. G.: Metabolic studies in Wilson's disease using Cu-64. *J. Lab. clin. Med.* **45**:623, 1955.
4. Cartwright, G. E. and Wintrobe, M. M.: Copper metabolism in normal subjects. *Amer. J. clin. Nutr.* **14**:224, 1964.
5. Flinn, F. B. and Inouye, J. M.: Some physiological aspects of copper in the organism. *J. biol. Chem.* **84**:101, 1929.
6. Van Ravesteyn, A. H.: Metabolism of copper in man. *Acta med. scand.* **118**:163, 1944.
7. Owen, C. A., Jr.: Distribution of copper in the rat. *Amer. J. Physiol.* **207**:446, 1964.
8. Jeunet, F.; Richterich, R. and Aebi, H.: Bile et céruloplasmine étudé in vitro à l'aide de la perfusion du foie de rat isolé. *J. Physiol. (Paris)* **54**:729, 1962.
9. Matthews, W. B.: The absorption and excretion of radiocopper in hepatolenticular degeneration. *J. Neurol. Neurosurg. Psychiat.* **17**:242, 1954.
10. Zimdahl, W. T.; Hyman, I. and Cook, E. D.: Metabolism of copper in hepatolenticular degeneration. *Neurology* **3**:569, 1953.
11. Martell, A. E.: Some factors governing chelating tendencies and selectivities in the interaction of liquids with metal

ions. In "Biological Aspects of Metal Binding." *Fed. Proc.* **20:**35, (No. 3), Part II, (Supplement No. 10), 1961.

12. Owen, C. A., Jr.: Metabolism of radiocopper (Cu-64) in the rat. *Amer. J. Physiol.* **209**:900, 1965.

13. Owen, C. A., Jr.: Absorption and excretion of Cu-64 labeled copper by the rat. *Amer. J. Physiol.* **207**:1203, 1964.

14. Owen, C. A., Jr.: Copper metabolism and Wilson's disease. In "Dynamic clinical studies with radioisotopes: proceedings of a symposium held at the Oak Ridge Institute of nuclear studies, October 21-25, 1963." Kniseley, R. M.; Tauxe, W. N. and Anderson, E. B. (Editors), U.S.A.E.C., 581-606, 1964.

15. Gitlin, D.; Hughes, W. L. and Janeway, C. A.: Absorption and excretion of copper in mice. *Nature* **188:**150, 1960.

16. Scheuer, P. J. and Barka, T.: Effect of copper loading on uptake and excretion of copper-64 by rat liver. *Nature* **201**:1135, 1964.

17. Gaballah, S. S.; Abood, L. G.; Caleel, G. T. and Kapsalis, A.: Uptake and biliary excretion of Cu-64 in rabbits in relation to blood ceruloplasmin. *Proc. Soc. exp. Biol.* **120**:733, 1965.

18. Denny-Brown, D. and Porter, H.: The effect of BAL (2, 3-dimercaptopropanol) on hepatolenticular degeneration (Wilson's disease). *New Engl. J. Med.* **245**:917-925, 1951.

19. Aisen, P.; Morell, A. G.; Alpert, S. and Sternlieb, I.: Biliary excretion of caeruloplasmin copper. *Nature* **203**: 873-874, 1964.

20. Verschure, J. C. M.; Mijlieff, P. F.; Heufsmitt, F. M. and Nooter Van Hoeven, A. E.: The dominating macromolecular complex of human gall bladder bile. *Clin. chim. Acta* **1**:154, 1956.

21. Verschure, J. C. M.; DeWael, J. and Mijlieff, P. F.: Further investigations on the macromolecular complex in human bile. *Clin. chim. Acta* **1**:511, 1956.

22. Rawson, A.: Human bile proteins. I. Proteins identified by antibody to human serum. *Clin. Chem.* **8**:310, 1962.

23. Russell, I. S. and Burnett, W.: The proteins of human bile. *Gastroenterology* **45**:730, 1963.

24. Clausen, J.; Kruse, J. and Dam, H.: Fractionation and characterization of proteins and lipids in bile. *Scand. J. clin. Lab. Invest.* **17**:325, 1965.

25. Yoon, D. S.; Shim, B. S. and Kil, T. S.: Bile specific protein components in human hepatic bile. *J. Lab. clin. Med.* **67**: 640, 1966.

# Copper Proteins in Brain and Liver in Normal Subjects and in Cases of Wilson's Disease*

HUNTINGTON PORTER, M.D.**

Copper-protein combinations in brain and liver of cases of Wilson's disease have been compared with copper proteins which have been isolated from normal human brain, normal adult human liver and normal newborn human liver. In Wilson's disease brain, pathologic copper appears to be bound to normal soluble brain proteins which are normally copper free. In liver, some of the pathologic copper may be in a form similar to that in the normal newborn.

Copper proteins in human tissues can be divided into two groups: first, those copper proteins which possess known enzymatic activity but which account for a relatively small proportion of total tissue copper; and second, those copper proteins which account for major proportions of tissue copper but which have as yet no known enzymatic activity. The group having known enzymatic activity includes cytochrome oxidase[1] and tyrosinase,[2] in both of which copper participates directly in the enzymatic reaction. The group accounting for major proportions of tissue copper includes the soluble copper proteins cerebrocuprein I[3,4] from brain, human hepatocuprein[5] from adult human liver, and erythrocuprein[6,7] from human erythrocytes and also the insoluble copper protein neonatal hepatic mitochondrocuprein[8,9] from newborn liver. In both human brain and human liver, the subcellular soluble fraction copper accounts for more than 60% of the total tissue copper.[10] There is evidence that most of this soluble copper is represented by the copper proteins cerebrocuprein I and human hepatocuprein which we have isolated. Thus chromatography of whole sucrose extracts of normal human brain or normal human liver gives single copper peaks which correspond in location to the peak of the partially purified copper protein as illustrated in Figure 1.[5] Human brain and liver are relatively rich sources of such soluble copper proteins, having a soluble copper protein content two to three times greater than that of erythrocytes.[11] There is evidence that brain contains at

*These investigations were supported by research grant 5 R01 NB 01733 from the National Institute of Neurological Diseases and Blindness, United States Public Health Service.

**Neurologist, Department of Neurology, New England Medical Center Hospitals and Associate Professor, Department of Medicine (Neurology), Tufts University School of Medicine, Boston, Massachusetts.

### ABOUT THE AUTHOR

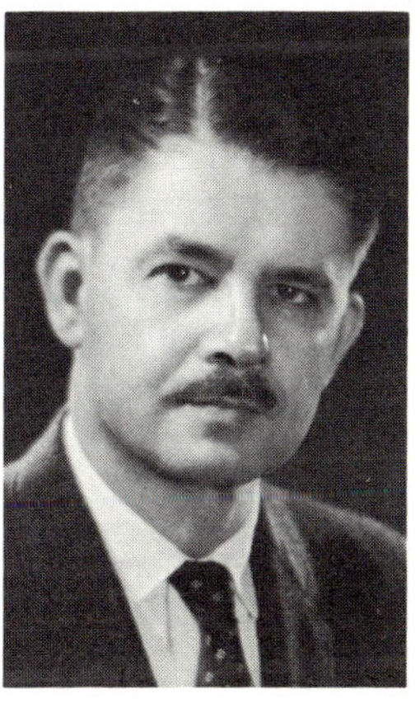

Dr. Huntington Porter was born January 26, 1919 in Boston, Massachusetts. He received a B.S. degree from Harvard College in 1941 and his M.D. degree from Harvard Medical School in 1944. He served as House Officer in the Neurological Unit at Boston City Hospital in 1944 and was Resident in Neurology at Massachusetts General Hospital in 1945.

Doctor Porter became a Research Fellow in Neurology at Boston City Hospital in 1949; Research Fellow in Neurochemistry 1949-1951; Scientific Research Assistant 1951-1954 and Assistant Biochemist 1955-1956, all at McLean Hospital. He was an Instructor in Neurology at Harvard Medical School from 1952-1958 and Assistant Neurologist at Massachusetts General Hospital 1955-1958. From 1958 to the present he has been Neurologist at the New England Medical Center Hospitals and Associate Professor of Neurology at Tufts University School of Medicine.

Doctor Porter is a member of the American Neurological Association, the American Academy of Neurology, the Association for Research in Nervous and Mental Disease and the International Society for Neurochemistry.

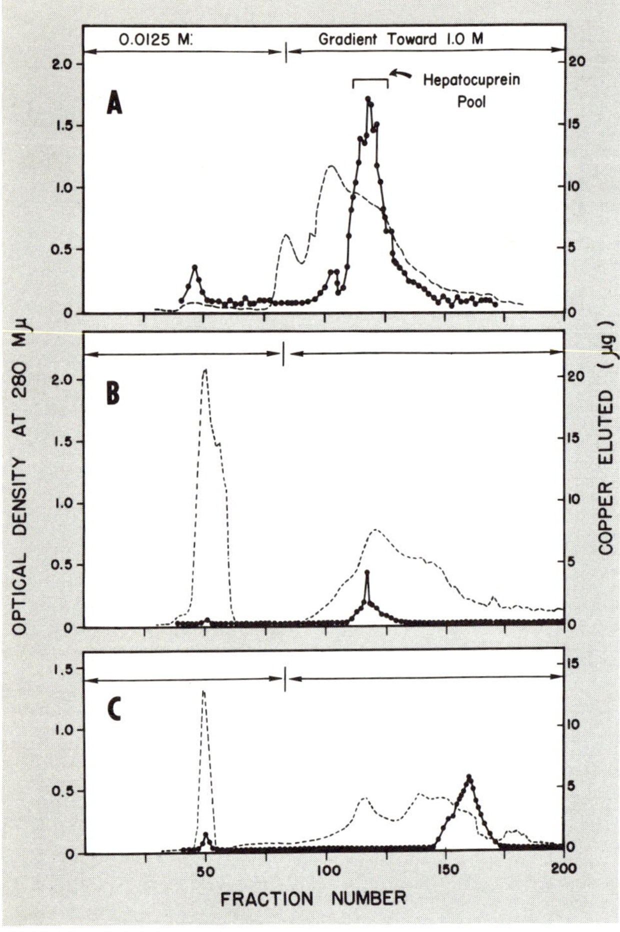


Fig. 1. Chromatographic separation of copper proteins of human liver and of human brain on DEAE cellulose eluted with ammonium bicarbonate in a linear gradient from 0.0125 toward 1.00 M. ---,Optical density at 280 mμ; •—•—•—,Copper eluted (μg). A, chromatography of partially purified hepatocuprein. B, chromatography of whole sucrose extract of liver. C, chromatography of whole sucrose extract of brain. Protein applied to the column was about 850 mg in A and 900 mg in B and C. (After Porter, Sweeney, and Porter.[5])

least three different types of copper protein including one other unknown copper protein in addition to cerebrocuprein I and cytochrome oxidase.[11,12] The procedure for isolation of cerebrocuprein I from the soluble Fraction I of human brain is illustrated in Table I.[4]

The soluble tissue copper proteins cerebrocuprein I from normal human brain, human hepatocuprein from normal adult human liver and erythrocuprein from human erythrocytes are all characterized by bluish-green color with an absorption spectrum showing a maximum in the visible range at 650 to 670 mμ, as illustrated in Figure 2. They are also similar in having a copper content of about 0.3%, ability to retain this copper at a pH as acid as 4.5 and a molecular weight of about 34,000. Their numerous similarities suggest that these soluble copper proteins isolated from the three different tissues may possibly be identical. This possibility is supported by the finding that both brain and liver contain material immunologically identical with purified erythrocuprein.[13,14] However, the quantitative immunologic data[13,14] and chromatographic studies[5] both suggest that there may be some differences between the soluble copper proteins from the three different tissues.

That normal newborn liver contains much larger concentrations of copper than other tissues has long been known.[15,16] We found the largest proportion of this physiologically increased copper of newborn liver to be localized in the mitochondrial fraction.[9,17] From the mitochondrial fraction of newborn bovine or human liver, we were able to obtain a subfraction containing more than 3% copper by successive differential centrifugations in different detergents, as illustrated in Table II.[8,9] The name neonatal hepatic mitochondrocuprein was suggested for the copper protein of immature liver mitochondria represented by this subfraction. Neonatal hepatic mitochondrocuprein differs from the soluble tissue copper proteins described in the preceding section in its extraordinarily high copper content which exceeds that of other known normal copper proteins by at least tenfold, in its failure to be extracted from the tissue in soluble form by either water or detergents and in its

**TABLE I**

## PURIFICATION OF HUMAN CEREBROCUPREIN I*

| Step | Fraction | Concentration of copper in fraction (%) | Yield per gm fresh tissue | |
|---|---|---|---|---|
| | | | Copper (μg) | Solids† (mg) |
| | Total human brain | | 4.2 | |
| 1 | pH 4.5 buffer extract | 0.008 | 2.38 | 30.00 |
| 2 | 75% acetone precipitate | 0.030 | 1.85 | 6.11 |
| 3 | 45-75% chloroform-ethanol precipitate | 0.095 | 1.24 | 1.31 |
| 4 | Undialyzable material | 0.17 | 1.31 | 0.78 |
| 5 | 50-75% acetone precipitate | 0.15 | 0.78 | 0.53 |
| 6 | Paper electrophoresis eluate | 0.29 | 0.15 | 0.05 |

*After Porter and Ainsworth.[4] †Based on dry weight.

TABLE II

## PREPARATION OF HUMAN CRUDE NEONATAL HEPATIC MITOCHONDROCUPREIN*

| Step | Fraction | Concentration of copper in fraction (%) | Yield per gm fresh tissue | |
|---|---|---|---|---|
| | | | Copper (μg) | Solids† (mg) |
| | Total immature liver | | 63.8 | |
| 1 | Mitochondria | 0.12 | 27.4 | 22.8 |
| 2 | Deoxycholate 14000 × g sediment | 1.5 | 21.8 | 1.5 |
| 3 | Tween 1600 × g sediment | 2.6 | 18.4 | 0.71 |
| 4 | Dodecylsulfate 1600 × g sediment | 4.4 | 15.4 | 0.35 |

*After Porter, Sweeney and Porter.[9] †Dry weight of acetone insoluble material.

amino acid composition. Crude neonatal hepatic mitochondrocuprein, both bovine and human, contains extremely large proportions of cystine which have averaged about 17% of the total amino acids recovered.[18] The copper in the neonatal hepatic mitochondrocuprein-containing subfraction was nondialyzable and appeared stable to acid pH but reacted directly with sodium diethyldithiocarbamate, although at an extremely slow rate. The copper in this subfraction and in the parent total mitochondrial fraction was insoluble in water over a wide pH range, in detergents and in a variety of organic solvents but could be quantitatively released into soluble form by treatment with trypsin. The copper-containing tryptic peptides of neonatal hepatic mitochondrocuprein contain large proportions of the amino acids lysine and arginine and are deep blue in color with an absorption maximum at 605 mμ (Fig. 3).[18] However, it is not certain that these blue peptides do not represent a rearrangement of copper from the type of copper-protein bond present in intact neonatal hepatic mitochondrocuprein. In the normal human, neonatal hepatic mitochondrocuprein appeared to be specific to the neonatal period. Thus yield of copper and concentration of copper in the neonatal hepatic mitochondrocuprein subfraction from newborn human livers averaged more than 80 times those in the corresponding material from adult human livers (Table III).[9] The extraordinarily high copper content of neonatal hepatic mitochondrocuprein compared to that of copper proteins known to have enzymatic activity and its other differences from such proteins suggest that neonatal hepatic mitochondrocuprein may have a storage function for copper in the immature animal analogous to that of ferritin for iron storage.

Among the manifestations of abnormal copper metabolism in Wilson's disease are two which are similar to the condition of the normal newborn infant; first, a reduced amount of normal plasma ceruloplasmin[19] and, second, a greatly elevated concentration of copper in the liver.[15,16] It therefore seemed of interest to investigate the possibility of a relationship between the type of copper protein formed by some of the pathologic hepatic copper in Wilson's disease and that formed by the physiologic increase in copper in newborn liver.

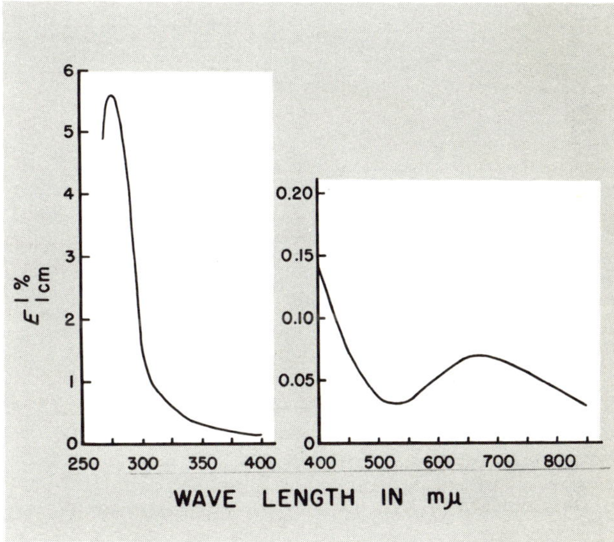


Fig. 2. Absorption spectrum of human hepatocuprein in barbital buffer pH 8.6; ionic strength 0.10 in visible range, 0.0244 in ultraviolet, read against buffer blank at the same concentrations. Protein concentrations at the time of measurement were approximately 5% for the visible range and 0.123% for the ultraviolet. (After Porter, Sweeney, and Porter.[5])

TABLE III

## Relation of Age of Subject to Yield of Human Crude Neonatal Hepatic Mitochondrocuprein*

| Age of Subject | Yield per g fresh tissue | | Concentration of copper in fraction |
|---|---|---|---|
| | Copper (μg) | Solids (mg) | (%) |
| Newborn† | 15.9 | 0.48 | 3.31 |
| Adult** | 0.15 | 0.63 | 0.02 |

*After Porter, Sweeney and Porter.[9]
†Average of three different preparations.
**Average of two different preparations.

TABLE IV

**Distribution of Copper Among Subcellular Fractions From Liver and Brain From Wilson's Disease, Liver and Brain From Normal Adults, and Liver From Newborn Infants****

| Tissue | Source | Fraction | | | | |
|---|---|---|---|---|---|---|
| | | Total Tissue | R-1 Nuclei | R-2 Mitochondria* | R-3 Microsomes | S Soluble |
| Liver | Wilson's disease | 103.1 | 28.6 | 36.5 | 10.1 | 27.7 |
| Liver | Normal adult† | 5.6 | 0.5 | 0.9 | 0.6 | 3.6 |
| Liver | Normal infant‡ | 73.3 | 14.1 | 29.6 | 5.4 | 21.4 |
| Brain | Wilson's disease | 64.7 | 9.1 | 4.9 | 5.6 | 44.7 |
| Brain | Normal adult† | 4.2 | 0.3 | 0.8 | 0.7 | 2.5 |

Copper expressed as $\mu$g/gm of fresh tissue.
*Mitochondrial fractions used in these experiments did not include washings from the nuclear residue. In newborn bovine liver, inclusion of these washings increased the yield of mitochondrial copper by about 20%.
†Average of two preparations from different subjects.
‡Average of three preparations from different subjects.
**After Porter.[10]

In an untreated case of Wilson's disease, a significant portion of the pathologic hepatic copper was found in the mitochondrial fraction (Table IV).[10] In a second case of Wilson's disease which had been vigorously treated and had a total liver copper content of only one-fourth of that shown for the untreated case in Table IV, 55% of the total hepatic copper was found in the soluble fraction. Copper in the mitochondrial fraction in this treated case was still more than five times that in normal human livers. In both cases of Wilson's disease, the mitochondrial copper was largely insoluble in detergents and could be concentrated by the procedure developed for concentration of neonatal hepatic mitochondrocuprein. In the two cases of Wilson's disease thus far investigated, yield of solids in the detergent-insoluble subfraction was much greater than the yield of solids in this subfraction obtained from normal newborn liver, suggesting that in Wilson's disease this subfraction contains some material other than neonatal hepatic mitochondrocuprein. Solution and further purification of this subfraction from normal newborn livers and from livers of cases of Wilson's disease and amino-acid analyses of the purified copper protein(s) obtained from the subfraction may provide further information as to whether or not some of the pathologic hepatic copper in Wilson's disease is bound in a form similar to physiologic neonatal hepatic mitochondrocuprein. Our laboratory does not as yet have any reproducible data on the types of pathologic copper protein present in the subcellular soluble fraction from livers of cases of Wilson's disease.

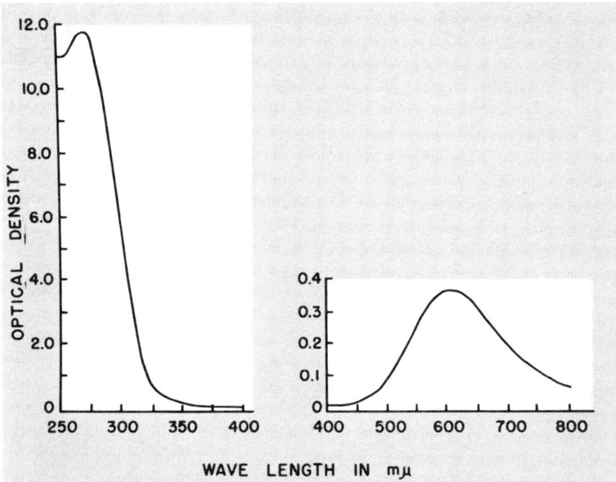


Fig. 3. Absorption spectrum of blue tryptic peptides of neonatal hepatic mitochondrocuprein in 0.1 M ammonium carbonate, pH 8.8, read against buffer blank at the same concentration. Protein concentrations at the time of measurement were estimated as approximately 0.32% for the visible range and 0.016% for the ultraviolet. (After Porter.[18])

In Wilson's disease brain (five cases), the largest proportion of the pathologic copper has consistently been found in the soluble fraction,[10,20] as illustrated in the case summarized in Table IV. Previous studies subjecting this soluble pathologic brain copper to the isolation procedure for the normal brain copper protein cerebrocuprein I have suggested that the quantity of normal cerebrocuprein I in the brain in Wilson's disease is probably not significantly increased.[21] On chromatography, the pathologic soluble copper proteins in the brain in Wilson's disease were found reproducibly spread over a very wide range of chromatographic fractions (Fig. 4).[10] This spread of pathologic brain copper over a wide range of eluent fractions, compared to the single well-defined copper peaks obtained from normal brain and normal liver, indicates that the pathologic copper in the brain in Wilson's disease is bound to a number of different proteins. The chromatographic pattern of elution of protein, as opposed to copper, appeared to be similar in Wilson's disease and normal brain. Both these results and our previous electrophoretic data[20] suggest that the pathologic copper in

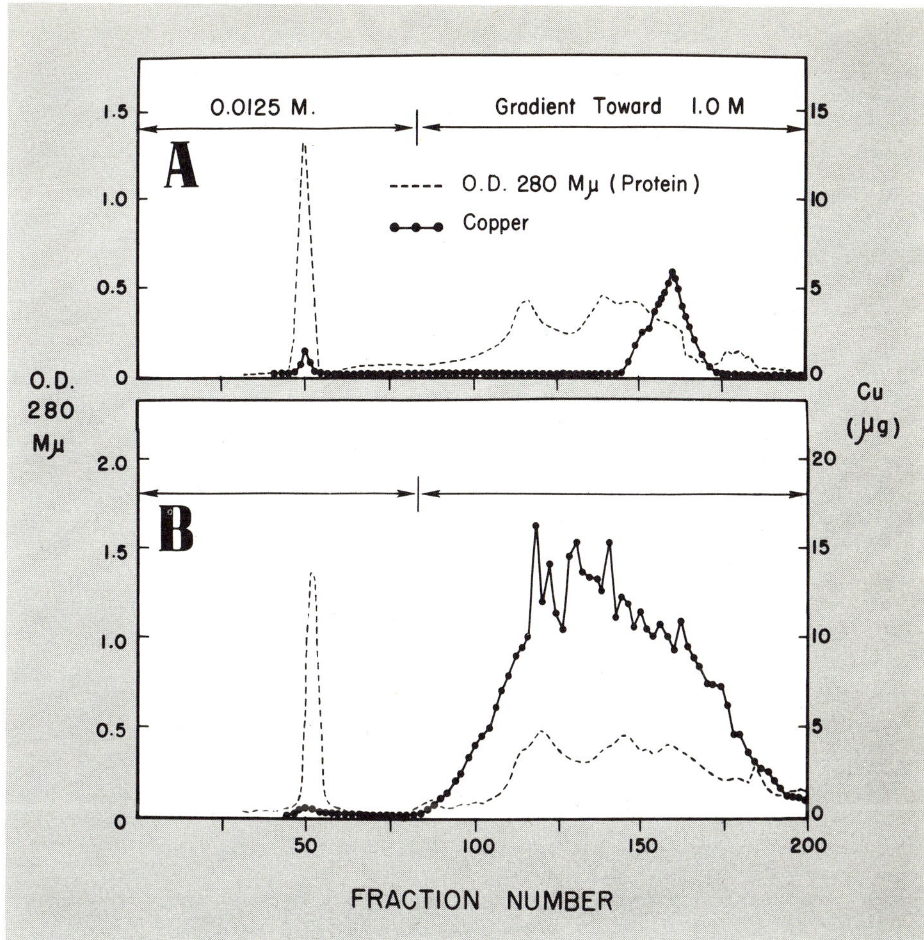


Fig. 4. Chromatographic separation of copper proteins of normal human brain and brain from case of Wilson's disease on DEAE cellulose eluted with ammonium bicarbonate in a linear gradient from 0.0125 M toward 1.00 M. ---, Optical density at 280 mμ; -•-•-, Copper eluted (μg). A, chromatography of sucrose extract of normal brain. B, chromatography of sucrose extract of brain from case of Wilson's disease. Protein applied to each column was about 900 mg. (After Porter.[10])

the brain in Wilson's disease becomes bound to normal brain proteins which are normally copper free.

The evidence that in Wilson's disease pathologic copper in both brain and liver is bound to a number of different proteins suggests that the evolution of the biochemical lesion may not represent solely the accumulation of increasingly larger amounts of a noxious copper protein. Rather, there may be a sequence of events as pathologic copper accumulates in the tissues with the formation of different tissue copper-protein combinations at different stages of the illness. Initial binding of pathologic copper in nontoxic form, for example a form similar to physiologic neonatal hepatic mitochondrocuprein, might help to explain the latent period between a disorder of copper metabolism present from birth and the hepatic, cerebral and renal deficits developing only after many years. These deficits may occur when pathologic copper later becomes bound to, and inhibits enzymatic activity of, other tissue proteins which are normally copper free. The finding of about 70% of the pathologic brain copper of Wilson's disease in the subcellular soluble fraction, as opposed to less than 10% of the pathologic brain copper in the mitochondrial fraction, suggests that the brain enzymes affected by copper in this disease are probably localized in the subcellular soluble fraction.

**Summary**

1. Copper proteins in the subcellular soluble fraction account for about 60% of the total tissue copper of normal human brain and normal human liver. The purified soluble copper proteins cerebrocuprein I from brain and human hepatocuprein from liver are characterized by a copper content of 0.3%, a molecular weight of about 34,000, bluish-green color with an absorption maximum at 650 to 670 mμ and ability to retain copper at a pH as acid as 4.5.

2. Neonatal hepatic mitochondrocuprein, which represents a major portion of the copper accumulating physiologically in newborn liver, differs from the soluble copper proteins in that it is localized in the mitochondrial fraction, has a copper content about ten times as great, has a very high cystine content, and is normally specific to the neonatal period.

3. In Wilson's disease liver, a significant proportion of the pathologic copper has been found in the mitochondrial fraction in detergent-insoluble form possibly similar to neonatal hepatic mitochondrocuprein.

4. In Wilson's disease brain, the major portion of the pathologic copper is in the subcellular soluble fraction and appears to be bound to a number of different normal brain proteins which are normally copper free.

## REFERENCES


1. Griffiths, D. E. and Wharton, D. C.: Studies of the electron transport system. XXXV. Purification and properties of cytochrome oxidase. *J. biol. Chem.* **236:**1850, 1961.

2. Brown, F. C. and Ward, D. N.: Studies on mamalian tyrosinase. II. Chemical and physical properties of fractions purified by chromatography. *Proc. Soc. exp. Biol.* **100:**701, 1959.

3. Porter, H. and Folch, J.: Cerebrocuprein I. A copper-containing protein isolated from brain. *J. Neurochem.* **1:**260, 1957.

4. Porter, H. and Ainsworth, S.: The isolation of the copper-containing protein cerebrocuprein I from normal human brain. *J. Neurochem.* **5:**91, 1959.

5. Porter, H.; Sweeney, M. and Porter, E.: Human hepatocuprein. Isolation of a copper protein from the subcellular soluble fraction of adult human liver. *Arch. Biochem.* **105:**319, 1964.

6. Markowitz, H.; Cartwright, G. E. and Wintrobe, M. M.: Studies on copper metabolism. XXVII. The isolation and properties of an erythrocyte cuproprotein (erythrocuprein). *J. biol. Chem.* **234:**40, 1959.

7. Stansell, M. J. and Deutsch, H. F.: Preparation of crystalline erythrocuprein and catalase from human erythrocytes. *J. biol. Chem.* **240:**4299, 1965.

8. Porter, H.; Johnston, J. and Porter, E.: Neonatal hepatic mitochondrocuprein. I. Isolation of a protein fraction containing more than 4% copper from mitochondria of immature bovine liver. *Biochim. biophys. Acta* **65:**66, 1962.

9. Porter, H.; Sweeney, M. and Porter, E.: Neonatal hepatic mitochondrocuprein. II. Isolation of the copper-containing subfraction from mitochondria of newborn human liver. *Arch. Biochem.* **104:**97, 1964.

10. Porter, H.: Tissue copper proteins in Wilson's disease, *Arch. Neurol.* **11:**341, 1964.

11. Porter, H. and Folch, J.: Brain copper-protein fractions in the normal and in Wilson's disease. *Arch. Neurol. Psychiat.* **77:**8, 1957.

12. Porter, H. and Ainsworth, S.: The intracellular distribution of copper in brain. *J. Neurochem.* **7:**20, 1961.

13. Shields, G. S.; Markowitz, H.; Klassen, W. H.; Cartwright, G. E. and Wintrobe, M. M.: Studies on copper metabolism. XXXI. Erythrocyte copper. *J. clin. Invest.* **11:**2007, 1961.

14. Stansell, M. J. and Deutsch, H. F.: Immunochemical studies of human erythrocyte proteins: erythrocuprein and catalase. *J. biol. Chem.* **241:**2509, 1966.

15. Bruckmann, G. and Zondak, S. G.: Iron, copper and manganese in human organs at various ages. *Biochem. J.* **33:**1845, 1939.

16. Butt, E. M.; Nusbaum, R. E.; Gilmour, T. C. and Didio, S. L.: Trace metal patterns in disease states. II. Copper storage diseases, with consideration of juvenile cirrhosis, Wilson's disease and hepatic copper of the newborn. *Amer. J. clin. Path.* **30:**479, 1958.

17. Porter, H.; Wiener, W. and Barker, M.: The intracellular distribution of copper in immature liver. *Biochim. biophys. Acta* **52:**419, 1961.

18. Porter, H.: The Biochemistry of Copper, J. Peisach; P. Aisan and W. E. Blumberg, (Eds.) Academic Press, New York. p. 159, 1966.

19. Scheinberg, I. H.; Cook, C. D. and Murphy, J. A.: The concentration of copper and ceruloplasmin in maternal and infant plasma at delivery. *J. clin. Invest.* **33:**963, 1954.

20. Porter, H.: Some properties of brain copper proteins in hepatolenticular degeneration. *Arch. Neurol.* **1:**544, 1959.

21. Porter, H.: Cerebrocuprein I copper in the brain in Wilson's disease. *Arch. Neurol.* **5:**197, 1961.

# Studies on Copper Metabolism in Wilson's Disease

Toshio Terao, M.D.*; Kazuteru Ogihara, M.D.* and Toshiji Mozai, M.D.*

Uptake of $^{64}Cu$ by erythrocytes was found to be lower in patients with Wilson's disease than in control subjects, following oral administration of $^{64}Cu$. The distribution of $^{64}Cu$ in the body was determined and residual radioactivity was measured. The effect of penicillamine on absorption of $^{64}Cu$ was also studied. The copper contents of hair and nails in control subjects and in patients with Wilson's disease was measured by neutron activation analysis.

An abnormality of copper metabolism has been reported by many workers as being one of the basic defects in Wilson's disease.[1] Recently, the use of radioisotopic copper has proved to be very helpful in the study of the disease and there have been numerous reports using this technic.

We have also conducted radioactive copper studies in cases of Wilson's disease in Japan, comparing the results with those reported in American and European countries.[2-8]

### Materials and Methods

Six cases of Wilson's disease were studied. Kayser-Fleischer corneal rings and hypoceruloplasminemia were present in all the cases. Three of those six cases showed mainly neurologic manifestations and the other three showed only abnormalities in liver function tests with a history of jaundice.

The control group altogether consisted of eight cases, of which three were normal, three had disorders of the nervous system without frank metabolic abnormalities, and two had liver cirrhosis. The specific activity of $^{64}Cu$ used was 0.4-0.5 mc/mg Cu. In each case 1-1.5 mc of $^{64}Cu$ (3 mg of copper) was administered as cupric chloride orally. In a few cases, however, up to 4 mc (8 mg of copper) was administered in order to follow the radioactivity in the blood for a longer period of time. The measurement of blood radioactivity was done in a well-type scintillation counter with a low background $\beta$-ray spectrometer, the latter being used particularly for the later period of diminished activity. With the use of this equipment it became possible to count under a background as low as 0.1 cpm for as long as 100 hours after administration of $^{64}Cu$.[9]

For external counting, a collimated scintillation counter with a thallium-activated sodium-iodide crystal of two inches diameter was used. The human counter with a plastic scintillator was used for whole body counting. A H.T.R. reactor was used for activation analysis with a flux of $1.7 \times 10^{12}$ neutrons/sec. cm$^2$ for five hours.

### Results

Figure 1 shows the total radioactivity in plasma after $^{64}Cu$ administration. As reported by others, the control group showed its peak in one to three hours, and the lowest level in four to six hours. The index proposed by Sternlieb,[7] namely the ratio of the plasma radioactivity of $^{64}Cu$ 48 hours after ingestion to the radioactivity at the initial peak in eight control subjects, averaged 1.22, while the corresponding value in six patients with Wilson's disease was 0.18. In Wilson's dis-

**ABOUT THE SENIOR AUTHOR**

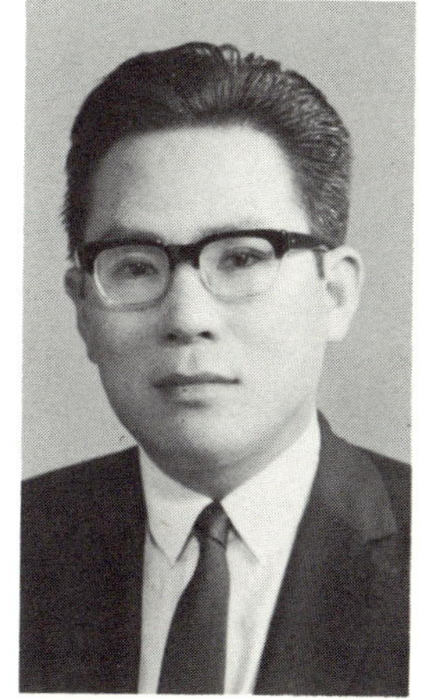

Dr. Toshio Terao, born in 1930, was graduated from the University of Tokyo, Faculty of Medicine in 1953. His internship was at the University of Tokyo Hospital from 1953 to 1954. He completed the courses of the Graduate School of the University of Tokyo, Division of Medical Sciences and received the degree of Doctor of Medical Sciences in 1960. Dr. Terao is a Fellow in the Third Department of Internal Medicine.

*Fellows, Third Department of Internal Medicine, University of Tokyo, Japan.

ease, the initial peak tended to be somewhat higher and slightly more delayed than that of normal, and in one of the cases the peak was considerably more delayed. The fall was slower than the controls' and the secondary rise could not be seen even when the measurement was continued for a long period. The radioactivity in plasma was confirmed to be mainly direct-reacting copper and only a small portion proved to be indirect-reacting copper. These results are in agreement with those of other reports.[2,4,7]

The radioactivity of whole blood and plasma was measured and packed cell radioactivity was calculated using the hematocrit value. The uptake of radiocopper by erythrocytes increased with time (Fig. 2) but in three of five cases of Wilson's disease it was lower than in the control subjects. Little difference was found in the corresponding stages in the other two patients.

Uptake of $^{64}Cu$ by liver, head, midthigh and calf was measured with a collimated scintillation counter. For

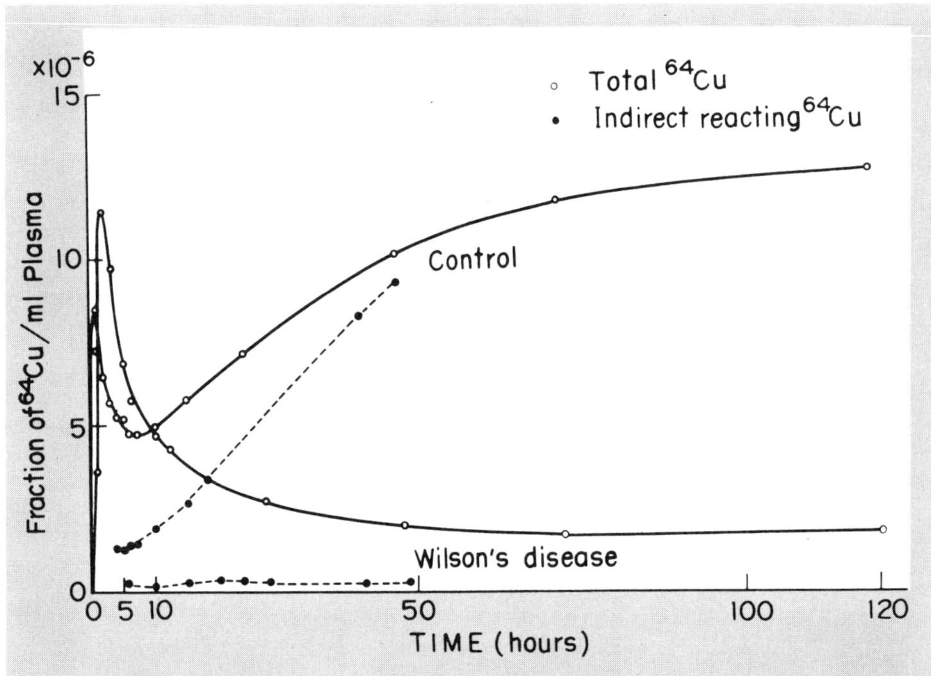


Fig. 1. Mean radioactivity in plasma of eight controls and six patients with Wilson's disease after oral administration of $^{64}CuCl_2$. Broken lines show indirect-reacting $^{64}Cu$.

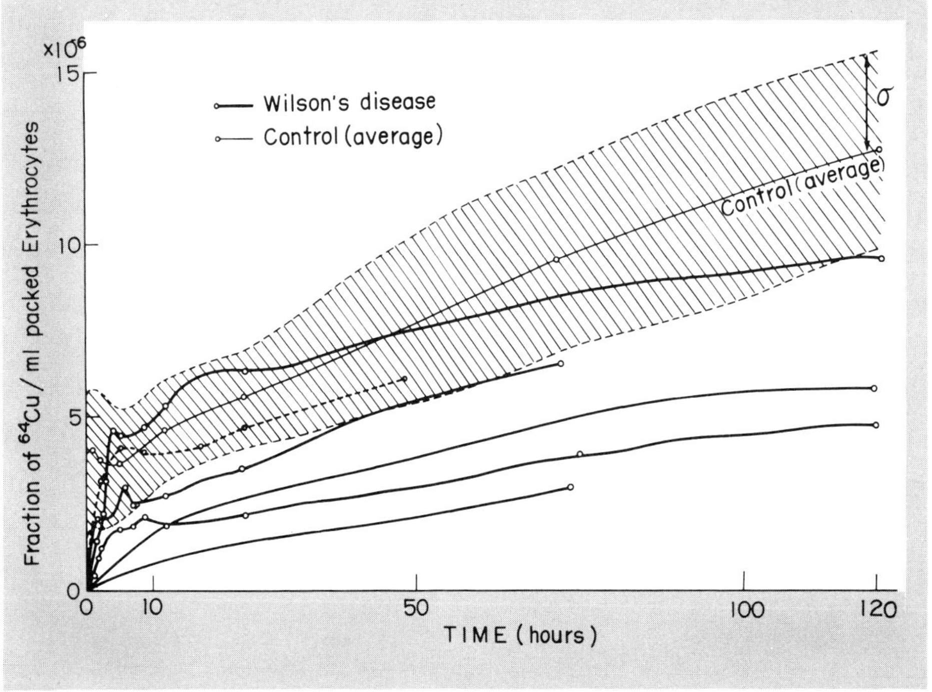


Fig. 2. Radioactivity in packed erythrocytes of eight controls (average $\pm$ $\sigma$) and five patients with Wilson's disease after oral administration of $^{64}CuCl_2$. The broken line in the figure shows the value of an instance of heterozygote (patient's mother).

the liver, the place and direction of maximal counting was selected and the region of the gallbladder was avoided. As pointed out by Walshe and others,[5,10-13] there were some cases with Wilson's disease in which the uptake in the head, calf or thigh was high. The radioactivity over the hepatic region exceeded that of the head or thigh. The solid lines in Figure 3 show the results obtained in Wilson's disease patients. In these patients the uptake by the liver was lower than in normal subjects. The uptake by the calf and head was higher.

The excretion of $^{64}Cu$ into urine and feces is illustrated in Figure 4. In the control group, the excretion of $^{64}Cu$ into urine was as low as 0.2% of the dose in 72 hours and a major portion of $^{64}Cu$ was excreted into feces, showing considerable variation. In patients with Wilson's disease, however, urinary excretion of $^{64}Cu$ was increased and fecal excretion was almost completed within three to four days. Therefore measurement of $^{64}Cu$ retained in the body with the human counter after the major portion has been excreted into feces seemed

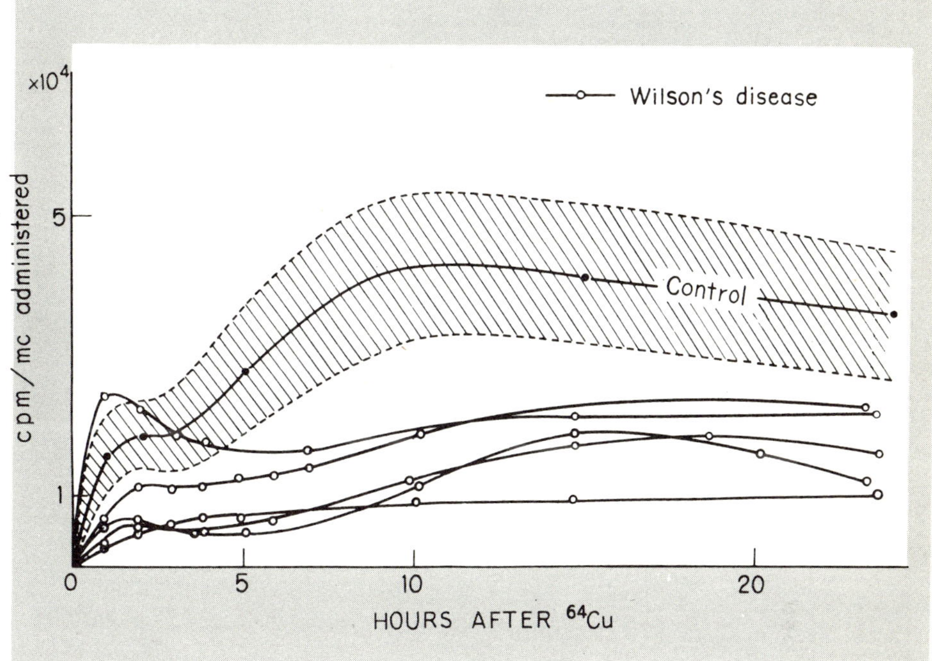


Fig. 3. Measurement of radioactivity over the hepatic region in patients with Wilson's disease (solid line). Average value in control subjects is shown as mean $\pm \sigma$ (shadowed area).

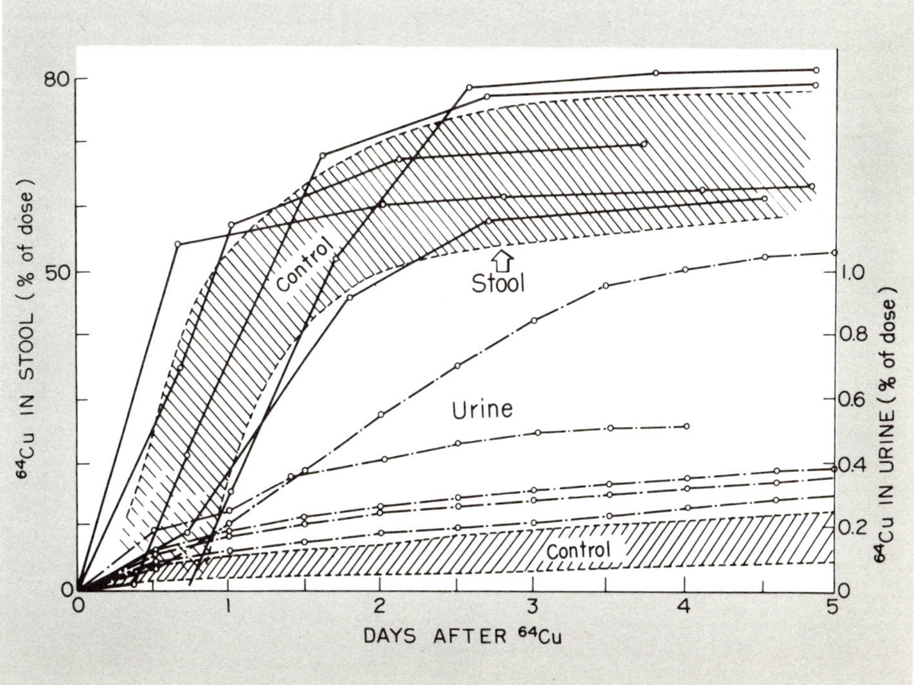


Fig. 4. Excretion of $^{64}Cu$ in urine and stools of patients with Wilson's disease following oral administration of $^{64}CuCl_2$.

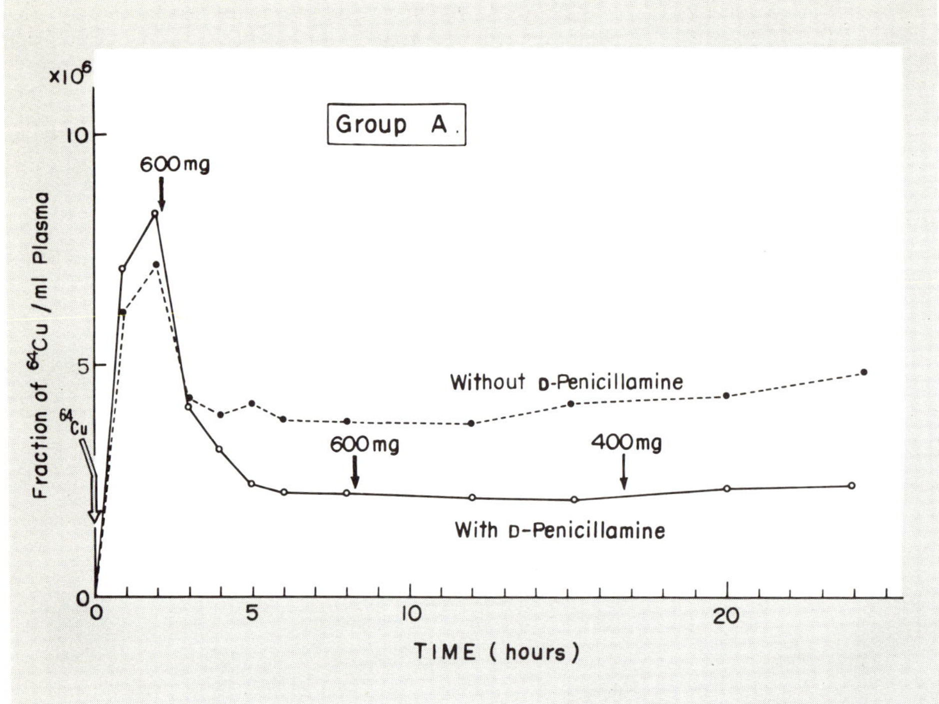


Fig. 5. Radioactivity in plasma in one subject from Group A given D-penicillamine two hours after $^{64}$Cu.

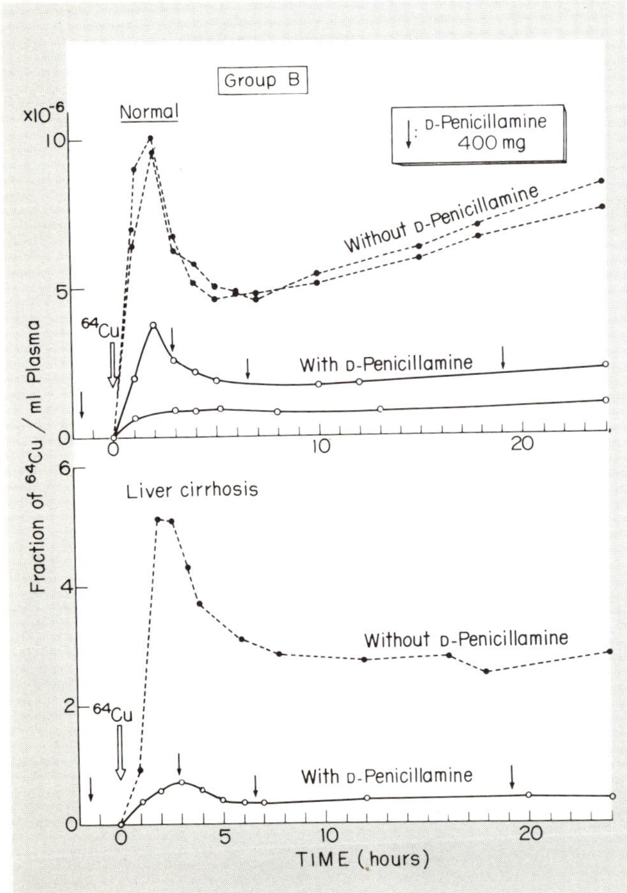


Fig. 6. Radioactivity in plasma after D-penicillamine (0.4g) given 1.5 hours before $^{64}$Cu (arrows).

of interest. In control subjects, total excretion of $^{64}$Cu up to the fifth day averaged approximately 77% into feces and 0.2% into urine. Of the remaining $^{64}$Cu, approximately 19% of the dose was measured by the human counter, but the remaining 4% could not be accounted for.

In four of the control subjects in whom the measurements were carried out one week after $^{64}$Cu administration by means of a human counter, 15.9% (14.6-16.9%) of the dose administered still was retained in the body, whereas in Wilson's disease, the remaining $^{64}$Cu was 16.6% (13.4-19.1%) with considerable variations.

We also studied the effects of administration of 1.2 g of penicillamine per day on $^{64}$Cu levels. The first dose of penicillamine was given to five of the control subjects immediately after $^{64}$Cu activity in plasma had reached its peak (group A). Figure 5 shows the change of radioactivity in plasma after penicillamine administration. The radioactivity in plasma after penicillamine is somewhat lower than the corresponding control value but uptake by the liver, assessed by external counting, did not change. Excretion of $^{64}$Cu into urine, however, was increased ten to 60 fold both in patients and in normal subjects.

Subsequently, we have given three of the control subjects the first dose of D-penicillamine 1.5 hours before the $^{64}$Cu administration so that penicillamine might exert its effect on $^{64}$Cu immediately after its intestinal absorption (group B). 0.4g of D-penicillamine was given before administration of $^{64}$Cu as shown by arrows in Figure 6. The level of $^{64}$Cu in plasma was markedly decreased in this group when compared with the radio-

**TABLE I**

**RETENTION RATE OF $^{64}Cu$ AFTER D-PENICILLAMINE TREATMENT FOR ONE WEEK EXPRESSED AS PERCENTAGE OF DOSE.**

*Each control subject was given 1.2g of D-penicillamine per day. Penicillamine treatment was started two hours after $^{64}Cu$ in group A, and 1.5 hours before $^{64}Cu$ in group B.*

| Case | Without D-penicillamine | With D-penicillamine | |
|---|---|---|---|
| | | 1st dose given 2 hrs. AFTER $^{64}Cu$ administration (A) | 1st dose given 1.5 hrs. BEFORE $^{64}Cu$ administration (B) |
| 1 | 14.6 | 13.9 | — |
| 2 | 16.5 | 15.0 | — |
| 3 | 15.9 | — | 5.8 |
| 4 | 16.9 | — | 4.1 |

(% of dose)

activity in plasma of the same subject without penicillamine (indicated by a dotted line). The uptake by the liver was also decreased. This was further confirmed by measuring the uptake with the human counter (Table I).

As described above, approximately 16% of the given $^{64}Cu$ remained at the end of the first week as shown in Table I. After one week, there was no difference in percentage retention between group A, given the first dose of penicillamine two hours after $^{64}Cu$ administration, and the group which received $^{64}Cu$ only. On the other hand, the percentage retention after one week in group B was markedly decreased.

Recent progress in neutron activation analysis enabled us to measure trace metals in hair and nails. We used this method to measure the copper in Wilson's disease. The results are shown in Figure 7. The copper in the hair of Japanese was less than that reported in other countries.[14] It varied considerably even in normal subjects. The copper in the hair and nails of patients with Wilson's disease was increased in some but normal in others. The open circles show the values in the cases to whom D-penicillamine was given intermittently for two years. The effect of penicillamine, however, was not striking.

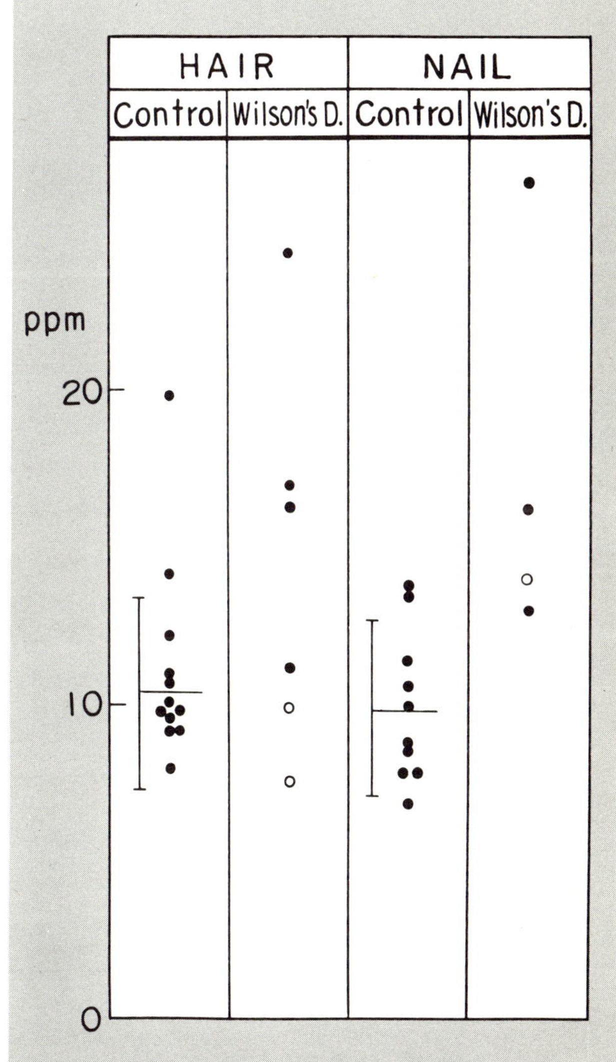


Fig. 7. Copper contents of hair and nails measured by neutron activation analysis. Open circles show the values in patients with Wilson's disease treated with D-penicillamine for two years. Horizontal lines show the mean value and vertical lines show the standard deviation in control subjects.

### Discussion

The distribution of $^{64}Cu$ in patients with Wilson's disease differs from that of normal subjects. The uptake by the liver is decreased, whereas the uptake by the head and thigh is increased; a large portion of radioactivity in the plasma is found as direct-reacting copper. It is interesting to note that incorporation into erythrocytes is decreased in most of our cases with Wilson's disease. Copper in erythrocytes is found mostly in the form of erythrocuprein. The amount of this copper protein in erythrocytes has been reported as not being decreased in Wilson's disease by Cartwright and others.[3,15] Further studies on this subject are desirable.

In addition, the remaining activity in the body after $^{64}Cu$ administration as determined by the human counter shows a reasonable agreement with the value calculated by subtracting the excretion into urine and feces from the given dose. Unexpectedly, the retention of $^{64}Cu$ in Wilson's disease and in the control subjects did not differ significantly.

Furthermore, a marked effect of penicillamine on retention and uptake of $^{64}Cu$ by the liver was demonstrated when the first dose of penicillamine was given before but not after $^{64}Cu$ administration. In interpreting these facts, we have considered the following two possibilities: either penicillamine chelates $^{64}Cu$ and suppresses its absorption or it promotes the excretion of newly absorbed copper, resulting in prevention of its deposition in the tissues.

**Summary**

1. The radioactivity of $^{64}Cu$ in plasma showed a decreased secondary rise in Wilson's disease.
2. In Wilson's disease, the uptake in the liver tended to be low, while that in the head, calf and thigh tended to be high.
3. The incorporation of $^{64}Cu$ into erythrocytes was lower in three of five patients with Wilson's disease.
4. a) Penicillamine given before $^{64}Cu$, was markedly effective in reducing the retention rate and the plasma level.

   b) The radioactivity in blood decreased to some extent when administration of penicillamine was started after $^{64}Cu$ administration, but the retention rate after one week did not differ from that without penicillamine.

**ACKNOWLEDGEMENTS**

We thank Prof. K. Nakao, and Prof. Y. Toyokura for their constant guidance and encouragement and Dr. T. Nagai for his assistance and technical advice.

## REFERENCES

1. Scheinberg, I. H.: Wilson's disease, some current concepts Blackwell Scientific Publications, Oxford, 4-17, 1961.
2. Bearn, A. G. and Kunkel, H. G.: Metabolic studies in Wilson's disease using $^{64}Cu$. *J. Lab. clin. Med.,* **45:**623-631, 1955.
3. Bush, J. A.; Mahoney, J. P.; Markowitz, H.; Gubler, C. J.; Cartwright, G. E. and Wintrobe, M. M.: Studies on copper metabolism. XVI. Radioactive copper studies in normal subjects and in patients with hepatolenticular degeneration. *J. clin. Invest.* **34:**1766-1778, 1955.
4. Earl, C. J.; Moulton, M. J. and Selverstone, B; Metabolism of copper in Wilson's disease and in normal subjects, studies with $^{64}Cu$. *Amer. J. Med.* **17:**205-213, 1954.
5. Maytum, W. J.; Goldstein, N. P.; McGuckin, W. F. and Owen, C. A., Jr.: Copper metabolism in Wilson's disease, Laennec's cirrhosis and hemachromatosis: Studies with radiocopper ($^{64}Cu$). *Proc. Mayo Clin.* **36:**641-660, 1961.
6. Sass-Kortsak, A.; Glatt, B. S.; Cherniak, M. and Cederlund, I.: Wilson's Disease, some current concepts. Blackwell Scientific Publications, Oxford, pp. 151-167, 1961.
7. Sternlieb, I.; Morell, A. G.; Bauer, C. D.; Combes, B.; de Bobes-Sternberg, S. and Scheinberg, I. H.: Detection of the heterozygous carrier of the Wilson's disease gene. *J. clin. Invest.* **40:**707-715, 1961.
8. Tauxe, W. N.; Goldstein, N. P.; Randall, R. V. and Gross, J. B.: Radiocopper studies in patients with Wilson's disease and their relatives. *Amer. J. Med.* **41:**375-380, 1966.
9. Tanaka, E.: A low background beta-ray scintillation spectrometer using a coincidence method with a Geiger counter. *Nuclear Instruments and Methods.* **13:**43-49, 1961.
10. Oldendorf, W. H. and Kitamo, M.: Increased brain radiocopper uptake in Wilson's disease. *Arch. Neurol.* **13:**533-540, 1965.
11. Osborn, S. B. and Walshe, J. M.: Effect of penicillamine dimercaprol on turnover of copper in patients with Wilson's disease. *Lancet,* **i:**70-73, 1958.
12. Osborn, S. B. and Walshe, J. M.: Wilson's disease, some current concepts. Blackwell Scientific Publications, Oxford, pp. 141-150, 1961.
13. Osborn, S. B. and Walshe, J. M.: Studies with radiocopper ($^{64}Cu$) in Wilson's disease; the liver thigh ratio. *Clin. Sci.* **27:**319-328, 1964.
14. Perkons, A. K. and Jervis, R. E.: Hair individualization studies, paper ICAA-II/54. 2nd International Conference on Modern Trends in Activation Analysis, 1965.
15. Cartwright, G. E.; Hodges, R. E.; Gubler, C. J.; Mahoney, J. P.; Daum, K.; Wintrobe, M. M. and Bearn, W. B.: Studies on copper metabolism. XIII. Hepatolenticular degeneration. *J. clin. Invest.* **33:**1487-1501, 1954.

# Contributions of Copper Balance Studies to Investigation and Management of Wilson's Disease*

RAYMOND H. WATTEN, M.D., Capt., MC**; JUN-BI TU, M.D., D.M.Sc.***; R. QUENTIN BLACKWELL, Ph.D.† and TSUNG-YUNG HOU, B.S.‡

Copper balance studies provide valuable information for diagnosis and management of Wilson's disease. For example, they provide reliable estimates of the dietary copper levels at which individuals are in copper balance and direct evaluation of the relative effectiveness of low copper diets alone in achieving copper balance. Furthermore, effectiveness of copper-removing agents can be directly assessed. Balance studies also help to distinguish heterozygous carriers of the gene for Wilson's disease from the asymptomatic homozygote who requires therapy.

## Introduction

The patient with Wilson's disease is prone to establish a positive copper balance at a dietary copper level with which the normal individual experiences no difficulty.[1-3] Although the biochemical nature of the disturbance in copper metabolism is poorly understood, it is known that the levels of plasma ceruloplasmin and total plasma copper generally are depressed, the rate of intestinal copper absorption increased, urinary excretion of copper elevated, and the deposition of copper in certain body tissues abnormally high.[2-7]

Attempts to treat the patient by replacement of the plasma ceruloplasmin were considered to be unsuccessful.[8] Instead of attempting to correct effects of the genetic defect, current therapy aims to diminish the effect of the environmental factor, the dietary copper. A number of copper-removing agents have been used as a means of preventing the continued accumulation of copper in the body and for the removal of copper already deposited in tissues, but the therapeutic results have been variable.[1,2,7-20] The apparent inconsistencies in clinical responses of patients to copper-removing therapy can be attributed to differences in the stage of the illness at which treatment began, and in some cases to an insufficient dosage of the drug to produce and maintain a definite negative balance.[15,16] In the few reports available concerning the use of copper balance determinations to follow the treatment of Wilson's disease, most of the investigators concluded that the analytical methods and results were unsatisfactory.[1,2,13-15] Some investigators considered the balance studies to be too difficult to carry out with sufficient accuracy to be meaningful. However, we have found that with proper facilities and sufficient technical personnel, copper balance determinations although tedious, are not too difficult. The principal problem complicating the determinations of daily copper balance is the daily variation in fecal copper levels which may be complicated further by bowel irregularity in some patients with Wilson's disease.

We have proposed a method for the calculation of daily copper balance which averages the daily fecal

---

*This work was accomplished under the Bureau of Medicine and Surgery Work Unit MR005.09-0040. The study was funded in part under U.S. Public Law, 480, Section 104(c) and in part by the Bureau of Medicine and Surgery, Department of the Navy, Washington, D.C. The opinions and assertions contained herein are those of the authors and are not to be construed as official or reflecting the views of the U.S. Navy Department or the U.S. Naval Service at large.

**Commanding Officer, U.S. Naval Medical Research Unit No. 2, Taipei, Taiwan, Republic of China.

***Research Associate, Department of Biochemistry, U.S. Naval Medical Research Unit No. 2, Taipei, Taiwan, Republic of China. Present Address: Department of Medicine, Kingston General Hospital, Kingston, Ontario, Canada.

†Head, Department of Biochemistry, U.S. Naval Medical Research Unit No. 2, Taipei, Taiwan, Republic of China.

‡Research Assistant, Department of Biochemistry, U.S. Naval Medical Research Unit No. 2, Taipei, Taiwan, Republic of China.

**TABLE I**

**RESULTS OF COPPER BALANCE DETERMINATIONS IN VARIOUS CONDITIONS**

| Clinical Status | Normal Control | Patients with Wilson's Disease | | | | | | | Heterozygous Carrier |
|---|---|---|---|---|---|---|---|---|---|
| | | Advanced | Advanced | Asymptomatic | Advanced | | | | |
| Subject | 1: TYH | 2: LCW | 3: TFC | 4: CFC | | | | | 5: TTC |
| Age and Sex | 28 M | 17 M | 11 F | 6 F | 8y. 6m. | 8y. 11m. | 9y. 2m. | 9y. 3m. | 40 F |
| Body Weight, Kg | 49 | 48 | 24 | 19 | 20 | 21 | 23 | 23 | 42 |
| Drugs Used During the Study Period | Nil | Nil | Nil | Nil | DL-penicillamine | Diethyl-dithio-carbamate | $K_2S$ | D-Penicillamine + $K_2S$ | Nil |
| Duration of Study, days | 14 | 6 | 14 | 14 | 10 | 15 | 15 | 15 | 14 |
| Mean Cu Intake, mg/day | 1.34 | 1.44 | 1.24 | 1.24 | 1.15 | 1.13 | 1.17 | 1.53 | 1.70 |
| Mean Cu Output, mg/day | | | | | | | | | |
| Urine | 0.02 | 0.09 | 0.25 | 0.13 | 2.68 | 0.12 | 0.18 | 3.13 | 0.02 |
| Stool | 1.20 | 0.52 | 0.40 | 0.50 | 0.50 | 0.57 | 0.67 | 0.68 | 1.11 |
| Total | 1.22 | 0.61 | 0.65 | 0.63 | 3.18 | 0.69 | 0.85 | 3.81 | 1.13 |
| Mean Cu Balance, mg/day; | +0.12 | +0.83 | +0.59 | +0.61 | −2.03 | +0.44 | +0.32 | −2.28 | +0.57 |
| mg/day/mg of Intake | +0.09 | +0.58 | +0.48 | +0.49 | −1.77 | +0.39 | +0.27 | −1.49 | +0.34 |

### ABOUT THE SENIOR AUTHOR

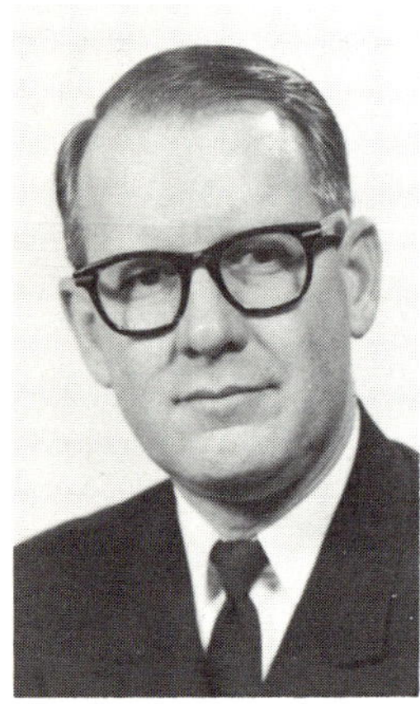

Dr. Watten, born in Minnesota, did undergraduate work at the University of Utah and the University of California and graduated from Stanford University, A.B. 1946, M.D. 1949.

As a Lieutenant (Junior Grade) in the Medical Corps Reserve he interned at the U. S. Naval Hospital, Long Beach, California. Commissioned in the regular navy in 1949, he was a medical resident at the U. S. Naval Hospital, Oakland, and was assigned to the Metabolic Research Facility there. His interests are clinical medicine and clinical research.

He reported to NAMRU-2 in July 1957 and served for a time as Executive Officer. He accompanied the U. S. Naval Medical Missions to East Pakistan and to Thailand in 1958, and was Medical Officer in Cholera Studies made by NAMRU-2 in Bangkok in 1958, 1959, and 1960.

In 1960, Captain Watten transferred to U. S. Naval Hospital, Oakland, as Director, Clinical Investigation Center until he received his present assignment as Commanding Officer of NAMRU-2 in October 1965.

copper excretion.[3] With this method copper balance studies have been made in advanced as well as in asymptomatic patients with Wilson's disease; in a heterozygous carrier of the abnormal gene, and in one normal control individual. This paper summarizes the results of the studies and illustrates the usefulness of copper balance determinations in the management of Wilson's disease.

**Materials and Methods**

Five subjects, including three patients with Wilson's disease, one heterozygous carrier of the abnormal gene, and one normal control subject are included in the present study (Table I). The three patients had the characteristic clinical and biochemical findings of the disease.[7]

The heterozygote, a 40-year-old woman, was the mother of four children affected with the disease. Her copper oxidase activity was 0.170 Ravin units (Normal, 0.217-0.686); total plasma copper was 70 $\mu$g per 100 ml (Normal, 86-170); and urinary copper level was 19 $\mu$g per day (Normal, 4-45).

Urine, stool, and dietary copper levels were determined by the method of Eden and Green.[21] The total daily copper intake was determined from aliquots of an homogenized duplicate diet. The total daily copper output was estimated as the sum of the 24-hour fecal and urinary copper excretions. A "corrected daily total output" of copper was estimated by combining the value for daily urinary copper excretion with the mean daily fecal copper excretion during the balance period.[3] The results of the mean copper balance of each determination were expressed in terms of mg/day as well as mg/day/

mg of intake. The daily copper balance was calculated by subtracting from the daily copper intake the corrected daily output; results are plotted in the figures. As shown in Table I, there was no remarkable difference between expression of the daily copper balance in absolute amounts and in proportion to each milligram of copper ingested. The results of each balance study were plotted, in terms of mg/day, as positive or negative values in the figures.

**Results and Discussion**

The material contribution to the understanding and therapeutic management of Wilson's disease provided by information from copper balance studies can be illustrated by a review of the present experimental results under those aspects of the disease to which they appear to contribute the most.

I. *Estimation of the Daily Requirement of Copper in the Normal Adult and the Dietary Copper Level at which the Patient with Wilson's Disease is in Balance.*

The minimal requirement of copper in the adult has been stated to be 2 mg a day.[22,23] This estimate was based on the results of previous balance studies which appear somewhat variable. Cartwright *et al*[2] reported that three normal controls were in balance with a copper intake of about 2.6 mg. Leverton and Binkley[24] found an approximate balance in 16 young women with a daily intake of about 1.6 mg. Recently, we determined the minimal copper requirement for a normal Chinese adult[3] to be about 1.2 mg (Fig. 1); balance studies of the female heterozygous carrier included in the present study also gave similar results (Fig. 1). This suggests that, at lower levels of intake, physiologic adjustments can be made to reduce copper excretion.

With respect to the relationship of daily copper intake to daily balances, remarkable differences exist between the normal subject and the patient with Wilson's disease. These are demonstrated in Figure 1 where it is evident from the separate curves that the minimal copper intake level above which the patient with Wilson's disease is in positive balance is much lower than the level for the normal subject. For our patients with Wilson's disease it was estimated[3] that the maximum allowable daily copper intake necessary to avoid a positive copper balance in the absence of binding agents was 0.6 mg. Since ordinary diets supply a copper intake of 2 mg per day or more,[22,23] patients are subject to high copper retention. Table I and Figure 2 demonstrate that patients with Wilson's disease always excrete smaller than normal amounts of copper via stool and larger than normal amounts in the urine. These data confirm previous reports[1,2] that the accumulation of copper is associated with a reduced fecal copper output. Balance studies alone cannot determine whether this reduction is due to increased absorption from the gut lumen, decreased excretion into the lumen, or both.

II. *Evalution of the Potential Usefulness of Low Copper Diet Therapy in the Treatment of Wilson's Disease.*

Many investigators have stressed the importance of a low copper diet in the treatment of Wilson's disease.[7,8] However, the effectiveness of such a diet cannot be established without balance studies. In this connection, a low copper diet is relative to the degree of copper balance

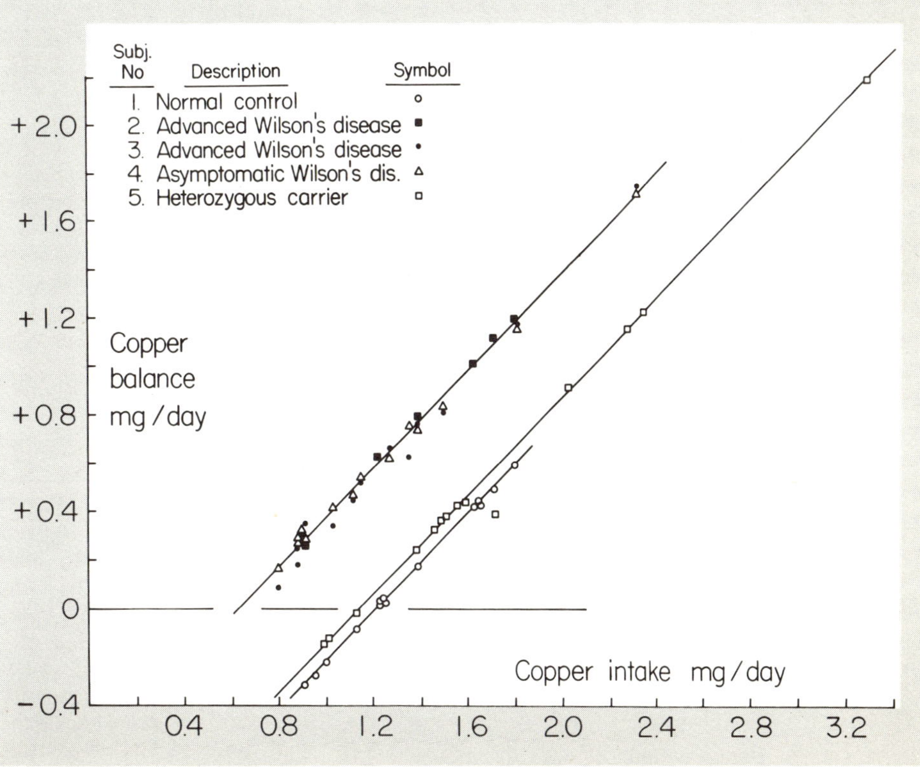


Fig. 1. Relationship of Daily Copper Intake to Daily Copper Balance.

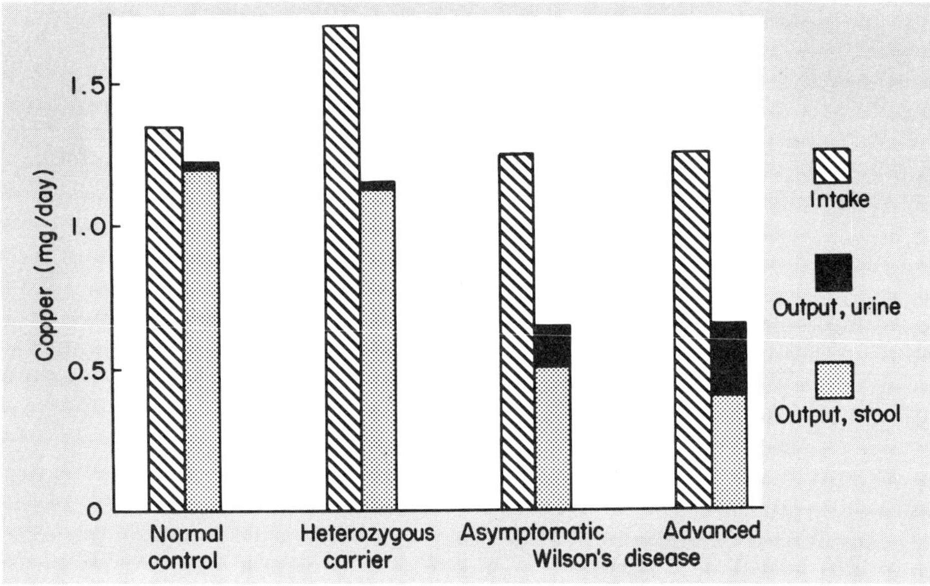


Fig. 2. Copper Balance Determinations in Various Conditions.

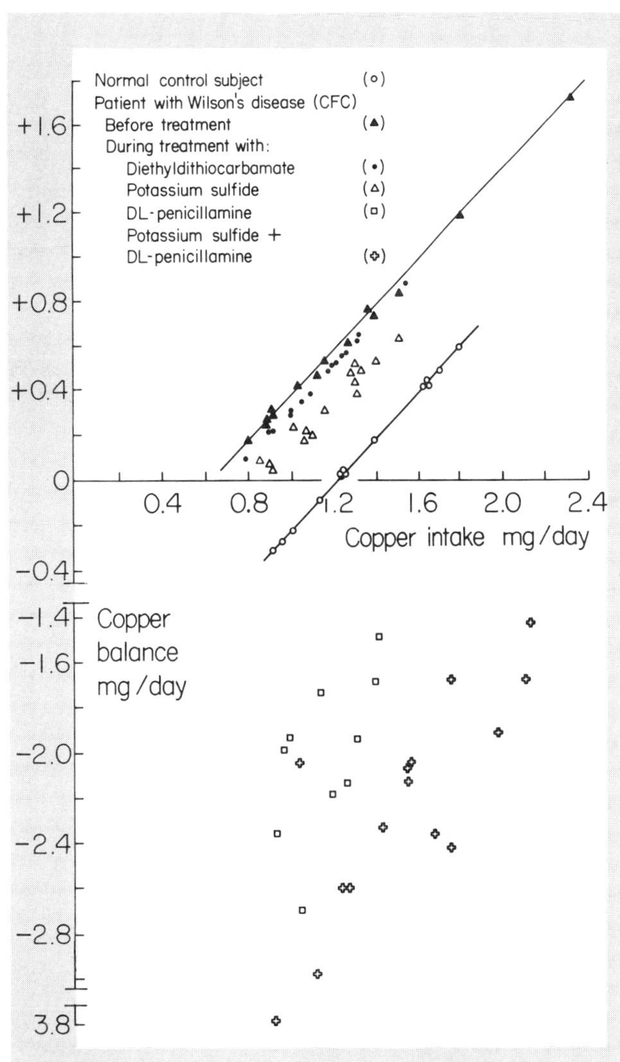


Fig. 3. Copper Balance Study at 6 Years of Age.

needed and differs considerably between normals and patients with Wilson's disease. As illustrated in Figure 1, a total daily intake below 1.2 mg produced a negative balance in our normal subject but for our patients with Wilson's disease it would require reduction to approximately 0.6 mg per day. From the results of the balance study it is clear that long-term management of Wilson's disease solely by means of a low copper diet is extremely unlikely. As many foods contain appreciable levels of copper it is very difficult to devise a low copper diet that is varied, interesting and sufficiently palatable for lifetime use. Therefore, a compromise must be made and diet therapy considered as an adjunct to drug therapy.

III. *Evaluation of the Relative Effectiveness of Various Copper-Removing Agents.*

A series of copper balance determinations were performed on a patient with Wilson's disease for the purpose of comparing several copper-removing agents. Each study lasted about two weeks with periods of several weeks or longer between studies during which no chelating agents were given. Results are summarized in Figures 3 and 4.

The first balance study was made when the patient was six years of age and asymptomatic and had not received any previous treatment. The marked positive balance found, as shown in Figure 3, was essentially the same as that noted in other patients with advanced Wilson's disease. The remaining balance studies were made when the patient was between the ages of eight and nine and had become symptomatic with extrapyramidal signs, evidence of mental retardation, and Kayser-Fleischer rings.

Administration of one gram DL-penicillamine daily in two divided dosages brought about a remarkable increase in the urinary excretion of copper associated with a marked negative balance. Fecal copper levels showed no remarkable change. Five months later,

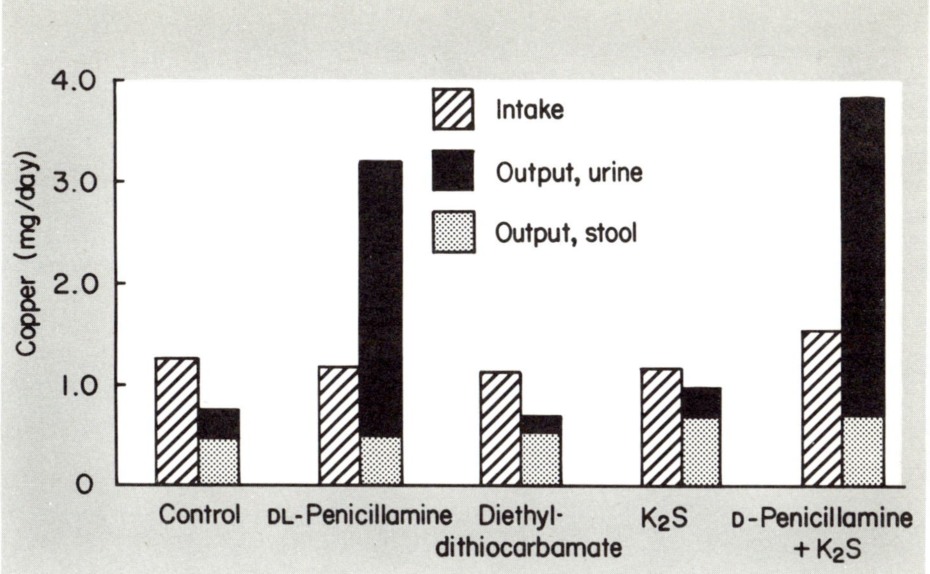


Fig. 4. Effect of Various Agents on Copper Balance of a Wilson's Disease Patient (CFC).

diethyldithiocarbamate was given orally with each meal in daily dosages of 35 mg per kg of body weight. This was followed three months later by the oral administration of potassium sulfide 20 mg three times daily. Both of the latter agents increased the fecal excretion of copper and thereby diminished the positive balance to some extent, but there was no change of urinary copper levels and negative balance was not achieved. Quite possibly a negative balance would have resulted with the use of potassium sulfide and a lower copper intake as was observed by Cartwright *et al.*[2] Our results with the diethyldithiocarbamate do not agree with those of Sunderman *et al*[14] who reported, in a three-day balance period, a substantial negative balance in a patient with a similar dosage of the diethyldithiocarbamate while on a considerably higher level of copper intake.

The final balance study was made with the combined administration of one gram daily of oral DL-penicillamine and 20 mg of potassium sulfide at each meal. Both the fecal and urinary copper excretion levels were increased and the most negative balance was established over the period of observation. These results confirmed previous reports.[18, 19]

It is widely accepted that, in all therapy programs for Wilson's disease, the amount of dietary copper intake will influence the balance state, and further, that the effectiveness of copper-removing agents gradually decreases with long-term use.[3, 8, 15, 18, 19] Under these circumstances periodic copper balance studies appear to be desirable for assessing the efficacy of current treatment. Although such information is considered to be ideal for optimum evaluation of progress achieved in copper-removing therapy, it would not be realistic to recommend these detailed analytical procedures for routine use. A simplified estimate of copper balance can be made from urinary copper analyses alone combined with estimates of copper intake made from food tables. Both from the present and from previous studies[2] it appears that patients with Wilson's disease have a net intestinal copper absorption of approximately one-half the dietary copper intake when the latter is approximately one to two mg per day (Table I, Figs. 2 and 4). Therefore, for purposes of the simplified estimate of copper balance, it can be assumed with no more than moderate error that one-half the estimated dietary copper intake is absorbed by the patient on such a dietary copper level. That amount subtracted from the daily urinary copper excretion would provide a simplified estimate of copper balance. These estimates do not take into account the effect of fecal copper-binding agents.

IV. *As a Diagnostic Aid to Distinguish the Heterozygote Carrier of Wilson's Disease Gene from the Homozygous Patient.*

The results of a balance study in a heterozygote who had a subnormal level of ceruloplasmin and low total plasma copper are shown in Figure 1. The balance line of the heterozygote appears to be slightly above that of the normal subject but much lower than that of the patients. This finding indicates that balance determinations may be useful in establishing a definite diagnosis of Wilson's disease under atypical conditions where some of the usual parameters such as ceruloplasmin, plasma and urine copper levels fail to differentiate the heterozygote from the homozygote.[25, 26, 27]

Since the disease is transmitted in an autosomal recessive manner[28] and is not expected to develop in the heterozygote, whereas the abnormal homozygote requires treatment by a lifelong regimen beginning as early as possible, the differentiation between these two genetic conditions is of great practical importance. Radiocopper studies have been used with some success for this purpose[29, 30]; recent work also has indicated the apparent usefulness of penicillamine-induced cupriuresis for the differentiation.[31] The present work suggests that copper balance determinations also may be useful.

**Summary**

Copper balance levels of patients with Wilson's disease were determined and compared with that of one heterozygote and one normal control subject. The results indicate that a decrease in copper intake is followed by a reduction in the amount of positive copper balance in all subjects. A daily dietary copper intake below 1.2 mg allowed a negative balance in the normal adult control but an amount below 0.6 mg was required to prevent positive balance in the patients.

The relative effectiveness of various copper-removing agents was evaluated by the copper balance determinations. Penicillamine in combination with potassium sulfide and a low copper diet established the best negative copper balance, which according to the current knowledge, appears to be most beneficial for the management of Wilson's disease. The usefulness of copper balance studies to evaluate the success of copper removal therapy was discussed and a simplified procedure for estimation of copper balance described.

The balance determinations disclosed a slight tendency for copper accumulation in a heterozygote. However, the distinct difference between the copper balances of the heterozygote and the patients suggests that such studies may provide an additional means to differentiate the heterozygote from the individuals who are homozygous for Wilson's disease gene.

## REFERENCES

1. Zimdahl, W. T.; Hyman, I. and Cook, E. D.: Metabolism of copper in hepatolenticular degeneration. *Neurology* **3**:569-576, 1953.
2. Cartwright, G. E.; Hodges, R. E.; Gubler, C. J.; Mahoney, J. P.; Daum, K.; Wintrobe, M. M. and Bean, W. B.: Studies on copper metabolism. XIII. Hepatolenticular degeneration. *J. clin. Invest.* **33**:1487-1501, 1954.
3. Tu, J. B.; Blackwell, R. Q. and Watten, R. H.: Copper balance studies during the treatment of patients with Wilson's disease. *Metabolism* **14**:653-666, 1965.
4. Scheinberg, I. H. and Gitlin, D.: Deficiency of ceruloplasmin in patients with hepatolenticular degeneration (Wilson's disease). *Science* **116**:484-485, 1952.
5. Cumings, J. N.: The copper and iron content of brain and liver in the normal and in hepato-lenticular degeneration. *Brain* **71**:410-415, 1948.
6. Matthews, W. B.: The absorption and excretion of radiocopper in hepato-lenticular degeneration (Wilson's disease). *J. Neurol. Neurosurg. Psychiat.* **17**:242-246, 1954.
7. Tu, J. B.: A genetic, biochemical and clinical study of Wilson's disease among Chinese in Taiwan. *Acta paediat.* Sinica **4**:81-104, 1963.
8. Scheinberg, I. H. and Sternlieb, I.: Environmental treatment of a hereditary illness: Wilson's disease. *Ann. intern. Med.* **53**:1151-1161, 1960.
9. Denny-Brown, D. and Porter, H.: The effect of BAL (2,3-dimercaptopropanol) on hepatolenticular degeneration (Wilson's disease). *New Engl. J. Med.* **245**:917-925, 1951.
10. Cumings, J. N.: The effect of BAL in hepatolenticular degeneration. *Brain* **74**:10-22, 1951.
11. Bearn, A. G. and Kunkel, H. G.: Abnormalities of copper metabolism in Wilson's disease and their relationship to the aminoaciduria. *J. clin. Invest.* **33**:400-409, 1954.
12. Walshe, J. M.: Penicillamine, a new oral therapy for Wilson's disease. *Amer. J. Med.* **21**:487-495, 1956.
13. Zimdahl, W. T.; Hyman, I. and Stafford, W. F.: The effect of drug upon the copper metabolism in hepatolenticular degeneration and in normal subjects. *J. Lab. clin. Med.* **43**:774 784, 1954.
14. Sunderman, F. W. Jr.; White, J. C. and Sunderman, F. W.: Metabolic balance studies in hepatolenticular degeneration treated with diethyldithiocarbamate. *Amer. J. Med.* **34**:875-888, 1963.
15. Tu, J. B.; Blackwell, R. Q. and Hou, T. Y.: Tissue copper levels in Chinese patients with Wilson's disease. *Neurology* **13**:155-159, 1963.
16. Scheinberg, I. H. and Sternlieb, I.: Wilson's disease. *Ann. Rev. Med.* **16**:119-135, 1965.
17. Bickel, H.; Neale, F. C. and Hall, G.: A clinical and biochemical study of hepatolenticular degeneration (Wilson's disease). *Quart. J. Med.* **26**:527-558, 1957.
18. Herring, V. G. III; Klatskin, G. and Brandt, I. K.: Hepatolenticular degeneration: Observations on a case treated with D-penicillamine. *J. Pediat.* **63**:550-560, 1963.
19. Goldstein, N. P.; Randall, R. V.; Gross, J. B. and McGuckin, W. F.: Copper balance studies in Wilson's disease. *Arch. Neurol.* **12**:456-462, 1965.
20. Playoust, M. R. and Dale, N. E.: Metabolic balance studies in a patient with Wilson's disease and hypercalcuria. *Metabolism* **10**:304-314, 1961.
21. Eden, A. and Green, H. H.: Micro-determination of copper in biological material. *Biochem. J.* **34**:1202-1208, 1940.
22. Darby, W. J.: Copper, *Handbook of Nutrition.* 108-110, 1951.
23. Cartwright, G. E. and Wintrobe, M. M.: The question of copper deficiency in man. *Amer. J. clin. Nutr.* **15**:94-110, 1964.
24. Leverton, R. M. and Binkley, E. S.: The copper metabolism and requirement of young women. *J. Nutr.* **27**:43-53, 1944.
25. Cartwright, G. E.; Markowitz, H.; Shields, G. S. and Wintrobe, M. M.: Studies on copper metabolism. XXIX. A critical analysis of serum copper and ceruloplasmin concentrations in normal subjects, patients with Wilson's disease and relatives of patients with Wilson's disease. *Amer. J. Med.* **28**:555-563, 1960.
26. Neale, F. C. and Fischer-Williams, M.: Copper metabolism in normal adults and in clinically normal relatives of patients with Wilson's disease. *J. clin. Path.* **11**:441-447, 1958.
27. Search for the heterozygote in Wilson's disease. *Lancet* **i**:812-813, 1963. (Anonymous)
28. Bearn, A. G.: Clinical studies. Genetic and biochemical aspects of Wilson's disease. *Amer. J. Med.* **15**:442-449, 1953.
29. Sternlieb, I.; Morell, A. G.; Bauer, C. D.; Combes, B.; De Bobes-Sternberg, S. and Scheinberg, I. H.: Detection of the heterozygous carrier of the Wilson's disease gene. *J. clin. Invest.* **40**:707-715, 1961.
30. Osborn, S. B.; Roberts, C. N. and Walshe, J. M.: Uptake of radiocopper by the liver. A study of patients with Wilson's disease and various control groups. *Clin. Sci.* **24**:13-22, 1963.
31. Tu, J. B.; Blackwell, R. Q.; Fresh, J. W. and Watten, R. H. In Birth Defects: Original Article Series, *Wilson's Disease.* The National Foundation, New York, Vol. IV, No. 2, pp. 114-121, April, 1968.

# Studies with Radiocopper ($^{64}$Cu and $^{67}$Cu): A Distinction Between the Hepatic and Neurologic Stages of Wilson's Disease

SIDNEY B. OSBORN, B.Sc., Ph.D.* and JOHN M. WALSHE, Sc.D., F.R.C.P.**

Conclusions reached after analyzing findings of 117 studies during the past ten years show clearly that patients in the early hepatic stage of Wilson's disease concentrate copper more readily in their livers than those in the late neurologic stages.

During the past ten years we have carried out 117 studies with intravenously administered radiocopper on patients with Wilson's disease and on suitable controls. It is our present object to report the conclusions we have reached following an analysis of our findings with particular references to the effect of 1) the specific activity of the radiocopper, 2) the duration and clinical type of the illness and 3) the part played by penicillamine on the handling of the injected radiocopper by the patients with Wilson's disease when compared with the various control groups.

## Methods

We have measured the uptake of copper by the liver, the ratio of activity in the liver to that in the thigh (L/T ratio), the plasma and red cell activity. From these data we have calculated the distribution of the injected copper, particularly that copper which cannot be accounted for as present in liver, blood, urine or stools. We have attempted to localize 'missing' radiocopper by profile counting with a whole body monitor and by the use of a Picker scintiscanner. We have also studied the effect of the synchronous administration of penicillamine together with the radiocopper, upon these various parameters.

For the purpose of this analysis we have subdivided our results as follows: normal controls (19), patients with chronic liver disease (16), patients with degenerative disease of the nervous system (6), individuals heterozygous for the Wilson's disease gene (11), patients in the hepatic stage of Wilson's disease (8), patients in the neurologic stage of Wilson's disease (19), subjects studied when penicillamine was given with the radiocopper (1 normal and 6 Wilson's disease patients). In all, 42 studies were made on the controls, 12 on the heterozygotes and 58 on the Wilson's disease patients. A number of studies made on patients with the mixed form of Wilson's disease have been omitted for the purpose of this analysis.

Details of the technics employed have been reported in our earlier communications.[1-6]

All patients in the neurologic stage of Wilson's disease had Kayser-Fleischer rings as did four of those in the hepatic stage; the remaining four did not have rings even when viewed under a slit lamp. In these four the diagnosis rested on a positive family history and on their inability to incorporate radiocopper into ceruloplasmin. The oxidase activity on the serum of the patients and the various controls is shown in Figure 1. The oxidase activity of the serum from all patients with Wilson's disease was significantly lower than for any of the controls; a relatively low value was found in the neurologic control cases but its significance was not immediately apparent. It should also be noted that patients in the hepatic stage of Wilson's disease had a serum oxidase significantly higher than those with the fully

### ABOUT THE SENIOR AUTHOR

Dr. S. B. Osborn is Director of the Department of Medical Physics at King's College Hospital and Medical School, London, and has worked on many applications of radioisotopes in medicine. He was formerly Physicist-in-Charge at University College Hospital, London, when his collaboration with Dr. Walshe began. He has also published widely in the field of radiation safety in medical practice.

*Director, Department of Medical Physics, Kings College Hospital and Medical School, London.

**Reader in Metabolic Disease, Department of Investigative Medicine, University of Cambridge, Cambridge.

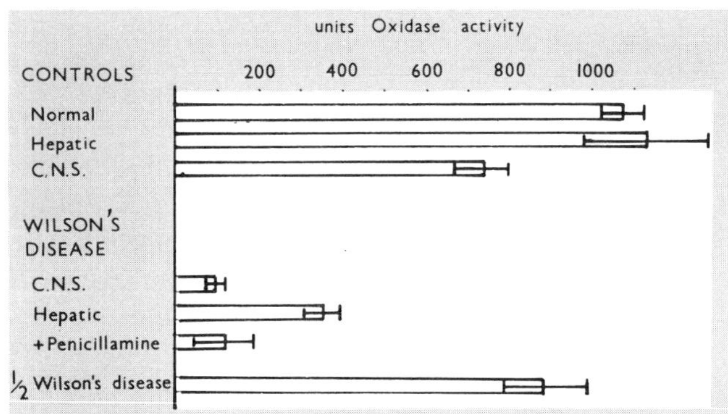


Fig. 1. This shows the mean oxidase activity (together with two standard errors), the control subjects and the various subgroups of patients with Wilson's disease and also the heterozygotes. Oxidase activity is expressed as arbitrary units; 800 are approximately equivalent to 30 mg/100 ml of purified ceruloplasmin.

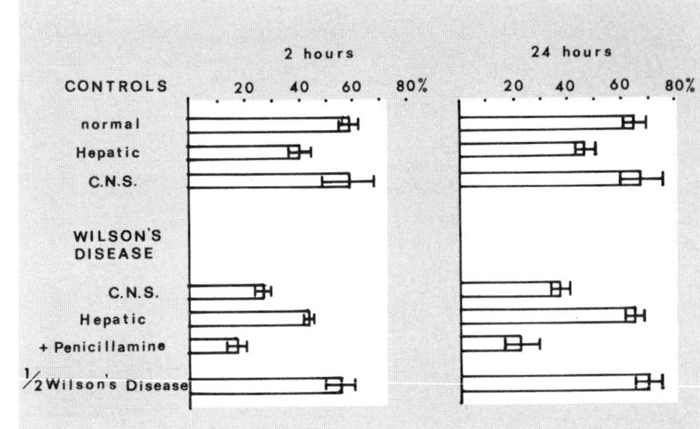


Fig. 2. This shows the mean results for uptake of radiocopper by livers of the various groups of controls and patients studied at two and 24 hours. Twice the standard error is shown for each mean.

developed neurologic lesion; nevertheless they had no greater ability to incorporate radiocopper into ceruloplasmin.

**Results**

*1. The role of specific activity of radiocopper.*

Data for the quantity of ionic copper injected were obtained on 65 occasions but seven of these have been omitted because the synchronous administration of penicillamine modified the hepatic uptake of copper; thus only 58 studies are here considered. A plot of liver uptake of copper against $Log_{10}$ ionic copper injected, over the range 2.5 to 610 $\mu$g $Cu^{2+}$, shows no negative correlation apparent between percentage uptake by the liver and amount of copper injected either for the controls or the patients with Wilson's disease. We have therefore concluded that our findings have not been influenced by this variable.

*2. Liver uptake of intravenously injected radiocopper.*

Although our most recent studies with $^{67}$Cu and with the larger doses of $^{64}$Cu now permitted (500 $\mu$c for patients) have enabled us to follow the fate of the metal for as long as 300 hours after injection, the majority of studies were limited to very much shorter periods by dose limitation (120 $\mu$c for both patients and controls). We have therefore confined ourselves to data available for all cases and have selected two fixed times of two and 24 hours after injection for the assessment of results. These are summarized in Figure 2. Among the controls nonspecific liver damage reduced the ability of the liver to concentrate copper at both two and 24 hours. Among the Wilson's disease patients the position was reversed, those with active liver damage having a significantly higher uptake of copper by the liver than those in the neurologic stage of the disease. The heterozygotes took up rather more copper in their livers, on average, than the controls though the difference was not significant.

*3. Liver/thigh ratio (L/T ratio).*

The L/T ratio was monitored continuously for the first 15 minutes after injection and at varying time intervals for 24 hours. The most significant variations were, however, found in the immediate post injection period and the findings at 15 minutes are summarized in Figure 3. Among the controls those patients with chronic liver damage had a reduced L/T ratio compared with the normals. The Wilson's disease patients again showed a separation into two groups, those with the neurologic lesion having a very low L/T ratio while cases with liver damage only had a moderate reduction of L/T ratio. Although the patients with Wilsonian liver damage had a lower L/T ratio (1.31 ± 0.37) than those with nonspecific liver disease (1.46 ± 0.045), the differences were not significant.

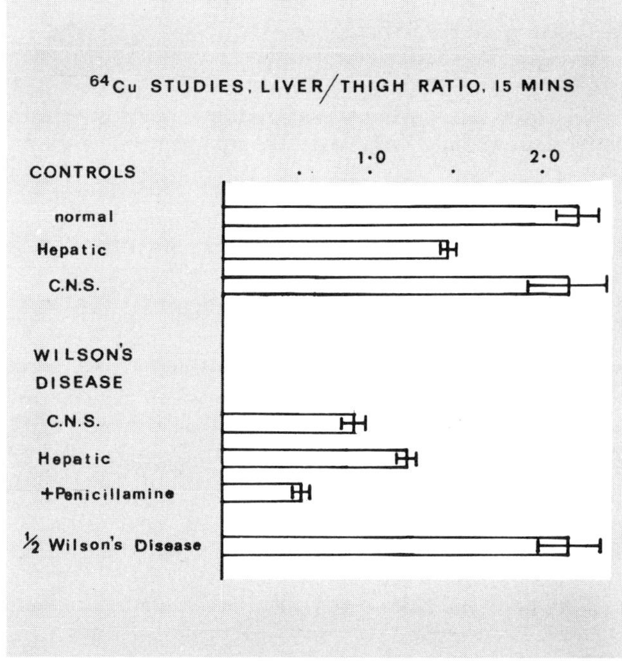


Fig. 3. Liver/thigh ratios calculated at 15 minutes after injection of radiocopper are shown for the various groups studied together with two standard errors. All figures were calculated for an arbitrary ratio of unity at zero time.

**TABLE I**

| | μg Cu | Liver uptake 2 Hr. | Liver uptake 24 Hr. | Plasma % 2 Hr. | Plasma % 24 Hr. | 24/2 | L/T (15) | Oxidase | Number 86 Cases | Number 112 Tests |
|---|---|---|---|---|---|---|---|---|---|---|
| **Controls** | | | | | | | | | | |
| Normal | 93±37 | 58.5±3.7 | 64.7±3.2 | 3.91±0.41 | 5.17±0.80 | 1.32 | 2.29±0.16 | 1070±54 | 19 | 19 |
| Hepatic | 50±20 | 39.7±3.7 | 46.3±3.8 | 3.32±0.30 | 3.95±0.63 | 1.19 | 1.46±0.05 | 1130±146 | 16 | 16 |
| C.N.S. | 114±90 | 57.9±8.4 | 66.2±8.4 | 3.52±0.81 | 4.73±1.14 | 1.34 | 2.27±0.26 | 728±61 | 6 | 6 |
| + Penicillamine | 4.1 | 35 | 26 | 3.6 | 2.8 | 0.78 | 1.55 | | 1 | 1 |
| **Wilson's Disease** | | | | | | | | | | |
| C.N.S. | 106±36 | 26.0±1.8 | 37.0±3.3 | 7.27±0.61 | 1.57±0.15 | 0.21 | 0.83±0.08 | 91.5±17.0 | 19 | 39 |
| Hepatic | 160±70 | 43.5±1.5 | 64.9±2.7 | 3.8±0.6 | 1.31±0.37 | 0.34 | 1.38±0.07 | 351±44 | 8 | 13 |
| + Penicillamine | 43±16 | 15.8±3.4 | 22.2±6.0 | 4.19±0.79 | 1.04±0.27 | 0.25 | 0.58±0.05 | 117±72 | 6 | 6 |
| **½ Wilson's Disease** | 211±97 | 55±5 | 70±4 | 3.07±0.06 | 2.11±0.44 | 0.69 | 2.31±0.22 | 890±100 | 11 | 12 |

*4. Plasma radioactivity.*

These results are summarized in Figure 4. The values for the percentage of the radioactivity retained in the plasma at two hours are very similar for all groups except for the patients in the neurologic stage of Wilson's disease where the plasma $^{64}Cu$ was markedly elevated corresponding with their inability to concentrate the metal in their livers. By 24 hours all the Wilsonian patients had very low values for plasma radioactivity and even those patients in the hepatic stage of the illness, with relatively high serum ceruloplasmin levels, were unable to incorporate radiocopper into this protein.

*5. Effect of penicillamine on radiocopper uptake.*

D-penicillamine HCl was given by mouth shortly before the radiocopper injection. One normal subject, who was also studied under basal conditions, was investigated by this technic together with three patients in the neurologic stage of Wilson's disease, two in the hepatic stage and one with a mixed lesion. In all subjects the liver uptake was greatly reduced (Fig. 2), the liver/thigh ratio was reduced (Fig. 3), as also was the percentage dose retained in the plasma at 24 hours. There was correspondingly an enormous increase in the excretion of radiocopper in the urine reaching as high as 87% of the dose in 24 hours in one patient compared with less than 3% in subjects who had not received penicillamine. In the normal individual the liver uptake was reduced from 68% to 30% by penicillamine and the liver/thigh ratio at 15 minutes from 2.4 to 1.5.

The means of all results together with twice the standard error of the mean are given in Table I.

**Conclusions**

These results make it clear that patients in the early hepatic stage of Wilson's disease concentrate copper more readily in their livers than those in the late neurologic stages. Presumably in the latter group the liver has become saturated with copper which is then allowed to spill over into the plasma and hence other tissues, principally the brain and kidneys, leading to the classical clinical picture of Wilson's disease. That this biochemical lesion is not simply the result of nonspecific liver damage is made apparent by reference to the con-

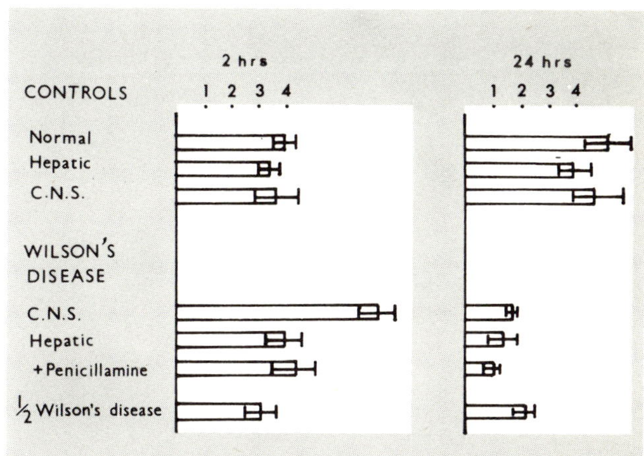


Fig. 4. The blocks represent the mean (plus or minus two standard errors) retention of radiocopper in the plasma at two and 24 hours after injection of the radioisotope. Plasma volumes were calculated from body weight according to figures given in Documenta Geigy, Scientific Tables, 6th Edition.

trol groups where those with chronic liver disease had a marked impairment of uptake of copper by the liver but no reduction in ability of incorporating the metal into ceruloplasmin. That these results are at variance with our earlier reports and those of other workers we are aware, but we believe that previously reported findings were based on small series of cases which did not permit breakdown into the clinical subgroups here used.

The predominance of neurologic cases in most reported series, therefore, gave a false impression of the fate of injected copper in this disease.

We now suggest the following natural history for Wilson's disease. In the early stages the liver concentrates copper as actively as normal; as the liver proteins become saturated with the metal there is a slowing down of uptake which is first seen in the immediate postinjection period and is manifest by the reduced L/T ratio. This is followed by, first, biochemical and then clinical liver damage as a result of which copper spills over into the tissues; the hepatic lesion becomes less active as excess copper is shed and regeneration is associated with an improvement of liver function in many cases, though others may die of subacute hepatic failure (when this is better recognized, the figure may prove to be as high as 50%). Eventually the cerebral proteins become saturated with excess copper and the full clinical syndrome of brain damage becomes apparent. Energetic treatment with penicillamine should reverse this sequence of events enabling the liver to recover its ability to concentrate copper. Data so far published suggests that this may take many years.

## REFERENCES


1. Osborn, S. B. and Walshe, J. M.: Effect of penicillamine and dimercaprol on turnover of copper in patients with Wilson's disease. *Lancet,* **i**:70-73, 1958.
2. Osborn, S. B. and Walshe, J. M.: Copper uptake by the liver: study of a Wilson's disease family. In *Wilson's disease: some current concepts.* Ed. Walshe, J. M. and Cumings, J. N.: Blackwells Scientific Publications, Oxford. 141-150, 1961.
3. Osborn, S. B.; Roberts, C. N. and Walshe, J. M.: Uptake of radiocopper by the liver. A study of patients with Wilson's disease and various control groups. *Clin. Sci.* **24**:13-22, 1963.
4. Osborn, S. B. and Walshe, J. M.: Filterable and non-filterable serum copper (2) Studies with $^{64}Cu$. *Clin. Sci.* **26**:213-217, 1964.
5. Osborn, S. B. and Walshe, J. M.: Studies with radiocopper ($^{64}Cu$) in Wilson's disease: the liver/thigh ratio. *Clin. Sci.* **27**:319-328, 1964.
6. Osborn, S. B. and Walshe, J. M.: Studies with radiocopper ($^{64}Cu$) in Wilson's disease: dynamics of copper transport. *Clin. Sci.* **29**:575-581, 1965.

# Turnover Studies of Intravenously Administered Radiocopper in Patients with Wilson's Disease: Effect of D-Penicillamine Therapy*

W. Newlon Tauxe, M.D., M.S.**; Norman P. Goldstein, M.D.***; John B. Gross, M.D., M.S.†
and Raymond V. Randall, M.D., M.S.†

Metabolic turnover studies were undertaken in 14 normal subjects and in 13 patients with Wilson's disease. Our findings support the concept that the liver trapping mechanism is quite avid in the presymptomatic group and that symptoms and signs develop as a result of tissue deposition of copper. After prolonged treatment with D-penicillamine, the liver counts remained low in the group of patients with residual symptoms but were relatively high in patients asymptomatic after prolonged therapy.

Although the basic mechanism of action remains unknown,[1] it is an accepted fact that the administration of D-penicillamine is of great benefit to patients with Wilson's disease. We have reported previously that, in a preliminary series of patients, D-penicillamine also has a profound effect on the kinetics of metabolism of intravenously administered radioactive copper ($^{64}$Cu).[2] Those studies suggested that, in addition to the distinction between normal and carrier states, four distinct patterns of copper handling could be observed in patients with Wilson's disease: 1) preclinical category before therapy; 2) symptomatic category before therapy; 3) during D-penicillamine therapy and 4) after temporary discontinuation of long-term therapy.

The purpose of this paper is to present results of an expanded series and to include data from longer periods of treatment.

## Materials and Methods

*Selection of Subjects.* – Studies of kinetics of metabolism of intravenously administered $^{64}$Cu were carried out 57 times, at approximately yearly intervals starting in 1958, in 13 patients with Wilson's disease. These results were compared with those observed in 18 normal subjects who had no familial history suggesting Wilson's disease.

*Protocols.* – As reported previously, total and bound radioactivity in plasma and radioactivity in urine and stools were determined after the intravenous injection of approximately 750 $\mu$c of $^{64}$Cu-labeled cupric acetate (Abbott Laboratories) in specific activities such that the amount of copper injected ranged from 0.006 to 0.44 mg with a mean of 0.101 mg. Blood samples were taken at 10, 20, 30, 45, 60, 120, and 200 minutes after injection, at six hours, and then twice daily until 72 hours. Radioactivity of the plasma was determined, along with an aliquot of the injected dose, in a well-type scintillation counter and expressed as percentage of the dose per liter of plasma; percentage of the dose in the entire plasma volume was calculated from regression equations of Retzlaff.[3] During the time of injection and continuously for the first two hours afterwards, a widely collimated probe was placed over the liver for monitoring by a method similar to that described by Osborn and Walshe.[4] The liver was also counted at all subsequent sampling times. Counts were corrected for background and physical decay of the radionuclide and expressed as counts per second/100 $\mu$c injected and in various other ways.

The rest of the data were derived in a manner similar to that described previously.[5]

## Results

Typical plasmatic disappearance curves of $^{64}$Cu in a patient with Wilson's disease and in a normal subject

*This investigation was supported in part by Research Grant NB-3655 from the National Institutes of Health, Public Health Service.

**Consultant, Section of Clinical Pathology, Mayo Clinic; Associate Professor of Clinical Pathology, Mayo Graduate School of Medicine (University of Minnesota); Rochester, Minnesota.

***Consultant, Section of Neurology, Mayo Clinic; Professor of Neurology, Mayo Graduate School of Medicine (University of Minnesota); Rochester, Minnesota.

†Consultants, Section of Medicine, Mayo Clinic; Associate Professors of Medicine, Mayo Graduate School of Medicine (University of Minnesota); Rochester, Minnesota.

TABL

| | Urine (%D) | | | Stool (%D) | | | Plasma (* | |
|---|---|---|---|---|---|---|---|---|
| | 24 hr. | 48 hr. | 72 hr. | 24 hr. | 48 hr. | 72 hr. | 24 hr. | 48 |
| Before Rx; before clin. N = 2 | 0.96<br>0.48 | 1.13<br>0.61 | 1.38<br>0.88 | 0.00<br>0.00 | 0.20<br>0.00 | 0.60<br>0.57 | 0.48<br>0.22 | 0<br>0 |
| Before Rx; clin., mean ± SD N = 5 | 1.80<br>±0.54 | 2.45<br>±0.75 | 3.49<br>±1.38 | 0.13<br>±0.13 | 0.35<br>±0.19 | 0.48<br>±0.26 | 1.91<br>±1.10 | 1<br>±0. |
| During Rx; mean ± SD N = 28 | 17.2<br>± 8.7 | 20.2<br>±10.3 | 22.3<br>±11.2 | 0.10<br>±0.14 | 0.57<br>±0.92 | 0.98<br>±1.09 | 0.91<br>±0.52 | 0.<br>±0. |
| Off Rx; mean ± SD N = 28 | 0.97<br>±0.56 | 1.24<br>±0.71 | 1.46<br>±0.81 | 0.18<br>±0.19 | 0.58<br>±0.42 | 1.10<br>±0.48 | 1.03<br>±0.46 | 0.<br>±0. |

*Total accounted for is sum of radioactivity, as percent of dose, in urine, stool, and plasma.

## ABOUT THE SENIOR AUTHOR

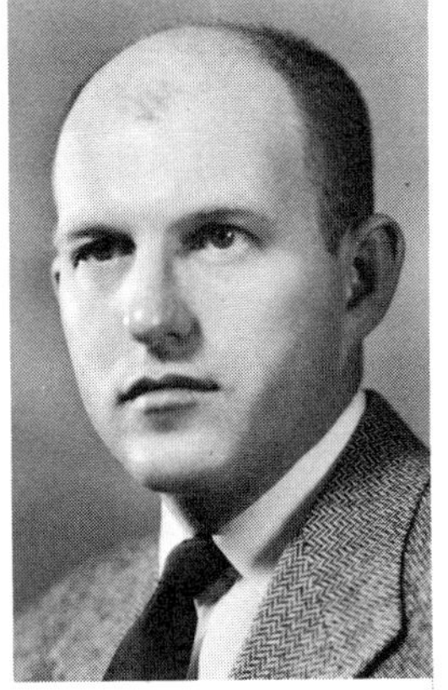

Dr. W. Newlon Tauxe, a member of the Section of Clinical Pathology of the Mayo Clinic, and associate professor of clinical pathology in the Mayo Graduate School of Medicine, University of Minnesota at Rochester, was born in Knoxville, Tennessee in 1924.

He obtained the degrees of bachelor of science in 1948 and doctor of medicine in 1950 from the University of Tennessee. He was an intern in the John Gaston Hospital in Memphis, Tennessee, in 1950, and was associated with the Oak Ridge National Laboratory of the Atomic Energy Commission at Oak Ridge, Tennessee, from 1951 to 1953.

He is a member of the Society of Nuclear Medicine, and the American Society of Clinical Pathologists, the American Medical Association, the Minnesota Society of Pathology, the Minnesota State Medical Association, the Zumbro Valley Medical Society, the Society of the Sigma Xi, the Phi Rho Sigma professional medical fraternity and the Delta Tau Delta social fraternity.

In 1963 Dr. and Mrs. Tauxe jointly received from Medical International Cooperation a MEDICO award "in grateful recognition of outstanding and meritorious service to MEDICO, a service of CARE, in the advancement of worldwide medical assistance." Dr. and Mrs. Tauxe went to Algeria in March, 1963, where they aided in setting up basic medical routines in hospitals there after many European physicians, nurses and technicians had left the country subsequent to the independence of Algeria.

are shown in the Figure. In both curves there is a rapid clearance of the copper from the plasma, followed, in the normal subject, by a gradual return of radioactivity as ceruloplasmin-bound copper, beginning after approximately three hours. This return was not seen in any patient with Wilson's disease nor was any effect on incorporation of copper into ceruloplasmin detected during or after treatment with D-penicillamine.

The data for normal subjects and the four categories of Wilson's disease are shown in the Table as means ± SD.

Prior to treatment the urinary values in the preclinical group were only a little higher than normal (not statistically significant at the 5% level) but they were significantly lower than the values in the symptomatic group prior to therapy. The most striking differences between these two groups were in the liver counts; the differences between these means at 24, 48, and 72 hours were 6.3, 5.9, and 8.8 SE. The highest liver counts of all categories were found in the preclinical group, averaging $194 \times 10^2$ cps/100 $\mu$c of injected dose. Radioactivity in the liver almost always increased during the period between 24 and 48 hours after injection in patients with Wilson's disease, frequently reaching a plateau between 48 and 72 hours; in normal subjects, radioactivity over the liver decreased between 24 and 72 hours after injection.

In all cases, the urinary excretions were markedly increased by D-penicillamine, reaching 51.6% of the dose at 72 hours in one case. No significant changes were produced by the therapy except that the liver counts became lower but still showed an increase in activity from 24 to 72 hours.

After temporary cessation of therapy of at least a year's duration, urinary excretion decreased to values still significantly above normal but significantly below pretreatment values. In general, liver counts increased during the course of treatment, attaining values in the

## URNOVER OF $^{64}$CU AFTER INTRAVENOUS INJECTION

| | Liver (cps/100 $\mu$c) x 10$^2$ | | | Total accounted for* | | | Total in body (%D) | | |
|---|---|---|---|---|---|---|---|---|---|
| 2 hr. | 24 hr. | 48 hr. | 72 hr. | 24 hr. | 48 hr. | 72 hr. | 24 hr. | 48 hr. | 72 hr. |
| .42<br>.30 | 163.0<br>22.9 | 187.2<br>27.6 | 194.2<br>17.7 | 1.44<br>0.70 | 1.81<br>0.83 | 2.40<br>1.75 | 99.04<br>0.48 | 98.67<br>0.61 | 98.03<br>1.45 |
| .27<br>.27 | 55.3<br>±12.3 | 62.4<br>±17.6 | 62.1<br>±18.5 | 3.63<br>±0.86 | 4.38<br>± 0.92 | 5.73<br>± 1.59 | 97.88<br>±0.37 | 96.95<br>± 0.75 | 95.60<br>± 1.38 |
| .50<br>.36 | 50.0<br>±18.0 | 51.4<br>±18.1 | 51.8<br>±18.9 | 18.26<br>±8.70 | 21.39<br>±10.50 | 23.79<br>±11.55 | 82.65<br>±8.69 | 79.26<br>±10.37 | 76.87<br>±11.23 |
| .77<br>.41 | 66.6<br>±29.2 | 72.3<br>±30.5 | 74.4<br>±31.8 | 2.16<br>±0.78 | 2.79<br>± 0.80 | 3.25<br>± 0.77 | 98.89<br>±0.57 | 98.16<br>± 0.78 | 97.39<br>± 0.93 |

range seen in the preclinical group in those patients who had become free of symptoms. In those patients who were studied more than once, all other values remained fairly constant during therapy as well as during temporary cessation of therapy. No significant differences (at the 5% level) in stool losses were observed among the categories and no changes were produced by treatment.

No differences between groups could be attributed to the amount of copper injected.

### Comment

Our data suggest that the liver is capable of trapping a fraction of intravenously administered copper in excess of what it normally traps, as reflected in the high liver counts seen in patients with preclinical Wilson's disease with low urinary values. Symptoms may develop as binding sites in the liver become saturated, as reflected by the observation of relatively low liver counts and relatively high urinary excretion values among the symptomatic patients studied prior to treatment with D-penicillamine.

Studies made while patients were on therapy yielded the expected efflux of injected $^{64}$Cu. However, when these patients were studied during temporary cessation of long-term therapy, total accountability values decreased markedly because relatively low values were found in plasma, urine, stool, and liver. Perhaps the injected $^{64}$Cu was seeking its former sites of deposition in the body, but by scanning technics we have been unable to observe anything but a generalized distribution.

The fact that the liver counts remained high in the asymptomatic group of patients studied during cessation of treatment suggests that the removal of copper from the binding sites in the liver is a slow process and that it may be associated with the gradual return to normal of severely afflicted patients on D-penicillamine therapy.

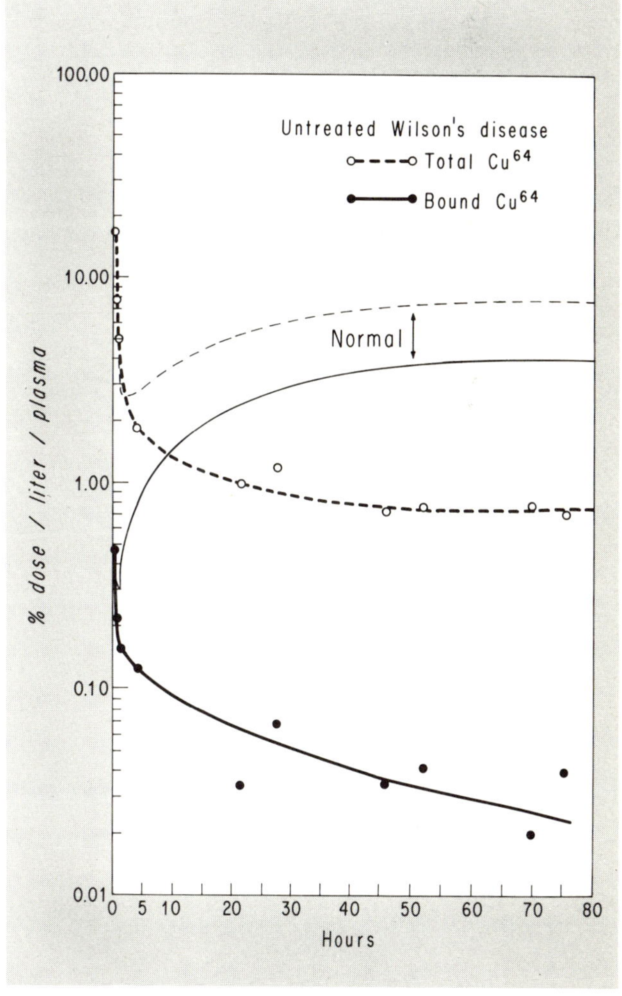


Fig. 1. Disappearance of $^{64}$Cu in homozygous normal subject and in untreated patient with Wilson's disease. (Modified from Tauxe, W. N.; Goldstein, N. P.; Randall, R. V. and Gross, J. B.: Radiocopper studies in patients with Wilson's disease and their relatives. *Amer. J. Med.* **41**:375-380, 1966.)

The fact that the radioactivity in the liver continuously increases over the 72-hour study period in the patients but decreases consistently in the normals suggests that, in the former, part of the hepatic binding process occurs at a slower rate or that copper is being withdrawn from some other pool which is not present in the normal subject.

#### Summary

Before the onset of symptoms of Wilson's disease, accumulation of injected $^{64}Cu$ in the liver is at a relatively high level, while urinary output is relatively low. After symptoms appear, however, hepatic uptake is relatively low and urinary activity is relatively high. Prolonged therapy with D-penicillamine might be expected to free hepatic binding sites for intravenously injected $^{64}Cu$, but it apparently does not readily do so unless the patients are asymptomatic. Curiously, intravenously injected $^{64}Cu$ also does not spill into the urine at pretreatment levels. Perhaps injected $^{64}Cu$ seeks extrahepatic binding sites in symptomatic subjects because hepatic sites are freed only slowly and are not readily available. The presence of symptoms and signs may in part be inversely related to the ready availability of hepatic binding sites.

## *REFERENCES*

1. McCall, J. T.; Goldstein, N. P.; Randall, R. V. and Gross, J. B.: Comparative metabolism of copper and zinc in patients with Wilson's disease (hepatolenticular degeneration). *Amer. J. med. Sci.* **254:**13-23, July 1967.
2. Tauxe, W. N.; Goldstein, N. P.; Randall, R. V. and Gross, J. B.: Radiocopper studies in patients with Wilson's disease and their relatives. *Amer. J. Med.* **41:**375-380, 1966.
3. Retzlaff, J. A.: Red cell volume, plasma volume, and lean body mass in healthy men and women: The development of a blood volume standard. Thesis, Graduate School, University of Minnesota, 1963.
4. Osborn, S. B. and Walshe, J. M.: Copper uptake by the liver. In Walshe, J. M. and Cumings, J. N.: Wilson's disease: some current concepts. Springfield, Illinois, Charles C. Thomas, Publisher, pp. 141-150, 1961.
5. Tauxe, W. N.; Goldstein, N. P.; Randall, R. V. and Gross, J. B.: Birth Defects: Original Article Series. *Wilson's Disease,* The National Foundation, New York, Vol. IV, No. 2, pp. 60-63, April, 1968.

# Ceruloplasmin as a Controlling Factor of the Hematopoietic System

MITIYUKI SHIMIZU, M.D.*

It is postulated that ceruloplasmin plays some role in the formation of erythropoietin. Normal rabbits were treated with ceruloplasmin and folic acid which resulted in the appearance of erythropoietin.

It has been elucidated that copper plays a role in erythropoiesis. It is postulated in our department that ceruloplasmin is a controlling factor[1] in the hematopoietic system, accelerating absorption and storage of iron and resulting in its increase in the liver.[2] Ceruloplasmin increases the number of young cells of erythropoietic system, especially polychromatic normoblasts, leading to a hyperplastic bone marrow. From these findings, we believe that ceruloplasmin has a relationship to the formation of erythropoietin.

The conditions that are known to increase erythropoietin in normal animals are anemia due to venesection,[3] anoxia,[4] and injection of cobalt.[5] The work described in this paper suggests that the repeated intramuscular injection of ceruloplasmin and folic acid also accelerates the formation of erythropoietin in normal animals.

## Methods and Materials

*Experimental Method*

Intramuscular injections of 3 mg of human or hog ceruloplasmin, 15 $\mu$g of folic acid and 30 $\mu$g of vitamin $B_{12}$ were given every day to rabbits for 16 weeks. The plasma was collected on the first, second, third and fourth week after injection and at regular intervals until the 16th week. The rabbits from which blood was collected were not used again. The plasma used for the determination of erythropoietic activity was made from the combined blood of three rabbits in each group to minimize individual variations. Control experiments were made with physiologic saline solution and with gamma globulin, which was used for checking the specific action of ceruloplasmin in forming erythropoietin.

*Measurement of Erythropoietic Activity*

Erythropoietic activity was assayed by measuring the incorporation of $^{59}$Fe into peripheral blood cells. Pure strain Wistar rats, weighing 150-200 g, were fasted for 24 hours, after which 2 ml of the test plasma was injected subcutaneously. Another 2 ml of the test plasma was injected subcutaneously 24 hours after the first injection. Forty-eight hours after the first injection, 1 $\mu$c ml of $^{59}$Fe was injected intraperitoneally. One ml of blood was collected from the orbital blood vessel, in a heparinized glass tube, 72 hours after the first injection of $^{59}$Fe.

Radioactivity of 0.5 ml of this blood was measured, using a well-type scintillation counter. The incorpora-

### ABOUT THE AUTHOR

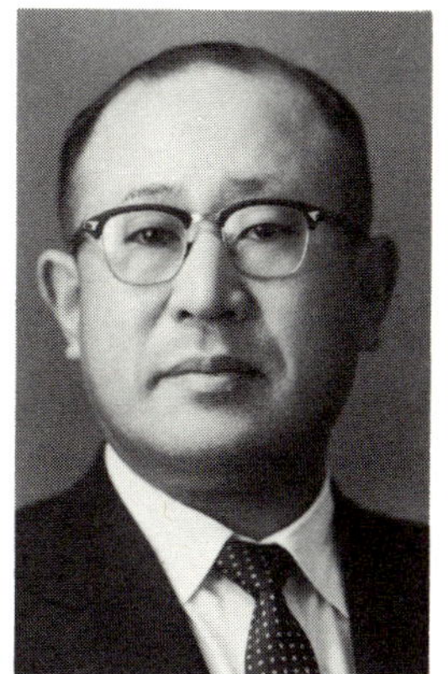

Dr. Mitiyuki Shimizu graduated from Tokyo University in 1941 and entered the Department of Internal Medicine, Tokyo University in 1942. He was a Research Fellow in the Department of Biochemistry, Tokyo University from 1947 to 1950. From 1954 to 1956 he was Research Fellow in the Department of Pathology, University of North Carolina, U.S.A. From 1956 to the present Dr. Shimizu has been Professor of Internal Medicine, Showa University Medical School, Tokyo.

*Professor of Medicine, Department of Medicine, Showa University Medical School, Tokyo, Japan.

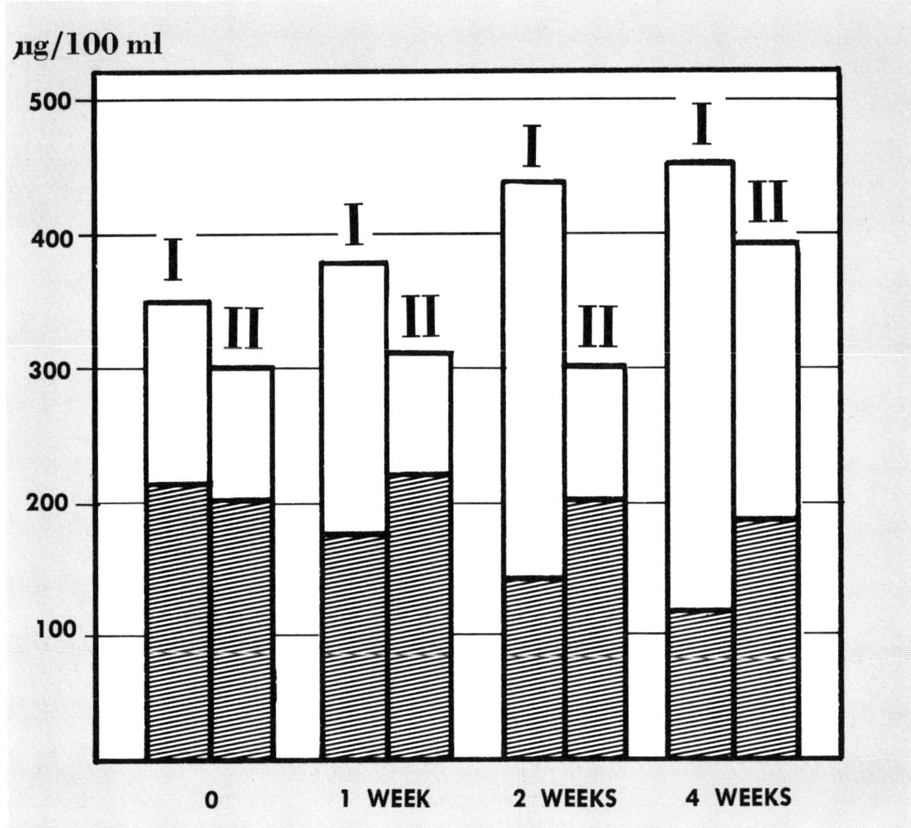


Fig. 1. Bars show total iron binding capacity. Diagonally lined bar shows serum iron level.
I: Treatment with ceruloplasmin and folic acid resulted in decrease of serum iron level and increase of unsaturated iron binding capacity.
II: Control.

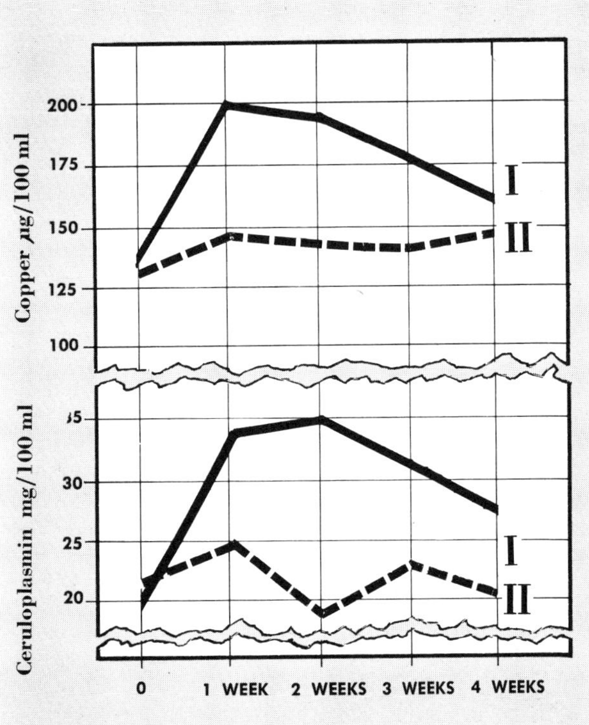


Fig. 2.
I: Serum ceruloplasmin and copper values increased rapidly after the injection.
II: Control.

tion of $^{59}$Fe into peripheral blood cells was calculated on the assumption that total amount of blood is 5% of body weight. A total of ten rats were used for one group. Control experiments were done for each test and the results were statistically evaluated.

### Experimental Results

As shown in Table I, intramuscular injection of ceruloplasmin and folic acid results in appearance of erythropoietin in rabbit plasma as early as the fifth day after the injection. Although the combined use of ceruloplasmin and folic acid increased erythropoietin in blood, ceruloplasmin or folic acid alone; ceruloplasmin and vitamin $B_{12}$; or vitamin $B_{12}$ alone failed to increase erythropoietin in blood. The same results were obtained on the 112th day after the injection. These values of $^{59}$Fe incorporation rate were two to three times that of the control.

In the next experiment, ceruloplasmin and folic acid were repeatedly injected every day, and $^{59}$Fe incorporation rate was checked at the times shown in Table II. The plasma collected at the first, second and fourth week after injection had erythropoietic activity of two to three times that of the control. This erythropoietic activity can be shown at any time after one week following the intramuscular injection. Erythropoietin activity was not increased by substituting $\gamma$-globulin for ceruloplasmin which seems to suggest that ceruloplasmin has some specific role in the formation of erythropoietin.

**TABLE I**

**ERYTHROPOIETIC ACTIVITY OF RABBIT PLASMA MEASURED BY $^{59}Fe$ INCORPORATION—EXPERIMENT I**

| Day After Injection | Group | Incorporation Rate (%) | Mean ±S.D. |
|---|---|---|---|
| 5th Day | C.P. Alone | 18.7<br>14.9<br>9.7<br>7.8 | 12.8±3.3 |
| | C.P. and F.A. | 28.4<br>20.7<br>23.8<br>16.5 | 22.7±4.4 |
| | C.P. and V.$B_{12}$ | 6.2<br>7.1<br>10.1 | 7.8±1.8 |
| | F.A. Alone | 8.1<br>11-1<br>8.9<br>9.6 | 9.4±1.1 |
| | V.$B_{12}$ Alone | 8.5<br>11.2<br>6.4<br>8.8 | 6.8±2.6 |
| 112th Day | C.P. Alone | 4.7<br>4.8<br>2.5<br>5.7 | 4.4±1.9 |
| | C.P. and F.A. | 14.4<br>32.3<br>15.2<br>16.7<br>6.6 | 21.3±9.4 |
| | C.P. and V.$B_{12}$ | 4.2<br>15.2<br>7.0<br>3.3 | 7.4±4.6 |
| | F.A. Alone | 11.9<br>9.5<br>5.6<br>11.7 | 9.7±2.5 |
| | V.$B_{12}$ Alone | 10.9<br>12.5<br>10.2<br>9.2 | 10.7±2.6 |
| Normal Plasma | | 16.5<br>12.5<br>9.7<br>4.3 | 10.7±3.8 |
| Physiological Saline | | 3.2<br>7.0<br>4.9<br>5.8<br>5.6 | 5.3±1.3 |

C.P.: ceruloplasmin. F. A.: folic acid.

**TABLE II**

**ERYTHROPOIETIC ACTIVITY OF RABBIT PLASMA MEASURED BY $^{59}Fe$ INCORPORATION—EXPERIMENT II**

| Day After Injection | Group | Incorporation Rate (%) | Mean ±S.D. |
|---|---|---|---|
| 7th Day | C.P. and F.A. | 22.6<br>21.1<br>27.4<br>25.9<br>22.1<br>30.0<br>12.5<br>19.1<br>29.9 | 23.4±5.3 |
| 14th Day | C.P. and F.A. | 17.0<br>10.9<br>20.9<br>19.8<br>21.3<br>23.9<br>18.4<br>21.4 | 20.0±3.7 |
| 28th Day | C.P. and F.A. | 17.3<br>19.4<br>39.2<br>16.7<br>28.6<br>21.9<br>10.0<br>20.8<br>55.8 | 25.5±8.7 |
| $\gamma$-Globulin and F.A. | | 16.7<br>3.4<br>5.0<br>8.2<br>16.2<br>3.5<br>10.3<br>6.5<br>5.1 | 8.3±4.8 |
| Normal Plasma | | 19.9<br>12.6<br>13.5<br>7.4<br>16.2<br>15.7<br>9.7<br>9.0<br>9.7 | 12.7±3.8 |
| Physiological Saline | | 2.7<br>13.6<br>10.0<br>7.0<br>7.0<br>5.6<br>7.0<br>8.7<br>10.0 | 7.9±2.9 |

C.P.: ceruloplasmin. F. A.: folic acid.

*Iron and Copper Metabolism, and Peripheral Blood Picture after Injection of Ceruloplasmin and Folic Acid*

Serum iron and copper metabolism were also investigated, checking the number of reticulocytes and erythrocytes and hemoglobin content.

Treatment with ceruloplasmin and folic acid resulted in a decrease of serum iron and increase of the total and unsaturated iron binding capacity of serum (Fig. 1). Serum ceruloplasmin and copper values increased rapidly after the injection (Fig. 2). With the increase of serum ceruloplasmin, reticulocytes in the peripheral blood showed a rapid increase, reaching a maximum in the fourth week (Fig. 3). Following this increase of reticulocytes, hemoglobin and erythrocytes increased from the fourth week, to a maximum at the eighth week (Fig. 4).

From these results, it was inferred that iron was utilized in erythropoiesis in the presence of erythropoietin produced by combined use of ceruloplasmin and folic acid.

Of the conditions known to increase erythropoietin in blood, both anemia due to venesection and anoxia are considered to aid the formation of erythropoietin by decreasing the supply of oxygen to tissues. This is said

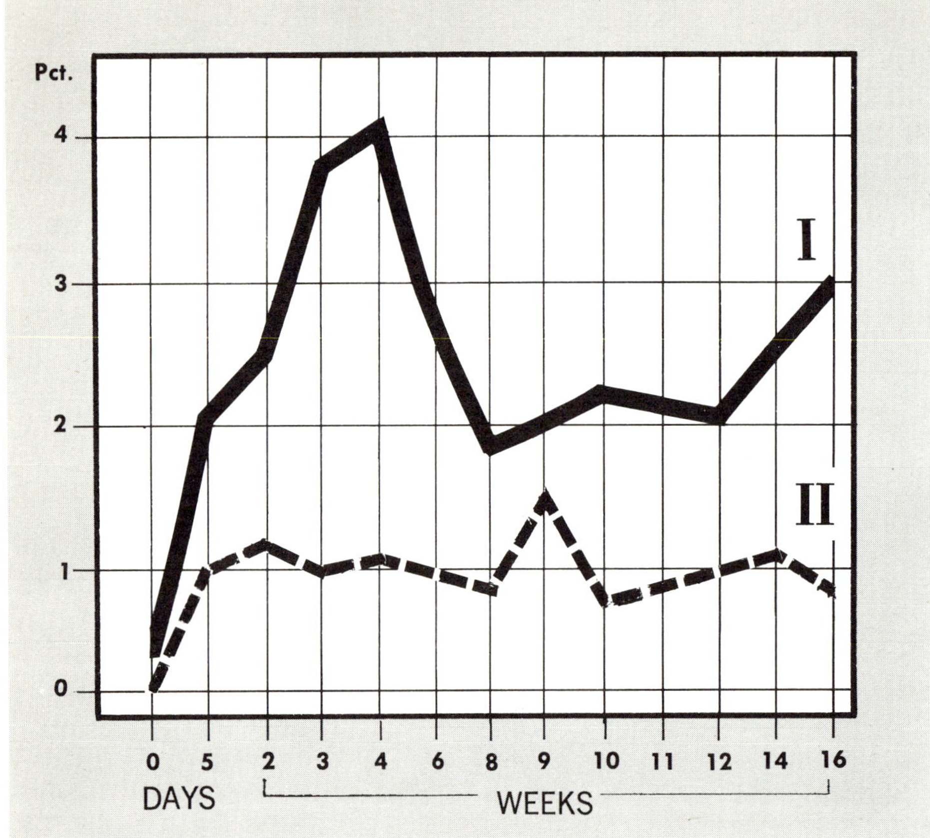


Fig. 3.
I: Reticulocytes showed a rapid increase, reaching a maximum in the fourth week.
II: Control.

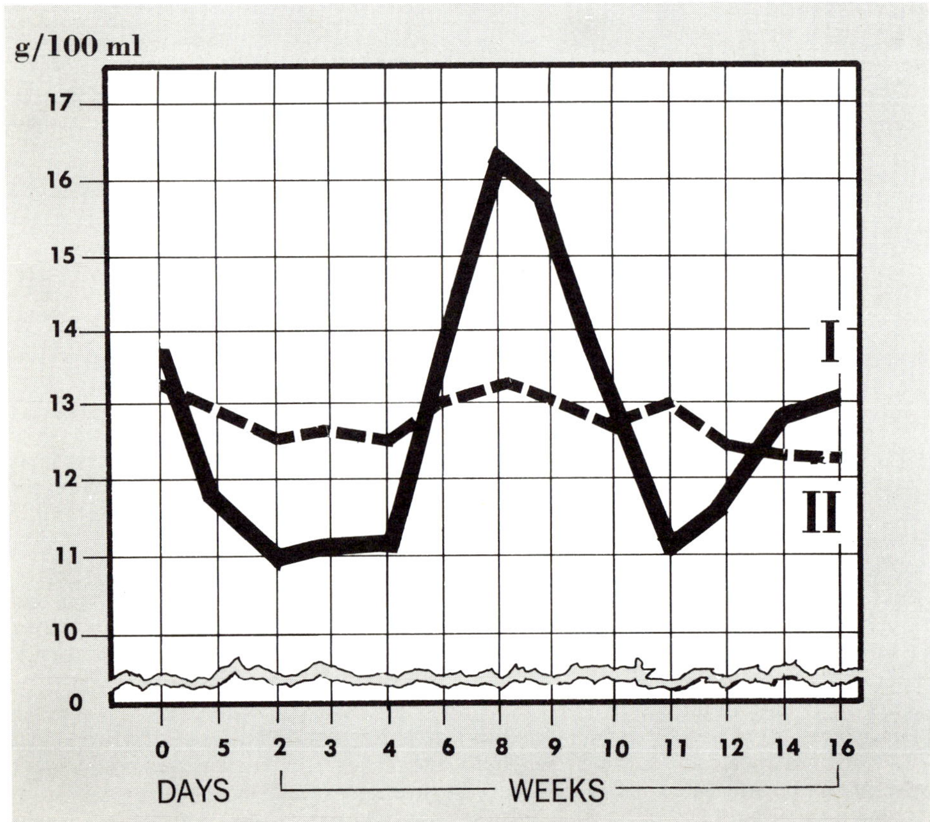


Fig. 4.
I: Hemoglobin increased from the fourth week, to a maximum at the eighth week.
II: Control.

to be supported by the fact that there is a correlation between the degree of anemia and the erythropoietic activity in blood or urine.[6,7,8]

On the other hand, the mechanism for accelerated formation of erythropoietin activity by injection of cobalt is still unknown, but it is thought that cellular anoxia, caused by the cobalt, plays a role in this mechanism.[9]

The results of the present series of experiments have shown a new condition which accelerates erythropoietin activity.

Recently in our department an erythropoietic stimulating substance was isolated from ceruloplasmin when a solution of ceruloplasmin was adjusted to pH 4.5 with hydrochloric acid.[10] This substance is thermostable, suggesting the possibility that ceruloplasmin is one of the source materials of erythropoietin. Ceruloplasmin can be divided into four fractions by DEAE cellulose column chromatography and the substance with erythropoietic activity was then isolated from the fourth fraction.[11] It has not been determined whether this substance is related to the form of erythropoietin in the experiments reported in this paper. Erythropoietin which appears in anemic patients is an $\alpha_2$-globulin, and it would seem that ceruloplasmin, also an $\alpha_2$-globulin, plays a role in the formation of erythropoietin.

**Summary**

Treatment of normal rabbits with ceruloplasmin and folic acid results in the appearance of erythropoietin. It seems that ceruloplasmin plays some role in erythropoietin formation.

## *REFERENCES*

1. Shimizu, M.: Clinical and experimental studies of ceruloplasmin as erythropoietic factor. *Proc. VIIIth International Congress of Hematology,* **ii:**979, 1960.
2. Takahashi, A.: Studies on influences of ceruloplasmin to catalase activity, copper and iron metabolism, and tissue respiration in liver. *Showa Medical Journal,* **20:**1450, 1961.
3. Carnot, P. and Deflandre, Cl.: Sur l'activité hémopoiétique des differents organes au cours de la régénération du sang. *C. R. Acad. Sci.,* **143:**384, 1906.
4. Förster, J.: Luftverdünnung und Blutregeneration durch "Hämopoietine". *Biochem. Z.,* **145:**309, 1924.
5. Goldwasser, E.; Jacobson, L. O.; Fried, W. and Plzak, L.: Mechanism of the erythropoietic effect of cobalt. *Science,* **125:**1085, 1957.
6. Lowy, P. H.; Keighley, G.; Borsook, H. and Graybiel, A.: On the erythropoietic principle in the blood of rabbits made severely anemic with phenylhydrazine. *Blood,* **14:**262, 1959.
7. White, W. F. and Josh, G.: Studies on erythropoietin. II. Production of high-titer plasma in sheep. *Proc. Soc. exp. Biol. Med.,* **102:**686, 1959.
8. Payne, R. W.: Plasma erythropoietin levels in anemia: Studies using an assay method in intact rats. *Brit. J. Haemat.,* **7:**285, 1961.
9. Laforet, M. T. and Thomas, E. D.: The effect of cobalt on heme synthesis by bone marrow in vitro. *J. biol. Chem.,* **218:**595, 1955.
10. Hatta, Y.; Maruyama, Y.; Tsuruoka, N.; Yamaguchi, A.; Ando, M.; Ueno, T. and Shimizu, M.: Studies on erythropoietin. III. Isolation of erythropoietin from ceruloplasmin molecule. *Acta haemat. jap.,* **26:**174, 1963.
11. Maruyama, Y.; Yuto, S.: Fujii, Y.; Mitsuoka, T.; Hojo, M.; Hatta, Y. and Shimizu, M.: Studies on erythropoietic substance. IV. Ceruloplasmin fraction and erythropoietic activity. *Acta haemat. jap.,* **28:**119, 1965.

# Genetic Studies of Wilson's Disease in Japan*

Masataka Arima, M.D.** and Isamu Sano, M.D.***

Wilson's disease is an inborn error of metabolism with various symptoms. This study was performed to clarify the characteristics of Wilson's disease in Japan, frequency of the gene, and factors determining the course and severity of the disease. Genetic factors appear to play an important role in determining the ages at onset and death, and the clinical forms.

It is generally accepted that the mode of inheritance of Wilson's disease is autosomal recessive.[1,2,3] Although the factors which determine the clinical course of the disease are not known, certainly both genetic and environmental factors have been incriminated.[4,5] In order to clarify the characteristics of Wilson's disease in Japan, the authors intended to study as many patients as possible from clinical and genetic standpoints.

### Materials

In cooperation with the departments of pediatrics, neuropsychiatry and internal medicine of about 60 large hospitals, 151 patients from 126 families were collected from all areas in Japan from 1955 through 1965. Only patients who exhibited evidence of abnormal copper metabolism such as Kayser-Fleischer rings, low ceruloplasmin levels, increased urinary copper excretion, and/or high copper contents in the liver were selected. These patients were classified as proved cases. In addition to these, by direct questioning of the relatives, 61 patients who had died of hepatic insufficiency or progressive neurologic symptoms, were found among the siblings of the proved cases. These 61 patients who had died were studied as probable cases of Wilson's disease.

### Age of Onset and Death

Age of onset of the disease ranged from four years to 41 years with the peak between six and 12 years of age (Fig. 1). The initial symptoms in cases with an earlier onset were mainly hepatic, such as jaundice, ascites and hematemesis, while in cases with late onset neurologic symptoms tended to be predominant (Fig. 2) as reported by several authors.[6,7,8,9]

The disease was classified as follows: the hepatic form, which shows predominant hepatic symptoms and insignificant neurologic symptoms throughout life; the hepatocerebral form in which there are mild or severe hepatic symptoms and marked cerebral symptoms; and the cerebral form in which predominantly neurologic symptoms without hepatic manifestations occur throughout most of life. As shown in Figure 3, the hepatic form had an earlier onset and death occurred sooner; in the cerebral form both onset and death were later. Therefore, from the clinical point of view, the hepatic form is the severest, the hepatocerebral form

## ABOUT THE AUTHOR

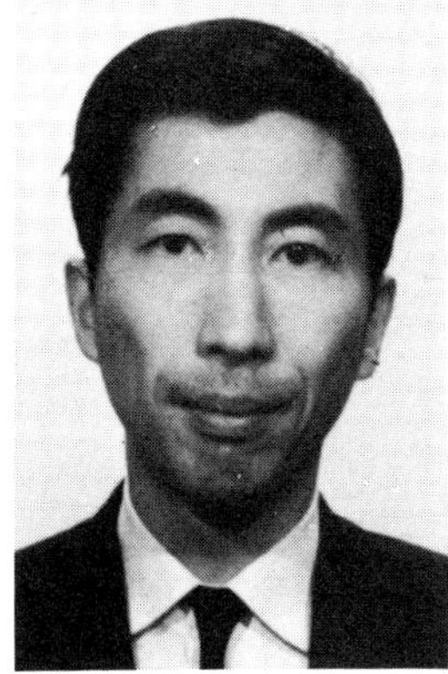

Born in 1929, Dr. M. Arima studied medicine at the University of Tokyo from 1949 to 1953 and then worked in the Department of Pediatrics of the University Hospital until 1964. He has paid special attention to neurologic diseases in childhood such as convulsive disorders, cerebral palsies and hereditary diseases of the central nervous system. His research and written articles cover the fields of pediatric neurology and medical genetics. Since 1964, he has been assistant professor of the Department of Pediatrics of the University of Toho, Tokyo, Japan.

*This study was supported in part by grants from NIH RG-9469 and Rockefeller Foundation RE:Ga MNS 62170.

**Assistant Professor, Department of Pediatrics, Toho University, Tokyo, Japan.

***Associate Professor, Department of Neuropsychiatry, Osaka University, Osaka, Japan.

follows it, and the cerebral form is the mildest form of the disease. The earlier onset of the disease in Japanese patients may be explained in part by the predominance of the hepatic symptoms.

### Sibship Studies

It is said that age of onset and clinical manifestations of a hereditary disease within sibships tend to be similar comparing those of the patients with other families.[4] In the sibships studied, differences in the age of onset between the first patients and their affected sibs ranged from 0 to 14 years with an average of 0.9 ± 3.2 years. The similarity in the age at onset in the sib pairs was highly significant ($p<0.005$) (Fig. 4).

In the sib pairs, the age at death was also very similar with a high coefficient of correlation ($p<0.005$) (Fig. 5).

Similarity in the form of disease of the propositi and in their affected sibs was also observed.

### Family Trees

Some examples of families with Wilson's disease were shown. In many families sib pairs showed a very similar course of the disease. However, in some families marked differences in the age at onset and death, as well as the clinical course of the disease, were observed. Three asymptomatic patients have had the preventive administration of penicillamine and a low copper diet during the last five years and are in good condition up to the present, which is several years past the ages at death of their affected sibs. These results appear to indicate the effectiveness of prevention which changes relevant environmental factors. Figure 6 shows a large kindred of Wilson's disease in Mikura Island with a population of only 300. (These families were investigated in cooperation with Drs. Mozai, Terao and Ogihara.) This island has been isolated from other areas for several hundred years.[10] In two families the disease developed in childhood and had a rapid course. On the other hand, two patients belonging to another family had a late onset with a mild course of the disease. Since the abnormal gene and environmental factors would probably be common to all patients, another factor such as a suppressor gene would appear to play an important role in the determination of the clinical course in these patients.

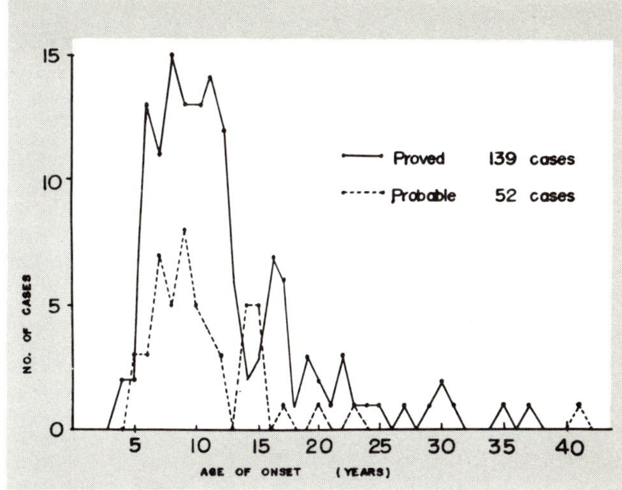


Fig. 1. Age of onset of symptoms in patients with Wilson's disease.

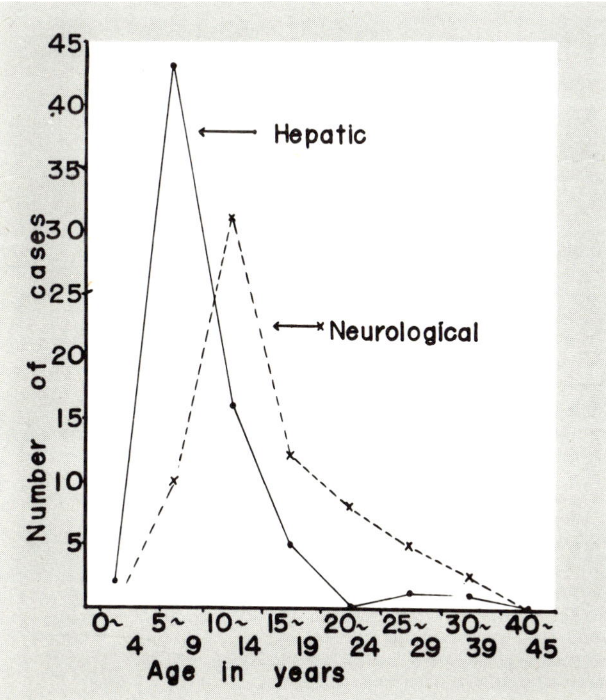


Fig. 2. Age of onset and initial symptoms in patients with Wilson's disease (136 proved cases).

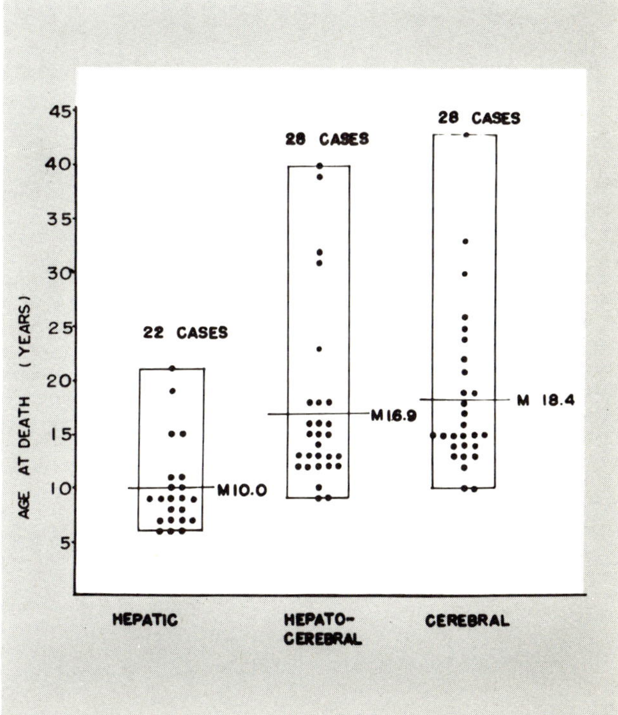


Fig. 3. Clinical form and age at death (78 proved cases).

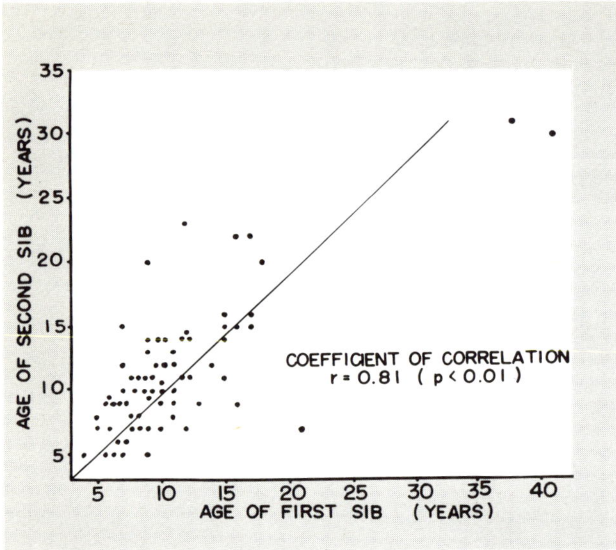


Fig. 4. Age of onset of symptoms in sib pairs with Wilson's disease (70 sibs).

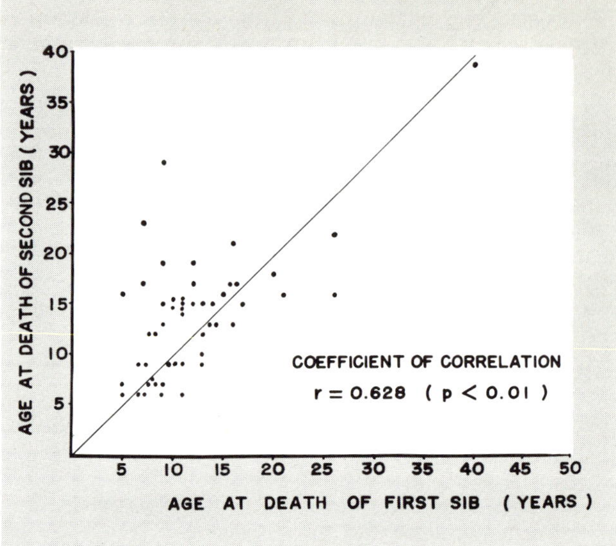


Fig. 5. Correlation of age at death in sib pairs (51 pairs).

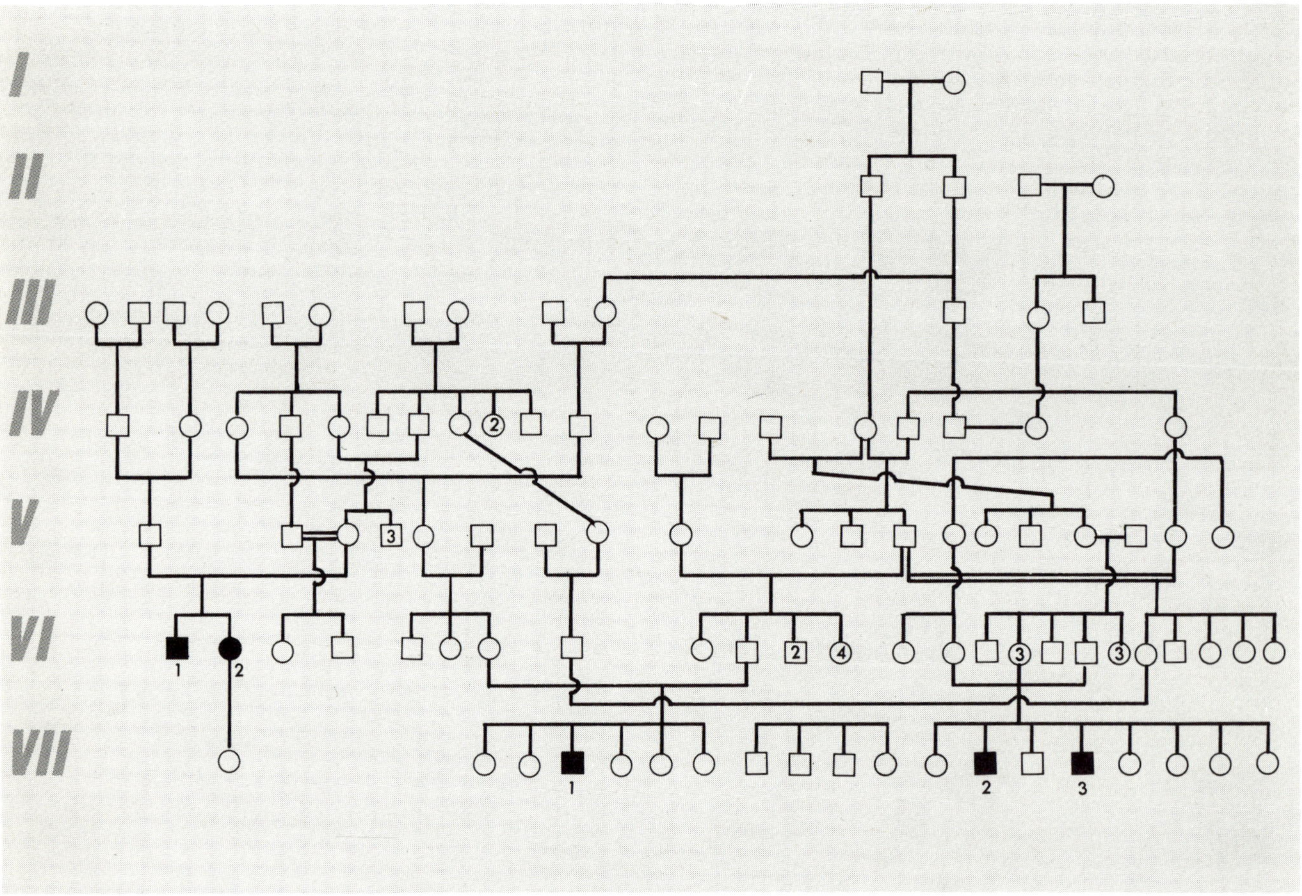

Fig. 6. Pedigree of families with Wilson's disease in Mikura Island: VI (1) Neurological symptoms at 37 years. Died at 40 years. Marked ceruloplasmin deficiency and K-F rings. VI (2) Bleeding tendency at 25 years. Neurological symptoms at 31 years. Died at 39 years. Ceruloplasmin deficiency and K-F rings. VII (1) Neurological symptoms at 11 years. Died at 12 years. Ceruloplasmin deficiency and K-F rings. VII (2) Hepatosplenomegaly at 9 years. Died of neurological symptoms at 11 years. Probable case. VII (3) Jaundice at 6 years 2 months. Died of hepatic insufficiency at 6 years 3 months. Copper in the liver markedly increased.

TABLE I

## AGE AT ONSET AND DEATH, AND CLINICAL FORM OF DISEASE, BY SEX

| Form | Proved | | | Probable | | |
|---|---|---|---|---|---|---|
| | Male | Female | Total | Male | Female | Total |
| Hepatic | 15 (29%) | 8 (28%) | 23 | 13 (50%) | 19 (73%) | 32 |
| Hepato-cerebral | 17 (33%) | 10 (34%) | 27 | 5 (19%) | 5 (19%) | 10 |
| Cerebral | 19 (37%) | 11 (38%) | 30 | 8 (31%) | 2 (8%) | 10 |
| Total | 51 (100%) | 29 (100%) | 80 | 26 (100%) | 26 (100%) | 52 |
| Age at Onset | | | | | | |
| Number of Cases | 87 | 52 | 139 | 26 | 26 | 52 |
| Range | 4-37 yrs. | 4-31 yrs. | | 6-41 yrs. | 5-23 yrs. | |
| Mean | 12.8 | 11.2 | 12.2 | 11.4 | 10.5 | 11.0 |
| Age at Death | | | | | | |
| Number of Cases | 58 | 29 | | 25 | 25 | |
| Range | 6-43 yrs. | 7-40 yrs. | | 6-44 yrs. | 5-29 yrs. | |
| Mean | 16.0 | 15.2 | 15.7 | 13.2 | 11.5 | 12.4 |

### Modifying Factors

*Sex:* In order to clarify the modifying factors, difference in the clinical course by sex was investigated. In the male patients, onset of the disease tended to be later than those in the female patients. The tendency of later onset in males was observed in both the proved and probable groups. Comparing the ages at death, the male patients tended to die later than the females in both the proved and probable groups. Frequency of each form of the disease was compared between the males and the females. No difference was proved in the definite cases. However, in probable cases, the females showed mainly the hepatic form, while the males showed a higher occurrence of the cerebral form. Although the difference in age at onset and death between the males and females was statistically significant, it was too slight to permit any definite conclusions to be drawn (Table I).

### Geographical Distribution

Families with Wilson's disease were commonly distributed in all areas of Japan. About half of the families were located in the Kanto, Tokyo and Kinki areas, where the population is large, and there are several large hospitals with well-equipped laboratories (Fig. 7). Thus, the predominance of the patients in these areas does not necessarily show a high frequency of the disease. The patients from the Kanto and Tokyo area tended to have an earlier onset and a predominance of the hepatic and hepatocerebral forms. However, in all areas, each form and all age groups were found. The difference by area was statistically insignificant. Thus, as far as the patients in Japan are concerned, a clear-cut difference by area in the clinical course has not been determined.

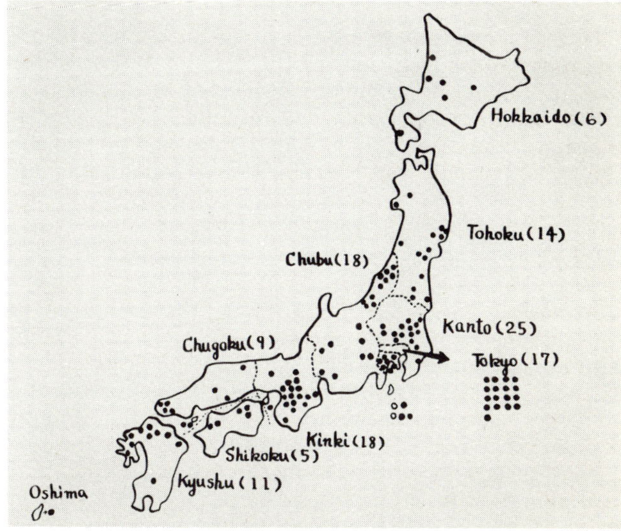


Fig. 7. Geographical distribution of families with Wilson's disease in Japan (123 families).

TABLE II

## Age at Onset and Consanguineous Marriage of Parents

| | Number of Patients | Range | Mean |
|---|---|---|---|
| Consanguineous | | | |
| a) Proved | 70 | 4-37 yrs. | 10.8 yrs. |
| b) Probable | 31 | 5-41 yrs. | 10.6 yrs. |
| Nonconsanguineous | | | |
| c) Proved | 62 | 6-35 yrs. | 13.0 yrs. |
| d) Probable | 21 | 7-23 yrs. | 10.7 yrs. |

a) — c) = $2.24 \pm 0.35$ ($p<0.01$)

### Consanguineous Marriage

Consanguineous marriage between the parents occurred in about half of the families. Although the ages of onset of the disease were similar in the consanguineous and nonconsanguineous groups, the mean age differed significantly. That is, the proved patients born from consanguineous unions tended to have an earlier onset compared with the patients from the nonconsanguineous group (Table II).

In our series, evidence of Wilson's disease was not found in members of any generation other than that of the propositus. Therefore, evidence for the presence of autosomal dominant or sex-linked recessive types of Wilson's disease has not been obtained. In addition, there has been no evidence that there are two or more kinds of a mutant gene in Wilson's disease. On the basis of these results, the differences between groups may be explained by some modifying factors working in a homozygotic condition.

### Gene Frequency

In a previous report, based on the author's personal experiences, the frequency of the gene of Wilson's disease in Japan was estimated to be between 0.0033 to 0.0066 by applying Dahlberg's formula.[11] In the present study, the mean rate of cousin marriage among the parents of patients was 0.34. However, a remarkable difference in the rate of consanguineous marriage was detected among families from large cities, small cities and rural areas. (Table III).

According to Dahlberg's formula, the incidence of consanguineous marriage among the parents of patients with an autosomal recessive disorder tends to be higher when the frequency of the abnormal gene is low and the incidence of consanguineous marriage in the general population is high. It has been estimated that the frequency of cousin marriages in the general population in Japan is 2 to 5 percent in large cities; 4 to 10 in small cities; 6 to 16 in rural areas. In our series, the lower incidence of cousin marriages among the parents of patients with Wilson's disease from large cities might have been caused by the lower incidence of cousin marriage in the general urban population. On the other hand, the relatively lower frequency of cousin marriages among the parents of patients in rural areas might indicate a higher frequency of the abnormal gene in these areas. It is assumed that the frequency of the gene in some rural areas in Japan is 0.01 or more as shown in Mikura Island.[10]

### Conclusion

Patients with Wilson's disease in Japan appear to have an earlier onset of the disease and death which is explained, in part, by the predominance of hepatic manifestations. It is possible that the Japanese diet, which contains much copper and relatively little protein, plays a role. However, genetic factors may also play an important role in the determination of the course and severity of the disease. In sibling groups, the age at onset and death, as well as the form of the disease, are significantly similar. In addition to the family background, consanguineous marriage between the parents plays a role in promoting the development of the disease. It is possible that another modifying gene is present. Females appear to have a little earlier onset and a predominance of hepatic symptoms which was not statistically significant. Differences in the course of the disease by area may be present but are also not significant. From the clinical point of view, as far as the patients in Japan are concerned, evidence of two or more kinds of mutant genes associated with Wilson's disease has not been obtained.

ACKNOWLEDGEMENTS

The authors express their appreciation to Professor T. Takatsu, Department of Pediatrics; Prof. K. Nakao; Prof. Y. Yoshitoshi; Dr. T. Mozai; Dr. T. Terao; Dr. K. Ogihara, Department of Internal Medicine; Professor J. Miyake; Dr. T. Shikata, Department of Pathology, Tokyo University; Prof. S. Katsuki, Department of Internal Medicine, Kyushu University and Prof. T. Inose, Department of Psychiatry, Yokohama University, and many other doctors for their kind cooperation and advice in the assessment of these families.

TABLE III

## Frequency of Consanguineous Marriage of Parents (120 Families)

| | Population | | | |
|---|---|---|---|---|
| | Urban | | Rural | Total |
| | >100,000 | <100,000 | | |
| First cousin | 9 | 14 | 18 | 41 |
| Second cousin | 3 | 1 | 4 | 8 |
| Other consang. | 2 | 1 | 6 | 9 |
| No consang. | 28 | 7 | 27 | 62 |
| Total | 42 | 23 | 55 | 120 |

## REFERENCES


1. André, M. J. and Bogaert L.: L'hérédité dans la dégénérescence hépato-lenticulaire et le probleme des rapports intrinsèques de la pseudo-sclérose de Westphal-Strumpell et de la maladie de Wilson. *Encéphale* **39**:1-34, 1950.

2. Bearn, A. G.: Wilson's disease. An inborn error of metabolism with multiple manifestations. *Amer. J. Med.* **22**: 747-757, 1957.

3. Sternlieb, I. and Scheinberg, I. H.: Detection of the heterozygous carrier of Wilson's disease gene. *J. clin. Invest.* **40**: 707-715, 1961.

4. Bearn, A. G.: A genetical analysis of thirty families with Wilson's disease. *Ann. hum. Genet.* **24**:33-43, 1960.

5. Denny-Brown, D.: Hepatolenticular degeneration (Wilson's disease). Two different components. *New Engl. J. Med.* **270**:1149-1156, 1964.

6. Scheinberg, I. H. and Sternlieb, I.: The dual role of the liver in Wilson's disease. *Med. Clin. N. Amer.* **47**:815-825, 1960.

7. Walshe, J. M.: Wilson's disease. The presenting symptoms. *Arch. Dis. Childh.* **37**:253-257, 1962.

8. Silverberg, M. and Gellis, S. S.: The liver in juvenile Wilson's disease. *Pediatrics* **30**:402-413, 1962.

9. Arima, M.; Komiya, K.; Kamoshita, S. and Mukai, N.: Clinical and pathological characteristics in Wilson's disease in cases under ten years of age. *Paediat. Univ. Tokyo.* **9**:17-22, 1963.

10. Arima, M.; Kamoshita, S.; Komiya, H. and Murokawa, H.: Genetical studies of Wilson's disease. 3. Genetical and epidemiological studies of Wilson's disease in Mikura Island. *Paediat. Univ. Tokyo* **10**:5-10, 1964.

11. Arima, M. and Kurumada, T.: Ibid. 2. Mode of inheritance and gene frequency in Japan. *Paediat. Univ. Tokyo* **7**:7-12, 1962.

# Copper Metabolism in Carriers of Wilson's Disease: Analysis of Kinetics of Intravenously Injected Radiocopper as a Means of Detecting the Carrier State*

W. NEWLON TAUXE, M.D.**; NORMAN P. GOLDSTEIN, M.D.***; RAYMOND V. RANDALL, M.D., M.S.† and JOHN B. GROSS, M.D.†

Metabolic turnover tests were performed in 18 normal subjects and in 13 heterozygous carriers. Our data support the concept that copper trapping by the liver is approximately the same in the two groups. Initial plasmatic disappearance rates are not significantly different, but radiocopper remains in the liver longer in the carriers as reflected by the higher liver count rates. It is transferred to blood more slowly, and excretion into the stool in the carrier is also considerably slower.

Up to the present the only definite means of distinguishing the carrier of Wilson's disease (hepatolenticular degeneration, HLD) from a normal person involves kinetic studies using radioactive copper. Numerous reports suggest that the defect of Wilson's disease is carried as an autosomal recessive trait. On this basis, both parents and all offspring of patients with homozygous Wilson's disease are certain to be carriers. However, only by positive identification of the carrier can the genetic pattern be determined reliably. The work of Sternlieb and coworkers[1] suggests that a defect exists in the liver in carriers of the disease, which results in altered kinetics of metabolism of labeled copper administered orally.

Preliminary data reported by us suggested that several criteria could be used to establish heterozygosity in patients who were given radioactive copper intravenously. It is the purpose of this paper to present $^{64}$Cu turnover data obtained from normal subjects, from definitely identified carriers, and from siblings of patients with Wilson's disease.

## Materials and Methods

We performed 38 metabolic turnover tests, by previously described technics,[2] after intravenous injection of approximately 750 $\mu$c of $^{64}$Cu in 18 normal subjects, in 12 persons who were parents of patients with Wilson's disease and in one son of a patient with the disease. None of the subjects had any symptoms or signs suggestive of Wilson's disease. Seven siblings of patients with definite Wilson's disease were studied; none of these subjects had any symptoms suggestive of Wilson's disease, but two of them had slightly enlarged livers (one fingerbreadth below the right costal margin). The test was repeated twice in one subject and once in another.

Radioactive copper ($^{64}$Cu) was obtained as cupric acetate in various specific activities so that the actual amount of copper injected ranged from 0.014 to 1.2 mg with a mean of 0.15 mg.

After intravenous injection of the $^{64}$Cu, plasma samples were obtained at 10, 20, 30, 45, 60, 120 and 180 minutes and at 24, 32, 48, 60 and 72 hours. Radioactivity was expressed as percent of dose per liter in total copper and in ceruloplasmin-bound copper after separation with diethyldithiocarbamate (Morell's method).[3] These values were plotted on semilogarithmic paper, and, from this curve, 20-, 30-, 100- and 200-minute values (total) were read and ratios based on them were derived. The minimum was found and the time of its appearance was

*This investigation was supported in part by Research Grant NB-3655 from the National Institutes of Health, Public Health Service.

**Consultant, Section of Clinical Pathology, Mayo Clinic; Associate Professor of Clinical Pathology, Mayo Graduate School of Medicine (University of Minnesota), Rochester, Minn.

***Consultant, Section of Neurology, Mayo Clinic; Professor of Neurology, Mayo Graduate School of Medicine (University of Minnesota), Rochester, Minn.

†Consultants, Section of Medicine, Mayo Clinic; Associate Professors of Medicine, Mayo Graduate School of Medicine (University of Minnesota), Rochester, Minn.

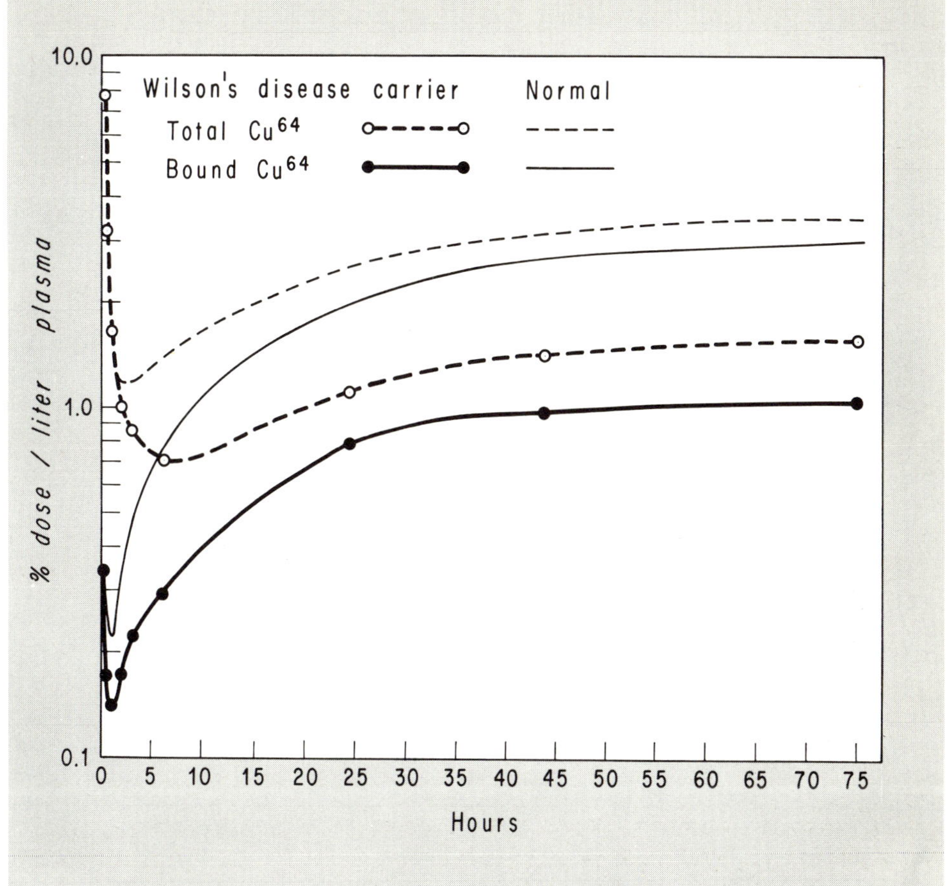


Fig. 1. Plasmatic disappearance of $^{64}Cu$ in a heterozygous carrier of Wilson's disease. Injected copper returns to circulating plasma as bound copper, in contrast to situation in homozygous Wilson's disease patient, but reappearance of $^{64}Cu$ is slower than that in homozygous normal, typical curves which are superimposed here as fine lines. (From Tauxe, W. N.; Goldstein, N. P.; Randall, R. V. and Gross, J. B.: Radiocopper studies in patients with Wilson's disease and their relatives. *Amer. J. Med.* **41**:375-380, 1966. By permission of the publisher, The Reuben H. Donnelley Corporation.)

determined. All urine and stools were collected for each day of the three-day period and analyzed separately. Cumulative radioactivity in both these excreta was expressed as percent of dose (%D) at 24, 48 and 72 hours. External counting over the liver was carried out by a method similar to that of Osborn and Walshe[4]; a widely collimated probe was in place in standardized position during the injection and for the subsequent two hours, and it was carefully replaced for the 6-, 24-, 32-, 48-, 60- and 72-hour measurements. All counts were corrected for background and radioactive decay and were plotted on semilogarithmic paper as counts per second per 100 $\mu$c of $^{64}Cu$ injected.

Plasma volumes were estimated by using regression equations based on height, weight, and age, as derived by Retzlaff,[5] and plasma values were expressed as %D on the basis of the plasma volume estimate.

Although the data points represent too short a period of observation for kinetic analysis, an effort to derive some expression of kinetics was made by deriving 30-minute:20-minute and 200-minute:100-minute plasma ratios and by calculating the 24-to-48 hour, 48-to-72-hour and 24-to-72-hour values of urinary and fecal excretion, total and bound plasma copper, and liver counts. The datum, total percent of dose accounted for, was derived by subtracting from 100% the sums of cumulative urine, stool and plasma percentage values.

The total amount of $^{64}Cu$ present in the body was calculated by subtracting urinary and fecal excretion, as percentage of dose, from 100%.

### Results

A typical plasmatic disappearance curve in a normal subject is compared with that in a carrier of Wilson's disease in the Figure. In both curves there is a phase of rapid clearance of $^{64}Cu$ from the blood, followed by a slower incorporation phase. In the case of the heterozygous carrier this latter phase is slower and the minimum is deeper and appears later; the differences between normal and carrier are significant at the 1% level for both values. The bound radioactivity roughly paralleled the total and approached it closely at 72 hours. A small percentage of radioactivity appeared as bound activity on the initial segment of the curve, but this probably represents incomplete removal of the free activity.

The results are summarized in Table I. No significant differences were noted in the urinary excretion values. The most significant differences between the two groups (normals and carriers) were the total accountability data, $t$ values being 6.0, 9.2 and 8.4, respectively, for the three intervals. The $t$ values for total retained dose also reached 5.1 and 6.3 at 48 and 72 hours, respectively.

**TABLE I** **TURNOVER OF $^{64}$CU A**

| | Urine (%D) | | | Stool (%D) | | | Plasma | |
|---|---|---|---|---|---|---|---|---|
| | 24 hr. | 48 hr. | 72 hr. | 24 hr. | 48 hr. | 72 hr. | 24 hr. | 48 |
| Normals, mean ± SD N = 18 | 0.20 | 0.26 | 0.32 | 1.9 | 5.8 | 12.2 | 6.0 | 7 |
| | ±0.08 | ±0.09 | ±0.11 | ±1.54 | ±2.97 | ±4.20 | ±2.70 | ±3 |
| Carriers, mean ± SD N = 13 | 0.18 | 0.24 | 0.33 | 0.5 | 1.6 | 3.1 | 2.2 | 2 |
| | ±0.12 | ±0.13 | ±0.23 | ±0.43 | ±0.74 | ±1.36 | ±0.87 | ±1 |
| Probable carriers N = 3 | 0.29 | 0.34 | 0.39 | 0.1 | 0.3 | 0.5 | 0.59 | 0 |
| | 0.034 | 0.40 | 0.46 | 0.0 | 0.2 | 2.0 | 0.59 | 0 |
| | 0.030 | 0.36 | 0.40 | 0.3 | 1.5 | 2.2 | 0.57 | 0 |
| Mean ± SD | 0.31 | 0.36 | 0.42 | 0.1 | 0.67 | 1.5 | 0.58 | 0 |
| | ±0.03 | ±0.03 | ±0.04 | ±0.15 | ±0.72 | ±0.89 | ±0.01 | ±0 |
| Probable normals N = 4 | 0.11 | 0.13 | 0.16 | 0.0 | 10.0 | 11.8 | 5.7 | 6 |
| | 0.24 | 0.31 | 0.33 | 1.0 | 3.8 | 10.0 | 8.4 | 10 |
| | 0.11 | 0.15 | 0.20 | 2.8 | 6.0 | 9.0 | 3.7 | 4 |
| | 0.28 | 0.53 | 0.88 | 1.7 | 5.8 | 7.5 | 3.3 | 4 |
| Mean ± SD | 0.19 | 0.28 | 0.39 | 1.38 | 6.40 | 9.58 | 1.17 | 1 |
| | ±0.09 | ±0.19 | ±0.33 | ±1.18 | ±2.60 | ±1.80 | ±0.10 | ±0 |

*Total accounted for is sum of radioactivity, as percent of dose, in urine, stool, and plasma.

Neither the 30:20 nor the 200:100 plasma ratios demonstrated significant differences between the groups. However, marked differences between stool values were found and there was no overlap between groups for the 48-hour and 72-hour values. Differences between the means of the two values were 5 and 6.3 SE, respectively. Significant differences were also noted in both total and bound plasmatic counting rates, *t*-test values being slightly higher for the former. Differences between the respective means for total plasma $^{64}$Cu were 6.6, 6.8 and 8.4 SE. Mean values of ceruloplasmin-bound radioactivity were 1.39, 1.81 and 1.94%D/liter of plasma for normal and 0.46, 0.71 and 1.04 for carriers; means were 5, 4.7 and 4.2 SE apart. Although there was considerable overlap, the differences in external counting rates over the liver were significant between the two groups.

No significant effects of the variations in specific activity of the injected $^{64}$Cu were demonstrable in these subjects.

Data on seven subjects thought not to have Wilson's disease are also presented in the Table, along with means and standard deviations. Significant differences at the 1% level were noted in all categories presented except urinary $^{64}$Cu and liver counts.

## Comment

Our data suggest that the copper trapping rates in liver are approximately the same in carriers and normals. Initial (30:20 ratios) plasmatic disappearance rates are not significantly different between the two groups. Higher liver count rates suggest that $^{64}$Cu remains in the liver longer in the carriers. Net transfer to blood and to the gut occurs more slowly in the carrier, as reflected by the slower incorporation rates, deeper and delayed minima and slower excretion rates in the carriers.

All of these points would support the concept that, although the liver traps copper at a normal rate, it discharges it at rates which are slower than normal. This suggests tests of heterozygosity. Sternlieb and coworkers[1] have developed such a test based on oral administration of $^{64}$Cu. The data presented here suggest that heterozygosity may be detected accurately after intravenous injection, thereby eliminating questions of variations in gastrointestinal absorption.

Complete separation between the two groups was obtained on the basis of the fecal excretion alone. Since this might be difficult to apply in the field, the combination of the other parameters would seem to be equally effective. Values for the total body retention of $^{64}$Cu were derived in the hope that use of whole-body radiation counters would help to distinguish the two groups without requiring assays of plasma, stool, and urine. These data and preliminary clinical tests suggest that this value for total body retention of $^{64}$Cu would be valid and has the further advantage of not being limited to the 72-hour count. Later counts may

## 'RAVENOUS INJECTION

| | Liver (cps/100 $\mu$c injected) x $10^2$ | | | Total accounted for* (%D) | | | Total in body (%D) | | |
|---|---|---|---|---|---|---|---|---|---|
| ır. | 24 hr. | 48 hr. | 72 hr. | 24 hr. | 48 hr. | 72 hr. | 24 hr. | 48 hr. | 72 hr. |
| 2 | 75.0 | 69.4 | 62.4 | 7.3 | 13.3 | 20.8 | 98.8 | 93.9 | 87.5 |
| 30 | ±23.41 | ±21.39 | ±19.22 | ±3.36 | ±3.34 | ±4.05 | ±1.55 | ±3.04 | ±4.29 |
| 4 | 79.8 | 80.5 | 77.1 | 2.9 | 4.7 | 6.7 | 99.4 | 98.2 | 96.6 |
| 44 | ±23.05 | ±23.25 | ±23.98 | ±0.92 | ±1.30 | ±2.43 | ±0.45 | ±0.69 | ±1.43 |
| 79 | 124.7 | 132.6 | 132.6 | 1.0 | 1.2 | 1.7 | 99.6 | 99.4 | 99.1 |
| 98 | 131.0 | 131.0 | 127.0 | 0.9 | 1.4 | 3.2 | 99.7 | 99.4 | 97.7 |
| .4 | 41.9 | 70.3 | 97.4 | 1.2 | 2.7 | 3.7 | 99.4 | 98.1 | 97.4 |
| 97 | 99.2 | 111.3 | 119.0 | 1.03 | 1.77 | 2.89 | 99.6 | 99.0 | 98.1 |
| .8 | ±49.68 | ±35.48 | ±18.93 | ±0.13 | ±0.82 | ±1.07 | ±0.14 | ±0.72 | ±0.91 |
| 5 | 77.4 | 54.4 | 48.5 | 5.8 | 16.4 | 18.6 | 99.9 | 89.9 | 88.0 |
| 3 | 82.3 | 79.8 | 61.7 | 9.6 | 14.1 | 21.7 | 98.8 | 95.9 | 89.7 |
| 9 | 87.9 | 85.3 | 72.3 | 6.6 | 11.0 | 15.1 | 97.1 | 93.9 | 90.8 |
| 3 | 70.4 | 63.6 | 56.9 | 5.3 | 10.6 | 13.2 | 98.0 | 93.7 | 91.6 |
| .7 | 79.5 | 70.8 | 59.9 | 6.84 | 13.03 | 17.13 | 98.4 | 93.3 | 90.0 |
| 01 | ± 7.44 | ±14.40 | ± 9.83 | ±1.94 | ±2.75 | ±3.75 | ±1.18 | ±2.51 | ±1.55 |

be more decisive in their separation, but we have too few data to make a report at this time.

Application of discriminant functions based on the data derived from known carriers and normals divides the seven siblings tested into two clearly defined groups —three carriers and four normals. Unfortunately, we have not had the opportunity of performing similar tests in their offspring in an effort to determine the zygosity of these subjects.

The initial rapid incorporation rates and the overall low total accountability values (maximum, only 30%) suggest that the copper is being incorporated rapidly up to a point and is being distributed rapidly through the body, but the relatively unchanging liver counts observed throughout the course of study suggest that some significant fraction of the liver activity stays there, possibly in some special pool within the liver, and that this pool is somewhat larger in the carrier than it is in the normal.

Our findings do not suggest any mechanism to explain these data, but trapping rates are probably related to the binding capacity of Morell and coworkers'[3] CuLP.

### Summary

Carriers of Wilson's disease seem to trap intravenously administered copper in their livers at rates indistinguishable from those observed in normal subjects, but the discharge rates into plasma and stool are lower. These rates may be used as a test to separate the two groups. In the future, probably the easiest way to separate the two groups will be by whole-body counting or by determining the percentage of dose circulating at 72 hours after intravenous injection of $^{64}$Cu.

## REFERENCES

1. Sternlieb, I.; Morell, A. G.; Bauer, C. D.; Combes, B.; De Bobes-Sternberg, S. and Scheinberg, I. H.: Detection of the heterozygous carrier of the Wilson's disease gene. *J. clin. Invest.* **40**:707-715, 1961.

2. Tauxe, W. N.; Goldstein, N. P.; Randall, R. V. and Gross, J. B.: Radiocopper studies in patients with Wilson's disease and their relatives. *Amer. J. Med.* **41**:375-380, 1966.

3. Morell, A. G.; Shapiro, J. R. and Scheinberg, I. H.: Copper binding protein from human liver. In Walshe, J. M. and Cumings, J. N.: *Wilson's disease: some current concepts.* Springfield, Illinois, Charles C Thomas, Publisher, pp. 36-42, 1961.

4. Osborn, S. B. and Walshe, J. M.: Copper uptake by the liver: study of a Wilson's disease family. In Walshe, J. M. and Cumings, J. N.: *Wilson's disease: some current concepts.* Springfield, Illinois, Charles C Thomas, Publisher, pp. 141-150, 1961.

5. Retzlaff, J. A.: Red cell volume, plasma volume, and lean body mass in healthy men and women: the development of a blood volume standard. Thesis, Graduate School, University of Minnesota, 1963.

# Comparative Neuropathologic Study of Wilson's Disease and Other Types of Hepatocerebral Disease

Hirotsugu Shiraki, M.D.*

Autopsied cases of Wilson's disease, in Japan, were compared with those of other types of hepatocerebral disease, i.e., Inose, pseudoulegyric and ischemic disorders. In addition to specific metabolic abnormalities, circulatory disturbances appear to play an etiologic role in each disease entity.

## Introduction

Wilson's disease belongs to the category of hepatocerebral diseases with interrelated pathology in both the central nervous system and liver. In this paper, the characteristics of Wilson's disease are compared with those of other types of hepatocerebral disease, since considerable knowledge of both disease groups, together with the central nervous system lesions in hepatic failure and experimental hyperammoniemia, has recently been accumulated. The following questions arise: what are the common pathomorphologic characteristics in each disease entity and how can Wilson's disease be differentiated from other types of hepatocerebral disease?

## Material

The material comprises 26 cases of hepatocerebral disease consisting of nine Inose; eight pseudoulegyric; and nine ischemic. In addition, 15 cases of Wilson's disease, of which 11 are hepatocerebral and four are abdominal; 98 cases of hepatic failure and 96 controls have been studied.

Since the three types of hepatocerebral disease, i.e., Inose, pseudoulegyric and ischemic, are not familiar to Western scientists, their clinico-pathologic features will be described in some detail.

## Findings

### *Inose Type of Hepatocerebral Disease (Hepatic Failure and Experimental Hyperammoniemia)*

In 1950 Inose[1] demonstrated the presence of carmine-positive granules in the enlarged astrocytic nuclei of cases of hepatocerebral degeneration. Despite the absence of those granules in the brains of Wilson's disease patients, he initially considered this a special type or variant of Wilson's disease. Subsequently, extensive work of this type has been carried out by Inose *et al*,[2-4] Shiraki *et al*,[5-7] and others, as a result of which the disease can be clearly differentiated pathologically from Wilson's disease. It is probable, we believe, that a great majority of the cases in the Western literature of "sporadic Wilson's disease" or Wilsonismus,[8] portal-system encephalopathies,[9] chronic portohepatic encephalopathies,[10] or acquired (non-Wilsonian) type of chronic hepatocerebral degeneration,[11] belong to this same category of disease and, thus, could better be called "Inose type."

*Clinical features.* Middle-aged individuals of 40 to 61 years with 51 as the average age of onset, sporadically developed the disease which had a duration of nine months to 16 years. Heredity apparently played no role; a previous history of liver disturbances was fairly common. In one case Banti's syndrome with splenectomy and an Eck fistula was noted seven years prior to the onset of the present illness.

From the initial to the terminal stage there were episodes of disturbed consciousness accompanied by neurologic deficits, such as tremor, dysphagia, dysarthria, nystagmus, hypotonia, impaired voluntary movements, hemiplegia, tic-like or choreoid hyperkinesia, hyperreflexia or hypersalivation. Those neurologic deficits, as a rule, disappeared with the termination of the bouts of disturbed consciousness. In some instances personality changes or slight dementia became manifest and persisted, particularly late in the illness.

Severe impairment of liver functions, such as ascites, edema, jaundice, caput medusae, hepatosplenomegaly or hemorrhagic diatheses as well as abnormal liver function tests were observed. Thrombus formation in the portal vein or in its branches and collateral circulation

*Professor of Neuropathology; Division of Neuropathology, Institute of Brain Research, School of Medicine, University of Tokyo, Japan.

were frequently encountered. No Kayser-Fleischer corneal rings were seen in any of the patients who were subjected to slit-lamp examinations.

Triphasic waves in electroencephalograms, aminoaciduria, increased amino acids in the spinal fluid or hyperammoniemia were present in the cases examined. Hypercupriuria was never found.

*Pathologic features.* Alzheimer type II glial nuclei were ubiquitously distributed in both cortices and subcortical grey matters (Fig. 1, A and G), while Alzheimer type I glial nuclei were consistently absent. Opalski cells were seen in only one case. A large number of carmine-positive granules of a glycogen nature were seen in the molecular layer, periadventitial spaces, neuropil, astrocytic nuclei and cytoplasmic processes, perineuronal spaces, and cytoplasm and nuclei of nerve cells (Fig. 1, B, C and D). Both Alzheimer type II glial nuclei and carmine-positive granules on the other hand were also visible in the 98 cases of different hepatic failure, with or without disturbed consciousness.[12-14] So these may represent nonspecific findings in the central nervous system due to liver damage of any cause. In contrast, experimentally-induced hyperammoniemia, by peroral and intraperitoneal administrations of $NH_4Cl$, and urease, respectively, in rats caused an enlargement of astrocytic nuclei in which no excess accumulation of glycogen granules (which are carmine-positive) occurred.[15]

Irregular-shaped, laminarly- or pseudolaminarly-distributed focal cortical necrosis (Fig. 1, F and G); spongy tissue disruption (Fig. 1E); deteriorated foci in the thalamus, in one case lateral geniculate body and fornix (Fig. 1K); and dissemination of ischemic nerve cells (Fig. 1A) were observed. Similar necrotic lesions in the cortices, diencephalon and brain stem were produced in dogs with intravenously-injected ammonium salt[16] (Fig. 2). Central pontine myelinolysis, which was first described by Adams *et al*[17] developed in three cases (Fig. 1J). The schematic distribution of the abovementioned foci was illustrated in Figure 1L.

Postnecrotic liver cirrhosis or fibrosis with intranuclear glycogen granules of hepatic cells (Fig. 1H), were always seen, and intra- and/or extrahepatic shunts due to thrombi of the portal vein, were sometimes present (Fig. 1I). No granules were found with the aid of copper stains and this negative finding was confirmed in one patient in whom tissue copper concentration was found to be in a normal range by using neutron activation analysis.

#### Pseudoulegyric Type of Hepatocerebral Disease

In 1962 and 1963 Shiraki and his associates[6,18,19] first described the pseudoulegyric type of hepatocerebral disease which, as far as known to us, has never been reported in Western literature. Although this disease shares many common features with the Inose type, it seemed differentiable from the latter on both clinical and pathologic grounds.

*Clinical features.* The disease sporadically occurred, chiefly in males about 20-40 years of age, with 28 as the average age. Males to females were seven to one. Duration of the illness was from eight months to six years.

During the initial stage episodes of disturbed consciousness and neurologic deficits similar to those of patients with the Inose type occurred and became persistent at the intermediate stage. At the terminal stage the patients developed an apallic syndrome or akinetic mutism as first described by Kretschmer[20] and Cairns,[21] respectively. The patients could not change their postures which were artificially induced and could not speak spontaneously except for occasional shouting or crying. Swallowing, urination and defecation were not disturbed, but they never responded adequately to external stimuli and could only follow intense light or noise with their eyes. They slept at night and opened their eyes in the daytime. They developed various primitive reflexes and there was blocking of highly integrated psychic functions, as expected. Progressive cachexia, epileptic convulsions or myoclonic jerks were observed during the course of illness. Corneal Kayser-Fleischer rings were never seen. Normal results were

## ABOUT THE AUTHOR

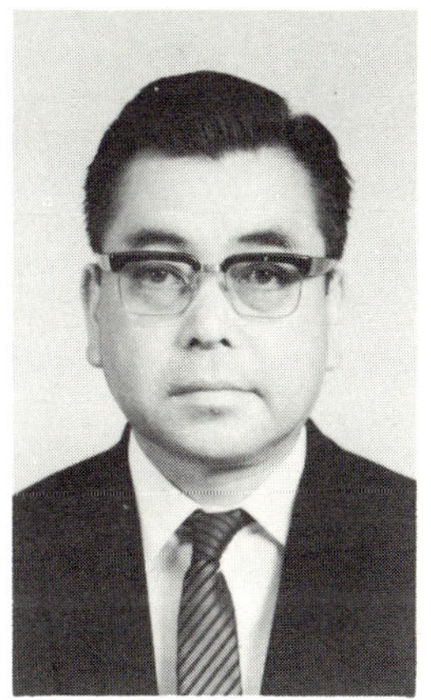

Dr. Hirotsugu Shiraki was born in Japan in 1917, received his medical degree from the University of Tokyo School of Medicine in 1941 and was drafted into the Japanese Navy as Super-Lieutenant Medical Officer in 1942. He is at present Professor of Neuropathology, Division of Neuropathology, Institute of Brain Research, School of Medicine, University of Tokyo, Japan.

Doctor Shiraki has held many positions including President and General Secretary of the Japanese Society of Neuropathology, Member of the Board of Directors of the Japanese Society of Neurology and the Japanese Society of Neurology and Psychiatry, Council of the Japanese Society of Neurosurgery and Member of a Special Committee of the South Pole, Science Council of Japan. His international positions are Vice President of the International Society of Neuropathology, Member of the Editorial Board of Acta Neuropathologica, Member of the Problem Commission of Neuropathology and Multiple Sclerosis Research Committee, World Federation of Neurology, Member of the International Brain Research Organization, Honorary Member of the French Association of Neurology. He is the author of many scientific papers.

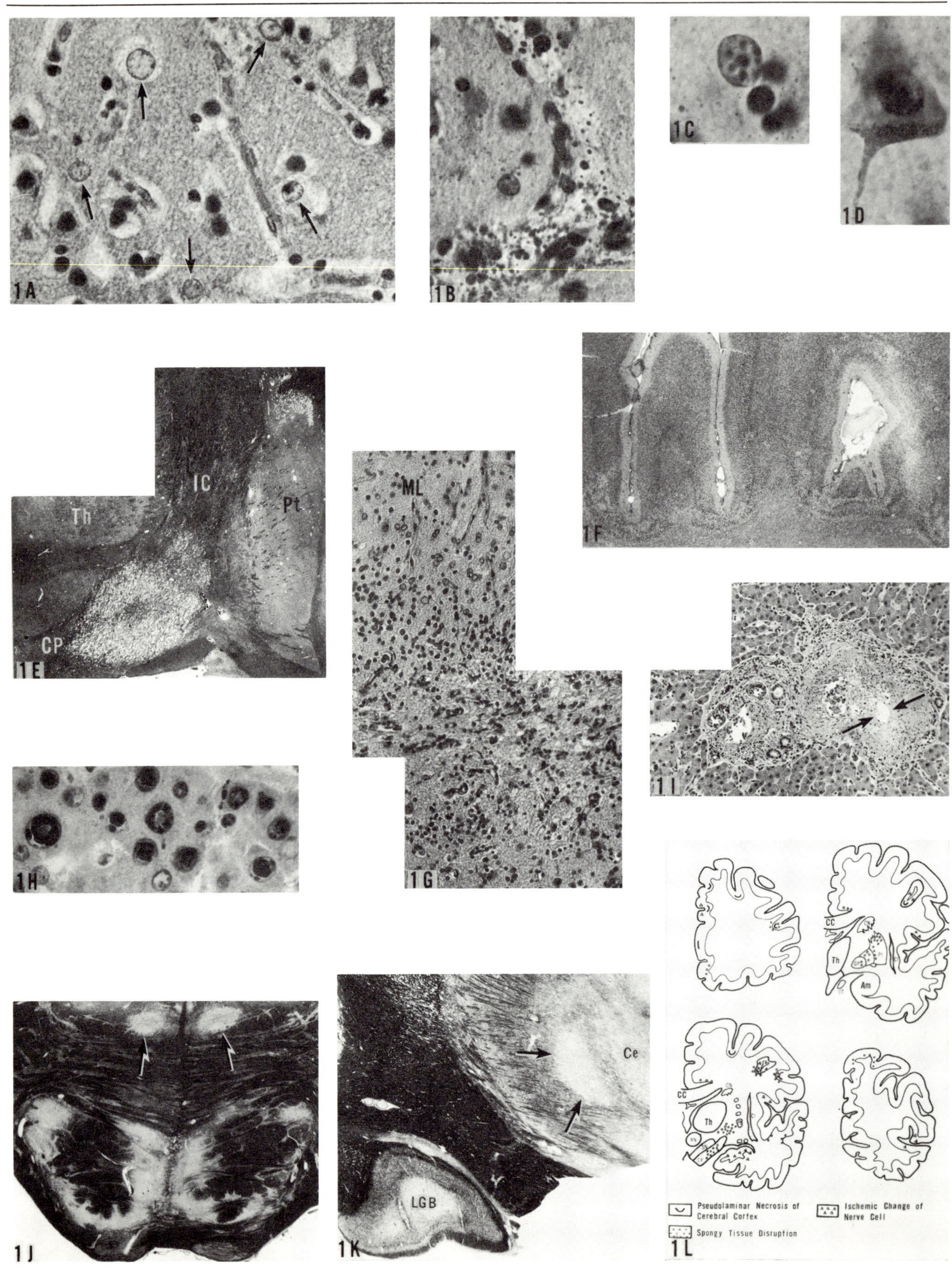
1A
1B
1C
1D
IC
Th
Pt
CP
1E
ML
1F
1G
1H
1I
CC
Th
Am
CC
Th
Ce
LGB
1J
1K
Pseudolaminar Necrosis of Cerebral Cortex
Ischemic Change of Nerve Cell
Spongy Tissue Disruption
1L

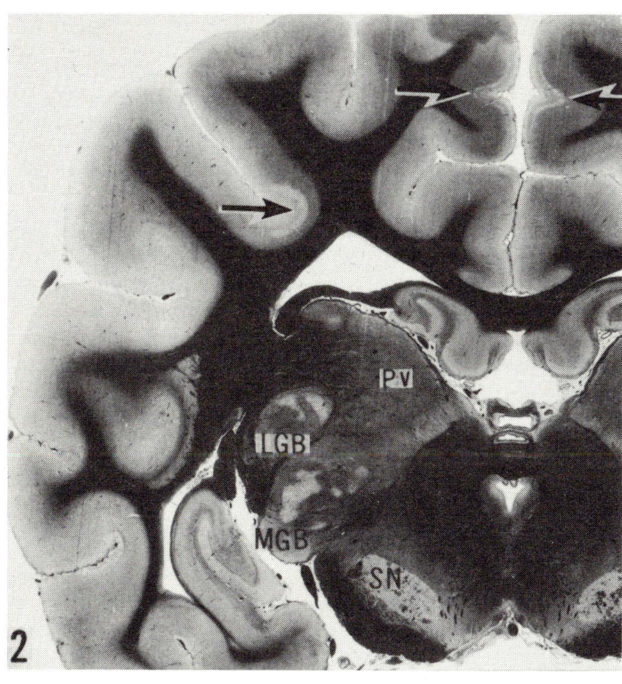


Fig. 2. **Experimental ammonium intoxication in dogs** (8 intravenous injections of 35 to 170 cc of ammonium phosphate by Ishii[16]). Coronal section through the posterior commissure. Variably sized, sharply demarcated, multiple or coalescent demyelinated foci in the substantia nigra (SN), medial and lateral geniculate bodies (MGB and LGB) and dorsal pulvinar (Pv). Hemorrhages predominate in the substantia nigra. Disintegration in a laminar fashion of the cortical myeloarchitecture predominant from the depth of the sulci (**arrows**). x 5.3. (Weil myelin.)

obtained in all those patients in whom urinary copper determinations were made.

There was minimal or slight disturbance of liver function, and portal hypertension was never present, constituting an important difference from the Inose type. Triphasic waves in electroencephalograms, hyperammoniemia or amino-aciduria were observed in the cases examined; hypercupriuria was never noted.

*Pathologic features.* Widespread, confluent necrosis and severe ulegyric atrophy involving both cortices and white matter were far more pronounced than in the Inose type, and predominated in the temporal, insular, frontal and lateral convexity of occipital gyri (Fig. 3, A, B, C and E). Both cleaning and organization processes, however, were inactive or even absent, as in the Inose type, and, thus, the name of "pseudoulegyric" could be derived from this observation. Spongy degeneration also involved the adjacent subcortical white matter, putamen and globus pallidus (Fig. 3E).

Alzheimer type II glial nuclei and glycogen granule accumulation in grey matter were essentially similar to those in the Inose type (Fig. 3, G and H). Ischemia, homogeneous appearance, vacuolization and edema of nerve cells suggested circulatory disturbance (Fig. 3, D, G, and I). The schematic distribution pattern of such foci is illustrated in Figure 3A. Generally speaking, ulegyric cortical atrophy, pseudolaminar cortical necrosis, spongy degeneration and diffuse demyelination of white matter were pronounced in the regions of ontogenetically recent origin and ischemic nerve cells and cortical deterioration of acute circulatory disturbance, in those of older origin. Minimal demyelination in the median rhaphae of the basis pontis was seen in one case.

Severe fatty infiltration of the liver occurred at the subacute stage and fatty cirrhosis or fibrosis subsequently (Fig. 3F). No copper-positive granules were found when staining methods were used. Extrahepatic shunts were never seen, and the liver in all other respects was similar pathologically to the Inose type.

Fig. 1. **Inose type of hepatocerebral disease.** A, E, H, I and L (56-year-old female, four years' duration). B (62-year-old male, one year and six months' duration). C (58-year-old female, one year duration). D (46-year-old male, one year and five months' duration). F, G, J and K (52-year-old female, two years' and six months' duration). **A** Third layer of the temporal cortex. Alzheimer type II glial nuclei (**arrows**) and ischemic shrunken nerve cells with dilated perineuronal space. x 530. **B** Third layer of the frontal cortex. Accumulation of tiny carmine-positive granules in the dilated periadventitial space of precapillary and the cytoplasmic processes of astrocytes. x 510. **C** Third layer of the occipital cortex. Multiple, coarse carmine-positive granules in the enlarged astrocytic nucleus and tiny ones in the adjacent parenchyma. x 1100. **D** Third layer of the frontal cortex. Tiny carmine-positive granules in the cytoplasm and axonal dendrite of a pyramidal cell, the nucleus of which also contains similar granules. x 900. **E** Coarse spongy tissue disruption in the dorsal putamen (Pt) and internal capsule (IC) down to the cerebral peduncle (CP). Th: thalamus. x 3.0. **F** Occipital gyri. Irregular, pseudolaminar, circumscribed or coalescent cortical necrosis predominant at the depth of the sulci. x 4.9. **G** Magnified area in F. Nerve cell disintegration with a few gitter cells and prominent vascular networks predominantly in the upper third layer. Numbers of Alzheimer type II glial nuclei in the molecular layer (ML). x 606. **H** Liver. Variably sized, multiple or single, carmine-positive granules in the enlarged nuclei of hepatic cells. x 475. **I** Liver. Organized thrombus with recanalization (**arrows**) in branch of portal vein. x 90. **J** Sharply-demarcated symmetrical demyelination restricted to the pontine basis, sparing the superior pontine fibres and the deeper regions of pyramidal tract. Smaller, though similar demyelination in the tegmentum (**arrows**). x 2.8. **K** Sharply demarcated demyelination in the lateral geniculate body (LGB) and the ventrolateral thalamic nucleus (**arrows**). Ce: centromedian. x 6.0. **L** Circumscribed, pseudolaminar cortical necrosis predominant at the depth of the sulci, spongy state in the subcortical white matter, cortex and basal ganglia, and dissemination of ischemic nerve cells in the cortex. (**A, E and I**, H.E.; **B, C, D and H**, Best carmine. **F and G**, Thionine. **J and K**, Woelcke myelin.)

### Ischemic Type of Hepatocerebral Disease

In 1964 Ando *et al*[22] first described one autopsy case in which heredity appeared to play a role, and in which pronounced ischemic nerve-cell changes, acute circulatory disturbances and Wilson pseudosclerosis were present. In 1966 Shiraki[23] summarized nine similar cases, and called them an ischemic type of hepatocerebral disease. No similar autopsy case has been reported in the Western literature.

*Clinical features.* The disease occurred sporadically in patients of 10 months to 53 years of age. Its duration was from four days to three years; generally, however, from three to six months. Heredity did not seem to play a role except for the case of Ando, *et al.*[22] It is of interest that in three patients hypophyseal or idiopathic dwarfism was present.

Bouts of disturbed consciousness, abnormal behavior and terminal coma were consistently observed; the apalic syndrome or myoclonic jerks were rare.

Liver function was minimally or slightly disturbed, resembling the situation in the pseudoulegyric type. Triphasic waves in electroencephalograms or hyperammoniemia were present in the cases examined.

*Pathologic features.* There were more ischemic and less of homogenous or edematous nerve cell changes. (Fig. 4, B and C). No remarkable damage of white matter occurred, and there was only occasional cortical necrosis or pallor (Fig. 4D). Such foci were almost symmetrically spread in both hemispheres and predominated in the cingulate, insular and temporal cortices (Fig. 4A). Fatty infiltration or fibrosis of liver (Fig. 4, F and G), was similar to those of the pseudoulegyric type. Even in the chronic case with a duration of three years, as well as in the infantile one with onset at ten months of age and a three months' duration, the hepatic changes were minor, resembling somewhat the cerebral type of Wilson's disease.

The ubiquitous distribution of Alzheimer type II glial nuclei (Fig. 4C), accumulation of glycogen granules (Fig. 4E) and spongy degeneration with inactive cleaning and organization processes were the same as in both Inose and pseudoulegyric types.

### Relationship of the Three Types of Hepatocerebral Disease to Hepatic Failures

The three types of hepatocerebral disease, Inose, pseudoulegyric and ischemic, had in common the following histopathologic characteristics: ubiquitous distribution of Alzheimer type II glial nuclei, abnormal accumulations of glycogen granules, spongy degeneration, absence of Alzheimer type I glial nuclei copper granules in liver, and inactive cleaning and organization processes. These findings, on the other hand, were also visible in the brains of patients with hepatic failure, and, thus, may indicate hepatogenic origin in which hyperammoniemia may play a role in the development of enlarged astrocytic nuclei (Fig. 7).

Clinico-pathologically, each type, however, had its own characteristics. For example,[12] in the pseudoulegyric type, the characteristic distribution pattern of the severest necrosis and the atrophy of both cortices and white matter coincided well with the severe neuropsychic deterioration, while ischemic nerve cells were visible in the mild foci. In the ischemic type, on the other hand, despite a similar distribution pattern of ischemic nerve cells, cortical necrosis was less severe and white matter was not affected. Minimal to slight impairment of liver function with fatty infiltration, fatty cirrhosis or fibrosis was common in both types, indicating a close relationship between the two, although the duration and age distribution of the patients varied conspicuously. In the ischemic type there was occasional dwarfism or retarded body development; these were absent in the pseudoulegyric type. In the Inose type, cortical lesions were mild and circumscribed, and liver function was severely disturbed and the patients' middle age contrasted with the youth of the males with the pseudoulegyric type.

### Wilson's Disease

In the 11 Japanese cases of hepatocerebral type of Wilson's disease the clinico-epidemiologic features were essentially the same as those in Caucasians.[7] Histopathologically, cavitary necrosis of the putamen developed in the seven cases in which both globus pallidus and caudate nucleus were less severely involved and occasionally were combined with cortical lesions, chiefly vascular, spongy degeneration and nerve cell disintegration. The latter findings were restricted, whether unilateral or bilateral, to the first and second frontal cortices and subcortical white matter, and were not visible in any of the four cases with simple atrophy of the putamen. Central pontine myelinolysis, with or without petechiae, was observed in three cases (Fig. 5A), while amyotrophic lateral sclerosis-like spinal lesions without gliosis, were seen in one case (Fig. 5B). In all cases, a few Alzheimer type I glial nuclei, a fair number of Opalski cells, ubiquitous distribution of Alzheimer type II glial nuclei, and spongy degeneration were noted. Intranuclear glycogen granules in astrocytes were scanty, however. Glial shrubberies in the cerebellar molecular layer (Fig. 5C), disintegrated Sommer's sector of Ammon's horn (Fig. 5D) and other cortical deterioration, indicating circulatory disturbances, were occasionally seen. Typical Wilson's cirrhosis, with intracytoplasmic copper granules and intranuclear glycogen granules, of hepatic cells, was pronounced. Activation analysis revealed an increased copper content in both grey and white matter, and in the liver.[5]

In the four cases of "abdominal" Wilson's disease[7] in Japanese children aged seven to nine with a positive family history, severe liver disturbance, characterized by epigastric pain, edema, ascites, jaundice, hepatomegaly or terminal coma; and decreased serum ceruloplasmin, hypercupriuria or Kayser-Fleischer corneal rings were noted. There was an excess proliferation of Glisson's sheaths and copper granules of hepatic cells were demonstrated histochemically (Fig. 6A). Ubiqui-

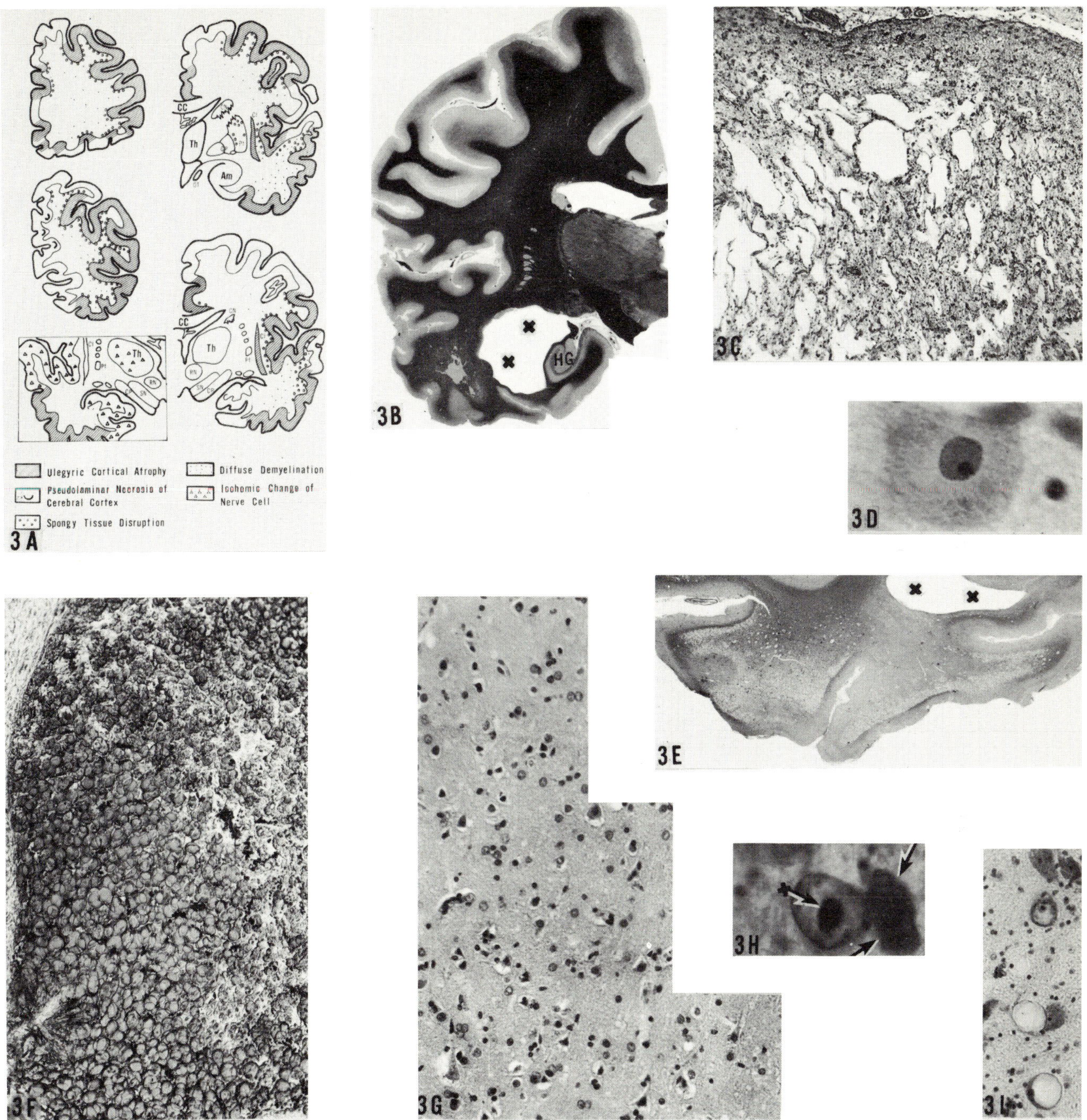


Fig. 3. **Pseudoulegyric type of hepatocerebral disease.** A, E, F and G (31-year-old male, eight months' duration). B, D and I (22-year-old male, two years' and eight months' duration). C (28-year-old male, six years' and seven months' duration). H (20-year-old male, one year and eight months' duration). A See text. B Severe cortical atrophy and demyelination of the white matter predominant in the temporal and insular gyri, sparing the hippocampal gyrus (HG). Conspicuously-dilated inferior horn of the lateral ventricle (**crosses**). x 1.0. C Conspicuous cystic softening of cortex and white matter of the temporal tip. x 115. D Putamen. Homogeneous change of large nerve cell with hyperchromasia at periphery of nucleus. x 1000. E Cortical atrophy and softening of the white matter predominant in the 2nd and 3rd temporal gyri, with conspicuous spongy state in the subcortical white matter. Crosses indicate the inferior horn of lateral ventricle. x 2.0. F Liver. Conspicuous fatty infiltration in the cytoplasm of all hepatic cells. x 82. G Parietal cortex. Dissemination of ischemic, shrunken nerve cells with eosinophilic cytoplasm and dilated perineuronal space, and Alzheimer type II glial nuclei. x 155. H Occipital cortex. One astrocytic nucleus filled with carmine-positive granules (**arrow**), and adjacent nucleus one with coarse central granule (**arrow with cross**). x 1000. I Abducens nucleus. Large single vacuole in the cytoplasm of nerve cell with eccentric nucleus. x 190. (B, Woelcke myelin; C, E and G, H.E.; D and I, Thionine; F, Sudan III; H, Best carmine.)

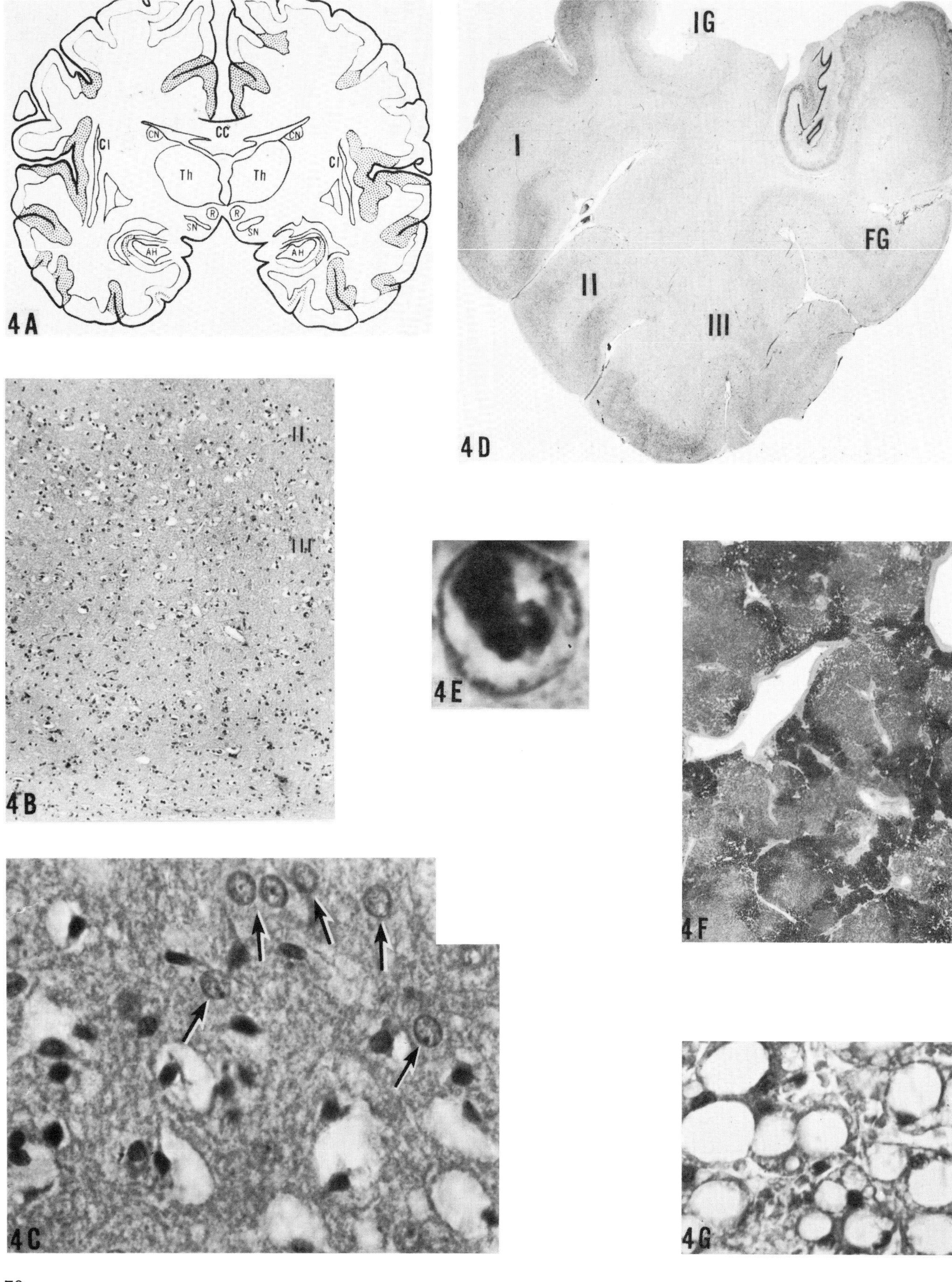
CC
CN
CN
Cl
Cl
Th
Th
R
R
SN
SN
AH
AH
4A
IG
I
II
III
FG
4D
II
III
4B
4E
4F
4C
4G

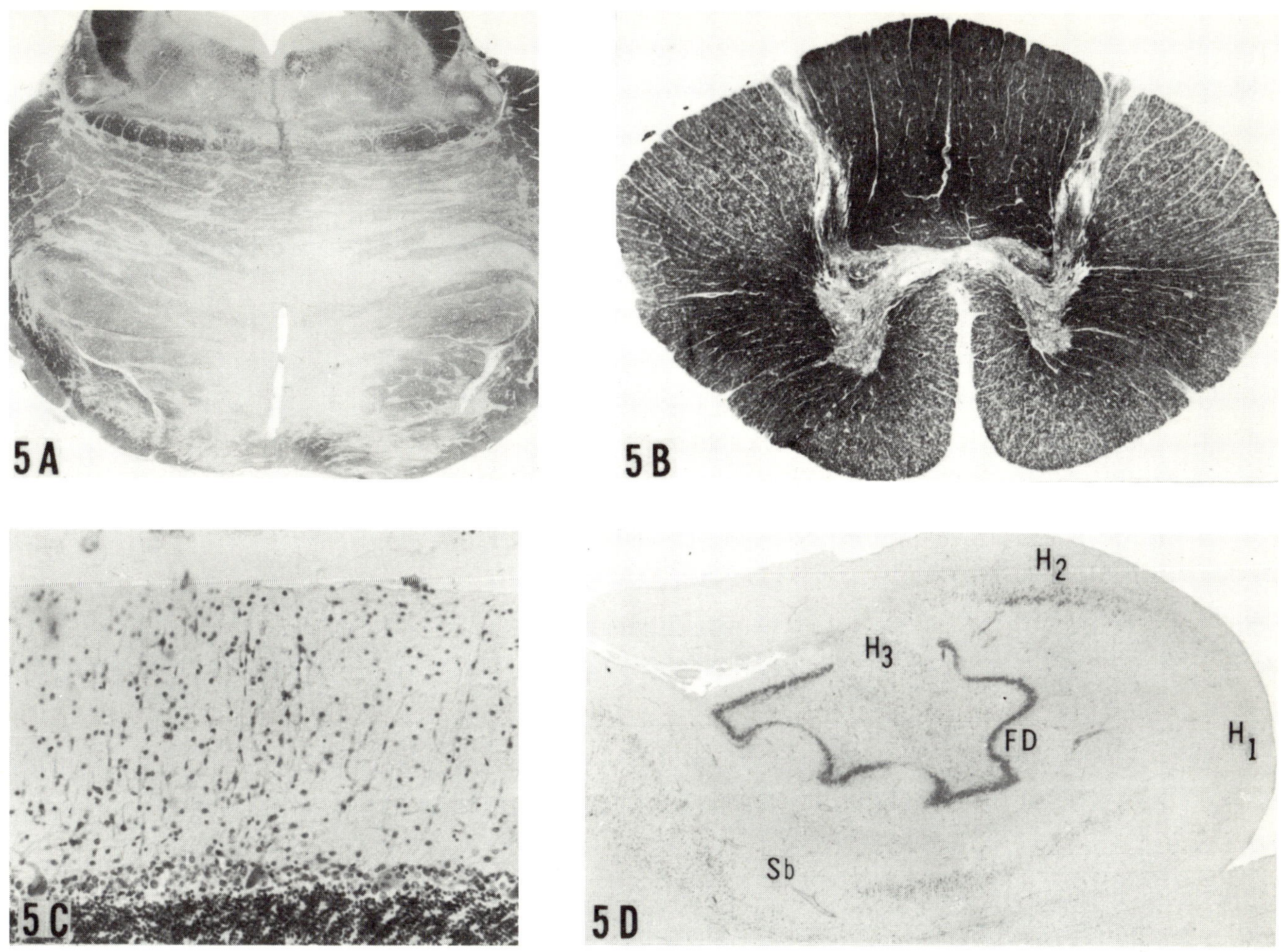


Fig. 5. **Hepatocerebral type of Wilson's disease.** A (14-year-old male, 10 months' duration). B (15-year-old male, two years' and four months' duration). C (22-year-old female, two years' and eight months' duration). D (15-year-old female, two years' and 11 months' duration). A Poorly defined, wing-like distribution of bilateral, symmetrical demyelination from the median raphe to the pontine basis, to some extent, spreading in the tegmentum as well. x 3.6. B Thoracic cord. Symmetrical demyelination bilaterally in the anterior and lateral columns. x 9.0. C Glial shrubs in the cerebellar molecular layer and preserved Purkinje cells with proliferated Bergman's glial nuclei. x 189. D Ammon's horn. Nerve cell disintegration predominant in the $H_1$ and $H_3$ areas, and subiculum (Sb), while absent in the $H_2$ area and fascia dentata (FD). x 8.4. (A and B, Woelcke myelin; C and D, Thionine.)

Fig. 4. **Ischemic type of hepatocerebral disease.** A-C (28-year-old male, three months' duration). D-G (30-year-old male, 2.5 months' duration). A Cortical foci **(dotted area)** with symmetrical, bilateral distribution in the temporal, insular and cingulate gyri, and Sommers sector of Ammon's horn (AH), and predominant at the depth of the sulci. CC: corpus callosum. Cl: claustrum. R: red nucleus. SN: substantia nigra. CN: caudate nucleus. Th: thalamus. B Ischemic, shrunken nerve cells predominant in the 2nd (II) and upper 3rd (III) layers of temporal cortex. x 125. C Magnified 3rd layer in B. Conspicuously shrunken nerve cells with darkly-stained nuclei, eosinophilic cytoplasm and dilated perineuronal spaces, sieve-like spongy tissue and Alzheimer type II glial nuclei **(arrows)**. x 710. D Temporal lobe. Cortical foci distributed in the 1st (I), 2nd (II) and 3rd (III) temporal, fusiform (FG) and insular (IG) gyri, and predominant at the depth of the sulci. x 2.8. E Cerebral cortex. Centrally-located, irregular coalescent, carmine-positive granules in Alzheimer type II glial nucleus with chromatin margination. x 2580. F Liver. Moderate fatty infiltration in several acini. x 10.3. G Magnified area in F. Vacuoles in the cytoplasm of hepatic cells corresponding to presence of fat granules. x 568. (B, C and G, H.E.; D, Thionine; E, Best carmine; F, Sudan III.)

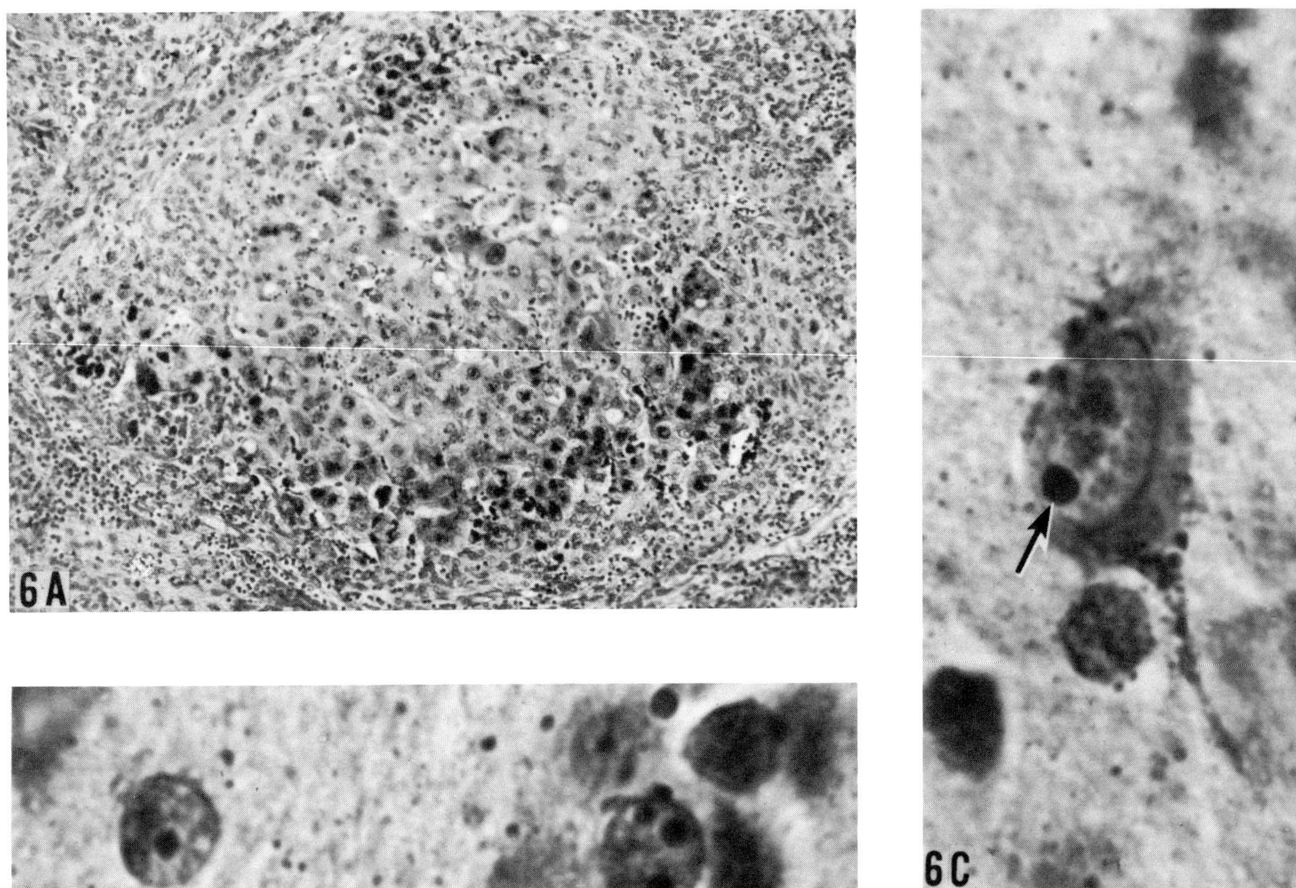


Fig. 6. **Abdominal type of Wilson's disease** (6-year-old male, 2.5 months' duration). A Liver. Copper granules in the cytoplasm of hepatic cells particularly at the periphery of the acinus. x 134. B Third layer of the occipital cortex. Multiple, tiny carmine-positive granules in the enlarged astrocytic nuclei and in the parenchyma. x 2325. C Third layer of the occipital cortex. Tiny carmine-positive granules in the cytoplasm and dendrites of the nerve cell as well as perineuronally. A larger granule is in the nucleus (arrow). x 2100. (A, Rhodanine; B and C, Best carmine.)

tous distribution of enlarged astrocytic nuclei and glycogen granules, on the other hand, were found in these brains (Fig. 6, B and C). Glycogen granules in the cortices were abundant, in contrast to their absence, or scanty distribution in the hepatocerebral type mentioned above.

It now seems obvious that three types of hepatocerebral disease, i.e., Inose, pseudoulegyric and ischemic, share such pathomorphologic characteristics as ubiquitous distribution of Alzheimer type II glial nuclei, abnormal accumulations of glycogen granules, spongy degeneration and inactive cleaning and organization processes (Fig. 7).

The hepatocerebral type of Wilson's disease, on the other hand, though also characterized by ubiquitously distributed Alzheimer type II glial nuclei, spongy degeneration, and inactive cleaning and organization processes, had a distribution of astrocytic glycogen granules which were extremely scanty. The latter, however, were conspicuously abundant in the brains of patients dying of "abdominal" Wilson's disease. Thus, abnormal metabolism of glycogen or carbohydrates, in each disease entity, should be investigated more carefully in the future.

The combination of Alzheimer type I glial nuclei, Opalski cells, a necrotizing process in the putamen and in certain frontal gyri, and copper granules in liver is specific and more or less characteristic of Wilson's disease. These findings differentiate it from other types of hepatocerebral disease. However, in some instances Wilson's disease develops without gyral lesions and with simple atrophy of the putamen without necrosis. A question then may arise as to whether such a difference in development could be related to abnormal copper or amino acid metabolism, hyperammoniemia, or other processes.

It is also true that both disease groups are more or less related through hepatic failure and occasional central pontine myelinolysis (Fig. 7).

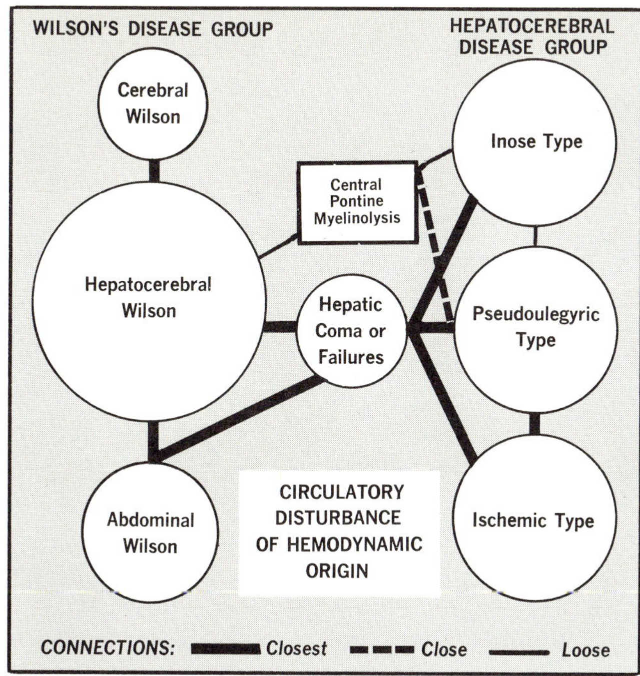


Fig. 7. Relationship of Wilson's and hepatocerebral disease groups, hepatic coma and central pontine myelinolysis, to circulatory disturbance of hemodynamic origin. See text.

## REFERENCES


1. Inose, T.: Contribution to pathology of extrapyramidal diseases. A specific form of hepatocerebral degeneration. *Psychiat. Neurol. jap.* **51**:245-271, 1950 (Jap. ed.).

2. Inose, T.: Hepatocerebral degeneration. A special type. *J. Neuropath. exp. Neurol.* **11**:401-408, 1952.

3. Inose, T.; Ichikawa Y. and Nomura, H.: Eine histochemische Studie bei den hepatocerebralen Degenerationen und bei Leberkrankheiten (Glykogenbefund). *Arch. Psychiat. Nervenkr.* **200**:509-519, 1960.

4. Inose, T.: Die Pathologie des extrapyramidalen Systems. *Rec. Adv. Res. Nerv. Syst.* **5**:57-71, 1960 (Jap. ed.).

5. Shiraki, H. and Yamamoto, T.: Histochemical aspects of hepatocerebral diseases with especial reference to inclusion bodies. *Rec. Adv. Res. Nerv. Syst.* **5**:73-101, 1960 (Jap. ed.).

6. Oda, M.: Ein Beitrag zu den klinischen und histopathologischen Problemen über die hepatocerebralen Erkrankungen, insbesondere über den "Pseudoulegyrie-Typ." *Psychiat. Neurol. jap.* **66**:892-931, 1964 (Jap. ed.).

7. Shiraki, H. and Oda, M.: Neuropathology of hepatocerebral disease with emphasis upon comparative studies. In *Neuropathology,* Vol I, J. Minckler (ed.). McGraw-Hill, New York, January, 1968.

8. Erbslöh, F.: Das Zentralnervensystem bei Leberkrankheiten. Hdb. d. Spez. Pathol. Anatomie u. Histologie. Springer, Berlin, Vol. XIII/2B, pp. 1645-1698, 1958.

9. Sherlock, S.; Summerskill, W. H. J.; White, L. P. and Phear, E. A.: Portal-systemic encephalopathy – Neurological complications of liver disease. *Lancet,* **ii**:453-457, 1954.

10. Baltzan, M. A.; Olszewski, J. and Zervas, N.: Chronic portohepatic encephalopathy. *J. Neuropath. exp. Neurol.* **16**:410-421, 1957.

11. Victor, M.; Adams R. D. and Cole, M.: The acquired (non-Wilsonian) type of chronic hepatocerebral degeneration. *Medicine (Baltimore)* **44**:345-396, 1965.

12. Harada, K.: Zur Histopatholgie des Gehirns bei Leberkrankheiten. *Brain and Nerve,* **13**:514-524, 1961 (Jap. ed.).

13. Oda, M. and Shiraki, H.: Uber die karmin-positiven Substanzen im zentralen Nervensystem. Ein Beitrag zue den Problemen der Glykogen-Stoffwechselstörung bei den hepatocerebralen Erkrankungen. *Adv. Neurol. Sci.* **4**:679-694, 1965 (Jap. ed.).

14. Stadler, H.: Histopathologische Untersuchungen zur Frage der Beziehung zwischen Leber- und Gehirnveränderungen. *Z. ges. Neurol. Psychiat.* **154**:626-657, 1936.

15. Suwa, N. and Saso, S.: Histochemical studies of glial nuclei in experimental ammoniemia of rats. *Adv. Neurol. Sci.* **4**:700-703, 1965 (Jap. ed.).

16. Ishii, T.: Neuropathological study of ammonia poisoning in dogs, with reference to pathogenesis of hepatocerebral disease (Inose type). *Psychiat. Neurol. jap.* **65**:667-685, 1963 (Jap. ed.).

17. Adams, R. D.; Victor, M. and Mancall, E. L.: Central pontine myelinolysis a hitherto undescribed disease occurring in alcoholic and malnourished patients. A. M. A. *Arch. Neurol. Psychiat.* **81**:154-172, 1959.

18. Shiraki, H.; Yamamoto, T.; Yamada, K. and Shikata, T.: An autopsied case of the "pseudoulegyria type" of the hepatocerebral disease. *Psychiat. Neurol. jap.* **64**:305-318, 1962 (Jap. ed.).

19. Takahashi, Y.; Oda, M. and Shiraki, H.: An autopsy case of the "pseudoulegyria type" of the hepatocerebral disease with a subacute clinical course. *Psychiat. Neurol. jap.* **65**:513-531, 1963 (Jap. ed.).

20. Kretschmer, E.: Das appalische Syndrom. *Z. ges. Neurol. Psychiat.* **169**:576-579, 1940.

21. Cairns, H.; Oldried, R. C.; Pennybacker, J. B. and Whitteridge, D.: Akinetic mutism with an epidermoid cyst of the third ventricle. *Brain,* **64**:273-290, 1941.

22. Ando, S.; Ohshima, Y. and Uryu, K.: A hepatocerebral disease. autopsy case having widespread incomplete cortical necrosis ("Erbleichung") making a special reference to the so-called pseudoulegyria type (Shiraki). *Psychiat. Neurol. jap.* **66**:498-510, 1964 (Jap. ed.).

23. Shiraki, H.: Suggestions on the metabolic studies of epilepsy from the neuropathological viewpoint. *Metabolism and Disease,* **3**:468-486, 1966 (Jap. ed.).

# Neuropsychiatric Manifestations In Wilson's Disease: Attacks of Disturbance of Consciousness

TADASHI INOSE, M.D.*

Changes in personality and psychoses may precede the appearance of neurologic manifestations in some patients with Wilson's disease. Disturbances of consciousness, however, predominate during late stages of the illness. No specific neuropathologic lesions in the central nervous system can be related to the psychiatric abnormalities which have been observed in three patients with Wilson's disease.

Some psychiatric problems in Wilson's disease will be described and discussed in this paper. In most cases of Wilson's disease morphologic changes are found in the central nervous system and some psychiatric changes can be seen. Because of the severe neurologic manifestations, psychiatric observation is not always performed sufficiently. Children with Wilson's disease usually visit pediatricians first, so psychiatrists have little chance to see the patient in an early stage. However, some cases are referred to psychiatrists because of disturbance of behavior, personality change and other psychiatric conditions.

It is well known that emotional instability and excitability are seen in most cases of extrapyramidal diseases. Besides these changes in mood, some patients are deeply despondent because of their fatal illness and suffer from impairment of motor activity. In this depressive state some patients are suicidal and one must be alert to avoid such accidents.

The most common psychiatric manifestation is a slowly progressive deterioration in the level of personality and intelligence. Patients are childish for their age, lose control, and often behave impulsively.

Two cases which the author treated and one which appeared in the literature are presented and discussed. The first case, a woman of 22 years of age was admitted to our hospital in July, 1959. Her family history showed nothing which would suggest hereditary disease. At the age of 13 one of her parents first noticed she ate too much. At 17 she manifested excitement, talked too much, became irritable, slept poorly and wandered around outside of her home. She was diagnosed "hypomanic" by a psychiatrist and received electroshock ther-

*Professor, Department of Psychiatry and Neurology, Yokohama University School of Medicine, Yokohama, Japan.

## ABOUT THE AUTHOR

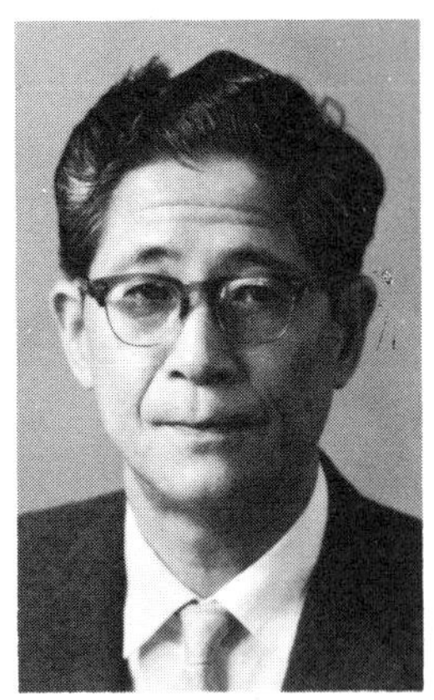

Professor Tadashi Inose, born in 1914, was graduated from the Medical School of Tokyo University in 1937, then studied psychiatry and neurology at the Department of Neuro-Psychiatry at Tokyo University. Professor Inose published a paper concerning hepatocerebral degeneration in *J. Neuropath. & exp. Neurol.* in 1952. In this work he proposed that a "special type" of hepatocerebral degeneration should be differentiated from Wilson's disease. This type of hepatocerebral disease has been called by his name in Japan.

Since 1954, he has been professor of psychiatry at Yokohama City University. His main research fields have been clinical and physiologic investigation of endogenous depression, clinical, neuropathologic and biochemical research on presenile dementia, neuropathologic and histochemical study of hepatocerebal diseases and lipid analysis of brains in lipidoses.

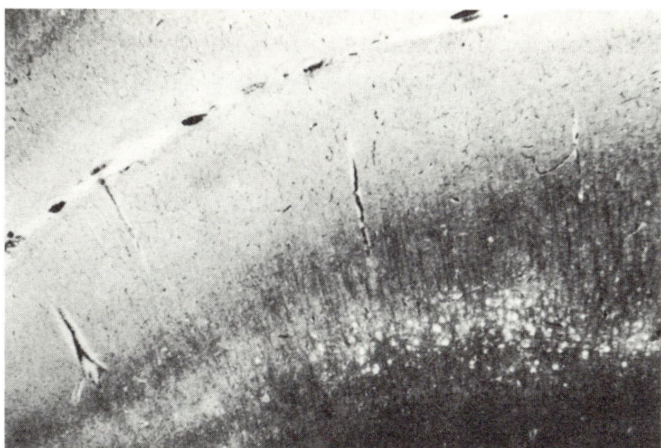

Fig. 1. Spongiform degeneration in the 5th layer of the occipital lobe. Case 2. Heidenhain-Woelke stain.

apy six times on an outpatient basis and improved. At the age of 20 her mother noticed a fine tremor in the fingers of both hands. Following this she became mute and spent most of her time in bed, which she sometimes wet.

At the age of 22 she recovered from this condition and could help with the housework. However, her handwriting deteriorated and she made errors in simple calculation. Rigidity and tremor appeared in the upper extremities. Two months later she became irritable and hostile, beat her mother and broke windows. She was admitted to our hospital on July 27, 1959. On admission her neurologic status was characterized by rigidity of all the muscles in her body and by contracture of the upper and lower extremities. She could not stand or walk. Anarthria, dysphasia and forced laughter were present. Tremor was seen in her lips and both extremities. Accordingly, Wilson's disease was suspected and was confirmed by the finding of corneal Kayser-Fleischer rings. She was bedridden with a high temperature until her death on the fourth day after admission. Thus there was no time to carry out liver function tests or estimations of ceruloplasmin of serum. Autopsy revealed incomplete softening of the putamen bilaterally and marked changes of astroglia. Alzheimer's glia cells type I and Opalski cells were seen in moderate amounts. This case indicates that Wilson's disease can manifest itself by a long period of mental disorder before the appearance of neurologic symptoms.

The second case, a 38-year-old man, was admitted to our institute in 1961. He was well until the age of 30 when he developed tremors in both hands and upper extremities, slight dysarthria and gait disturbance. At the age of 32, ascites and hydrocele were noted. At the same time a change in personality first appeared; there was considerable irritability and occasional violence. He had several episodes of delirium and coma for three months before his death at the age of 38 years. Moderate organic mental disturbance was noticed in the interval. Bilateral Kayser-Fleischer rings and cupriuria of 130 $\mu$g/liter were demonstrated. This patient expired eight years after the onset of the disease. Necropsy disclosed cirrhosis of the liver; brain sections showed moderate changes characterized by hepatogenic encephalopathy and mild changes of Wilson's disease. The neuropathologic findings of this case will be presented and discussed later.

The third case was reported by Okada *et al*[6] in 1960 in Japan. This was a man whose first trouble started with tremor of the right hand at the age of 25. The following year his handwriting, dressing and eating became difficult and tremor was found in the left hand also. Ophthalmologic investigation revealed corneal Kayser-Fleischer rings. Amnesia, slight dementia and euphoria developed. BAL was given and neurologic symtoms improved. Three years later ascites was noted and at the same time emotional irritability developed. At the age of 28 he complained of abdominal pain and fell into delirium. Soon after he was sent to a mental hospital because of prominent personality changes. For the first four months he was manic, then depressive and the alternation of manic and depressive states continued until three months before his death at the age of 29. In the last stage of his illness he had to be isolated because of disturbance of consciousness combined with manic excitement, marked dementia with emotional instability, attacks of anger and forced laughter and crying. Then he went into final coma.

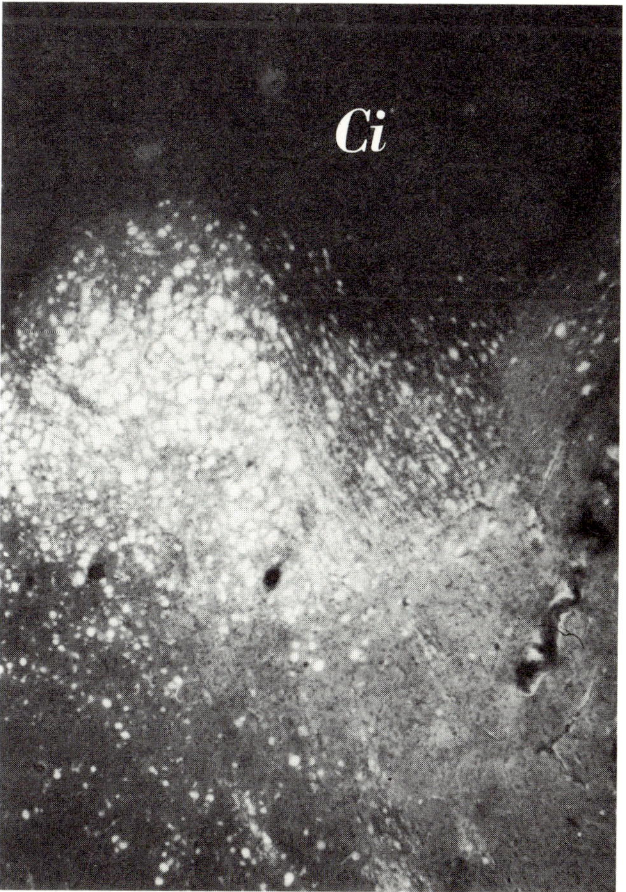


Fig. 2. Spongy state of the upper part of the putamen. Ci: internal capsule. Case 2. Heidenhain-Woelke stain.

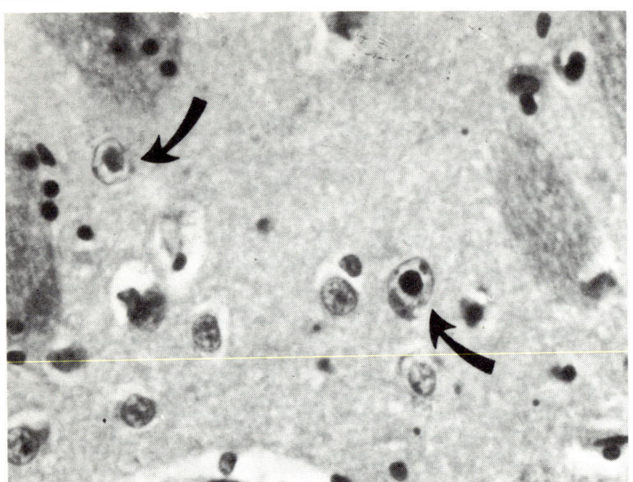

Fig. 3. Glycogen granule in the "naked glia" (arrows). Case 2. Best's carmine stain.

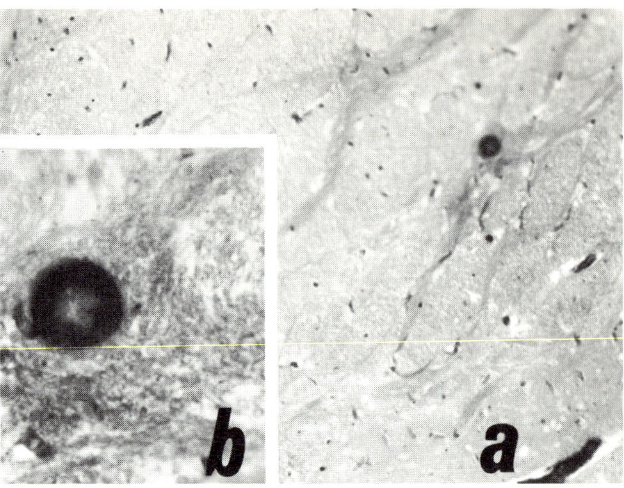


Fig. 4. Opalski cell in striatum (a). Higher magnification (b). Case 2. PAS stain.

In the last two cases there were no estimations of the blood ammonium level so that the presence of portosystemic shunts could not be ascertained.

If the neuropathologic findings of our two cases are compared, the difference between them is obvious. The neuropathologic feature of the second case consists of spongiform degeneration of cerebral parenchyma and abundant appearance of "naked glia," i.e. Alzheimer's glia cell type II. The former is found in the 3rd-5th layers of cerebral cortex in form of pseudolaminar arrangement, sometimes with capillary proliferation in the striatum and in the crus cerebri. Figure 1 shows spongiform degeneration in the fifth layer of the occipital lobe and the same change is found in the cortex of all other parts of the brain. The spongiform change in striatum is found at the upper part of the putamen which seems to be one of the characteristics of hepatoportal systemic encephalopathy (Fig. 2). Further, Best's carmine stain demonstrated glycogen granules in the nucleus of "naked glia" (Fig. 3). These findings were suggested as characteristic for the special type of hepatocerebral degeneration which was differentiated from Wilson's disease by the author.[2] Opalski cells which are stained by PAS-reaction (Fig. 4)[3,4] were also present. Further silver impregnation methods demonstrated morphologic changes of astroglial cells as severe as in Wilson's disease. This case, therefore, should be diagnosed as Wilson's disease although Alzheimer's glia cell type I could not be found with the Nissl preparation.[5]

In the third case neither spongiform degeneration nor carmine-stained glial nuclei could be found. The only point that suggests the difference from usual Wilson's disease is rarity of typical Alzheimer's glial cell type I.

From these results of the neuropathologic investigation no decisive evidence on the pathogenesis of the deterioration of consciousness could be derived. But it suggests the possibility that hepatoportal systematic encephalopathy could contribute to cerebral change in Wilson's disease.

## Conclusion

1) Psychiatrists can often observe adolescent or adult patients with Wilson's disease manifesting behavior and personality disturbances or psychotic states, including manic excitation.

2) Disturbances of consciousness can occur in the course of the illness, especially in the late stage and they are often predominant clinical symptoms.

3) A hepatogenous factor may play a role in the pathogenesis of disturbance of consciousness.

## REFERENCES

1. Baltzan, M. A.; Olszewski, J. and Zervas, N.: Chronic portohepatic encephalopathy. *J. Neuropath. exp. Neurol.* **XVI:**410-421, 1957.

2. Inose, T.: Hepatocerebral degeneration, a special type. *J. Neuropath. exp. Neurol.* **XI:**401-408, 1952.

3. Inose, T. *et al.*: Eine histochemische Studie bei den hepatocerebralen Degenerationen und bei Leberkrankheiten (Glykogenbefund). *Arch. Psychiat. Nervenkr.* **200:**509-519, 1960.

4. Inose, T.: Neuropathologie der hepatozerebralen Erkrankungen nebst einigen histochemischen Bemerkungen. *Proc. IV. int. Congr. Neuropath.* Georg Thieme, Stutgart, Vol. I, pp. 170-173, 1962.

5. Nakai, J.: *Morphology of Neuroglia.* Igaku Shoin, Tokyo, pp. 151-163, 1961.

6. Okada, R. *et al.*: A case of Wilson's disease – on its clinical picture and pathology.*Int. Med.* **5:**373-381, 1960 (Japanese).

# Psychiatric Aspects of Wilson's Disease: Results of Psychometric Tests During Long-Term Therapy*

NORMAN P. GOLDSTEIN, M.D.**; JOSEPHINE C. EWERT, M.A.†; RAYMOND V. RANDALL, M.D.‡ and JOHN B. GROSS, M.D.‡

Twenty-two patients with Wilson's disease have been studied. Thirteen of the 22 patients had no history or clinical evidence of psychiatric disease. Five of the other nine patients showed psychiatric improvement with treatment of hepatolenticular degeneration. Sixteen patients underwent psychometric testing. One patient was mentally retarded. Twelve patients were retested at various intervals after starting treatment with a low copper diet and penicillamine. The intelligence tests of all patients except the one who was mentally retarded showed slightly improved performance after long-term treatment.

Because of the lack of recent publications related to the psychiatric aspects of Wilson's disease and the paucity of reports of psychologic testing, we thought that a review of our experience and data in these areas was warranted. A total of 17 patients were studied with psychometric tests. In addition, we were able to follow the course of treatment with repeated testing in 13 of these patients, the treatment mainly consisting of oral administration of penicillamine (either DL- or D-) and a diet low in copper.

## Clinical Material and Methods

Twenty-two patients with Wilson's disease have been studied at the Mayo Clinic in the years 1952 through 1964 (Table I). Fifteen adult patients underwent psychometric testing which usually included the Wechsler Adult Intelligence Scale (WAIS), the Wechsler Memory Scale, the Bender-Gestalt test, the Shipley-Hartford tests, and the Minnesota Multiphasic Personality Inventory (MMPI). The two children were tested with the Wechsler Intelligence Scale for Children (WISC).

*This investigation was supported in part by Research Grant NB-3655 from the National Institutes of Health, Public Health Service.

**Consultant, Section of Neurology, Mayo Clinic; Professor of Neurology, Mayo Graduate School of Medicine (University of Minnesota); Rochester, Minnesota.

†Consultant, Section of Psychiatry, Mayo Clinic; Rochester, Minnesota.

‡Consultants, Section of Medicine, Mayo Clinic; Associate Professors of Medicine, Mayo Graduate School of Medicine (University of Minnesota), Rochester, Minnesota.

An opinion as to the psychiatric status of the patients was derived from interviews with the individual patients, history related by members of the family, and results of psychologic tests and clinical observation.

## Results

Of the 15 adult patients who had psychometric tests during the course of these studies, six of them were first tested after the start of treatment. The results of pretreatment psychometric testing in the remaining nine adult patients (cases 4, 7, 8, 9, 10, 13, 16, 17, and 22) are shown in Table II. The average scores of this group, based on age norms, appeared unremarkable and served as a reference for future testing.

Eight of these nine adult patients were tested again 16 to 30 months after start of treatment, and scores were higher on certain tests, presumably indicating an improved performance after this period of therapy. On the Wechsler Adult Intelligence Scale, improved performance was noted on information, comprehension, similarities, verbal scale IQ, and block design. On the Shipley-Hartford tests, no change was noted in vocabulary but there was definite improvement in concept formation and IQ. The Wechsler Memory Scale quotient also indicated an improved performance. The Bender-Gestalt results suggested that there was some improvement in tremor as well as improved recall.

Four of these eight patients (cases 4, 7, 16, and 17) were retested 63 to 73 months after start of treatment. Although the number of patients is small, the trend to-

TABLE I

# SUMMARY OF PATIENTS STUDIED

| Case | Sex | Age (yr.) At onset of symptoms | Age (yr.) At diagnosis | Age (yr.) At time of 1st psychometric tests | Education | Occupation | Psychiatric diagnosis |
|---|---|---|---|---|---|---|---|
| 1 | M | 37 | 39 | 45 | Grade 12 | Assembler | |
| 2 | M | 25 | 30 | 36 | Grade 10 | Laborer, State Highway Dept. | |
| 3 | M | 15 | 17 | 24 | Grade 12; electronics, 2 yr. | Helper in bowling alley | |
| 4 | F | 18 | 21 | 23 | College, 1½ yr. | Housewife | Hysterical personality (anxiety depression) |
| 5 | F | 14 | 16 | 28 | Grade 8 at 14 yr. | None; helped mother with housework | |
| 6 | F | 20 | 23 | .... | Grade 12 | Housewife and clerk | |
| 7 | M | 26 | 27 | 28 | Grade 9 | Bus driver | |
| 8 | M | Asymptomatic | 34 | 34 | Grade 11 | Milk route | |
| 9 | M | 15 | 16 | 16 | Grade 11 | High-school student | Neurosis-depressive reaction |
| 10 | M | 46 | 48 | 48 | Grade 8 at 15 yr. | Farmer | Confusional state |
| 11 | M | 29 | 30 | .... | Not known | Stock clerk | |
| 12 | F | 19 | 20 | .... | Grade 12 | Housewife | |
| 13 | M | 19 | 20 | 20 | Grade 12; technical school, ½ yr. | Farmer | |
| 14 | M | 23 | 27 | .... | B.A. | Office worker | Schizoid personality |
| 15 | M | 23 | 45 | 49 | Grade 5 at 14 yr. | Farmer | Hypomanic-paranoid reaction |
| 16 | F | 23 | 24 | 24 | College, 2 yr. & 3 summer sessions | School teacher | Depressive reaction |
| 17 | M | 39 | 40 | 40 | Business college, 2 yr. | Bookkeeper | Mixed psychoneurosis |
| 18 | M | 24 | 26 | .... | Not known | Welder | |
| 19 | M | 5 | 12 | 12 | Special education class | Student | Mental retardation with psychosis |
| 20 | F | Asymptomatic | 5 | 8 | Elementary school | Student | |
| 21 | M | 27 | 28 | 29 | Grade 12 | Factory worker | Mixed psychoneurosis with hysterical aphonia |
| 22 | F | 18 | 34 | 42 | Grade 12 & comptometer course, 8 mo. | Housewife | |

TABLE II

**Summary of Results of Psychometric Tests Before and After Treatment in Nine Adult Patients With Wilson's Disease**

| Test | Pretreatment test | | Tests 16 to 30 months later | | | Tests 63 to 73 months later | | |
|---|---|---|---|---|---|---|---|---|
| | No. of patients | Aver. | No. of patients | 1st test | 2nd test | No. of patients | 1st test | 2nd test |
| Wechsler (WAIS) | | | | | | | | |
| Information | 7 | 9.7 | 7 | 9.7 | 11.0 | 3 | 10.3 | 11.7 |
| Comprehension | 8 | 9.9 | 7 | 10.6 | 11.7 | 3 | 10.7 | 14.0 |
| Arithmetic | 8 | 11.1 | 6 | 11.5 | 11.0 | 3 | 10.7 | 11.3 |
| Similarities | 8 | 9.5 | 7 | 9.4 | 11.4 | 3 | 9.3 | 13.7 |
| Digit span | 8 | 9.0 | 7 | 8.7 | 8.4 | 3 | 8.3 | 9.0 |
| Verbal scale IQ | 8 | 99.0 | 7 | 100.0 | 104.4 | 3 | 99.0 | 112.3 |
| Block design | 8 | 9.4 | 7 | 9.6 | 10.3 | 2 | 10.0 | 10.5 |
| Shipley-Hartford | | | | | | | | |
| Vocabulary | 6 | 28.2 | 6 | 28.2 | 28.8 | 3 | 29.7 | 32.3 |
| Concept formation | 6 | 21.3 | 6 | 21.3 | 28.3 | 3 | 18.7 | 32.7 |
| IQ | 6 | 102.2 | 6 | 102.2 | 111.0 | 3 | 98.7 | 120.3 |
| Wechsler Memory Scale quotient | 6 | 103.8 | 6 | 103.8 | 111.3 | 3 | 107.0 | 121.7 |
| Bender-Gestalt | | | | | | | | |
| Tremor | 8 | 1.1 | 6 | 1.3 | 0.9 | 4 | 1.0 | 0.5 |
| Recall | 8 | 5.2 | 6 | 5.6 | 7.1 | 3 | 4.8 | 7.2 |

ward improvement seems clear (Table II). Noteworthy are the changes in the Wechsler verbal scale IQ, the Shipley-Hartford concept formation and IQ, and the Wechsler Memory Scale quotient. Again the Bender-Gestalt showed less tremor and improved recall.

Although the study of the group averages showed a trend toward improved performances, the group changes are less dramatic and perhaps less revealing than the test results for individual patients. This is especially true in case 7 (Table III; Fig. 1); this patient showed remarkable improvement in most portions of the Wechsler Adult Intelligence Scale, while the results on tests of block design were the same before and after treatment. On the Shipley-Hartford tests, the change in the vocabulary portion was not great but concept formation and IQ showed remarkable improvement. The improvement in the Wechsler Memory Scale quotient paralleled that in the Wechsler verbal scale IQ but there was no essential change on the Bender-Gestalt test. The pretreatment MMPI showed mild depression, mild suspiciousness, and some overemphasis of symptoms but no evidence of psychosis or crippling neurosis. With continued treatment of this patient, the MMPI showed improvement in mood with mild hypomania and emotional lability. On the last MMPI, in 1965, the patient seemed well adjusted although there was still some evidence of mild hypomania and immaturity.

Another patient (case 16) showed less striking improvement (Table IV; Fig. 2) over a five-year period. Of particular interest were the results of the second set of tests, at a time when the patient had relapsed clini-

## ABOUT THE SENIOR AUTHOR

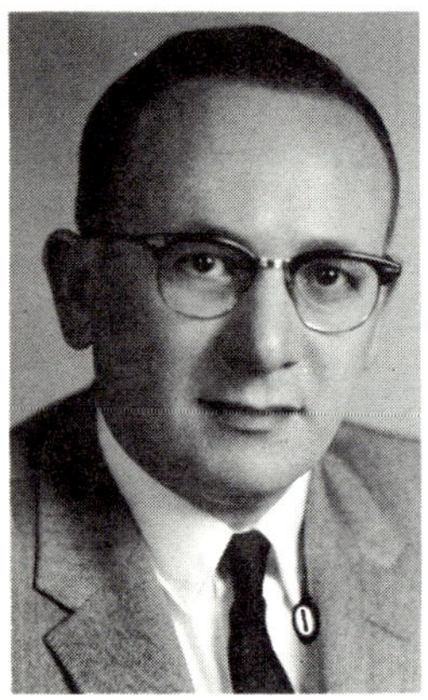

Dr. Norman P. Goldstein, head of a section of neurology in the Mayo Clinic, Rochester, Minnesota, and professor of neurology in the Mayo Graduate School of Medicine of the University of Minnesota at Rochester, was born in Brooklyn, New York in 1921. He received the degree of bachelor of arts *magna cum laude* from New York University in 1941; the degree of master of arts in biochemistry in 1942 from George Washington University and the degree of doctor of medicine *with distinction* in 1946 from the same university.

Dr. Goldstein was certified as a specialist in psychiatry in 1954, and as a specialist in neurology in 1956, by the American Board of Psychiatry and Neurology, Inc. He is a fellow of the American Academy of Neurology and a member of the American Neurological Association, the American Medical Association, the American Psychiatric Association, the American Academy for Cerebral Palsy, the Association for Research in Nervous and Mental Disease, the American Association for the Advancement of Science, the Central Society for Neurologic Research, the Minnesota State Medical Association, the Zumbro Valley Medical Society, the Society of the Sigma Xi, Phi Beta Kappa, the Phi Delta Epsilon professional medical fraternity, and the Alumni Association of the Mayo Graduate School of Medicine.

Dr. Goldstein has maintained a special interest in the neurochemical aspects of Wilson's disease, multiple sclerosis and the demyelinating diseases, cerebral edema, and in peripheral neuritis, and has contributed to the literature of his specialty. He is coauthor of the volume, *Clinical Examinations in Neurology*, published in 1956 and again in a new edition in 1963.

In 1967 he was appointed a professorial lecturer in neurology and neurologic surgery in the George Washington University School of Medicine.

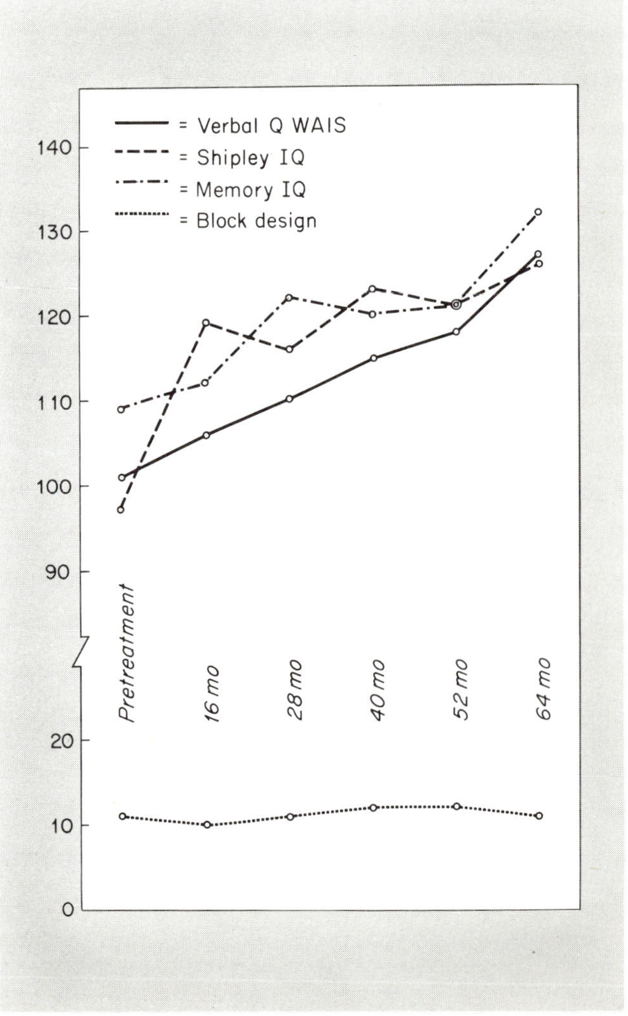


Fig. 1. Results of psychometric tests in case 7.

## TABLE III

## RESULTS OF PSYCHOMETRIC TESTS IN CASE 7

| Test | Nov., 1959 | 16 mos. | 28 mos. | 40 mos. | 52 mos. | 64 mos. |
|---|---|---|---|---|---|---|
| Wechsler (WAIS) | | | | | | |
| Information | 10 | 10 | 11 | 12 | 12 | 12 |
| Comprehension | 12 | 15 | 15 | 16 | 14 | 16 |
| Arithmetic | 11 | 10 | 10 | 12 | 16 | 15 |
| Similarities | 10 | 11 | 13 | 12 | 13 | 16 |
| Digit span | 9 | 10 | 10 | 11 | 11 | 14 |
| Verbal scale IQ | 101 | 106 | 110 | 115 | 118 | 127 |
| Block design | 11 | 10 | 11 | 12 | 12 | 11 |
| Shipley-Hartford | | | | | | |
| Vocabulary | 31 | 33 | 31 | 32 | 33 | 34 |
| Concept formation | 16 | 32 | 30 | 36 | 34 | 36 |
| IQ | 97 | 119 | 116 | 123 | 121 | 126 |
| Wechsler Memory Scale quotient | 109 | 112 | 122 | 120 | 121 | 132 |
| Bender-Gestalt | | | | | | |
| Tremor | ½ | ½ | 1 | ½ | ½ | ½ |
| Recall | 6 | 7 | 7½ | 7½ | 6 | .... |
| MMPI high scores | 2'90 | '193 | 9'21 | '95 30 | '95 40 | '9354 |

cally despite eight months of treatment. Part of the difficulty was the result of unrecognized bleeding from esophageal varices as well as a catatonic-like state produced by increased muscular rigidity. After splenectomy and construction of a splenorenal shunt and continued treatment with D-penicillamine, she showed a steady if moderate improvement. The first three MMPI results indicated that she was depressed, worried, hypochondriac, and basically immature; there was also evidence of a lack of drive and a tomboyish reaction. By the fourth test, there was evidence of rebelliousness which also showed up on later tests. However, the most recent tests showed absence of a hypochondriac reaction, and she tended to smooth over her own faults. She also seemed to be quite sensitive and projected her problems.

Another patient (case 17) also showed marked impairment on testing at the time of clinical worsening, eight months after start of treatment (Table V; Fig. 3). The pretreatment Wechsler verbal scale IQ and Memory Scale quotient dropped to 89 and 66, respectively, while the information and similarities scores on the Wechsler Adult Intelligence Scale showed little change; there was also little change on the vocabulary scale of the Shipley-Hartford tests. With continued improvement during six years of treatment, there was generally a better performance on the various subtests, except for decreased scores in arithmetic and digit span. The original pretreatment MMPI in 1960 confirmed the psychiatric history that the patient was anxious, depressed, immature, and hypochondriac; he was insecure about his masculinity and anergic. Despite the improvement in the neurologic status, the last MMPI in 1966 again confirmed the clinical impression that he basically was an immature, suspicious, hypochondriac man who was now handling his anxiety by denial; he still demonstrated poor masculine identification and marked passivity.

The five other adults (cases 4, 8, 9, 13, and 22) who were retested 16 to 30 months after start of treatment showed general improvement on the various tests. Four other patients (cases 1, 2, 3, and 5) were retested at various intervals for five to six years after start of treatment but unfortunately no pretreatment psychologic studies had been done; these patients also showed improvement in the various psychometric tests, which generally paralleled improvement in their neurologic status. Thus, a total of 12 adult patients were retested periodically, usually at 12-month intervals; eight of these patients were retested periodically for five to six years (cases 1, 2, 3, 4, 5, 7, 16, and 17) and all showed varying degrees of improvement, both clinically and on psychometric testing.

In contrast, the one child (case 19) who was retested at intervals during 38 months of treatment showed a gradual deterioration on the Wechsler Intelligence Scale for Children (Table VI; Fig. 4) despite definite improvement neurologically. This child was mentally re-

TABLE IV

## RESULTS OF PSYCHOMETRIC TESTS IN CASE 16

| Test | Oct.,* 1960 | 8 mos. | 14 mos. | 19 mos. | 30 mos. | 42 mos. | 52 mos. | 63 mos. |
|---|---|---|---|---|---|---|---|---|
| Wechsler (WAIS) | | | | | | | | |
| Information | 10 | 10 | 10 | 10 | 10 | 11 | 11 | 11 |
| Comprehension | 8 | 7 | 9 | 13 | 14 | 14 | 11 | 13 |
| Arithmetic | 7 | 6 | 9 | 7 | 9 | 8 | 7 | 9 |
| Similarities | 9 | 8 | 12 | 13 | 12 | 12 | 13 | 13 |
| Digit span | 7 | 6 | 7 | 7 | 7 | 7 | 7 | 7 |
| Verbal scale IQ | 90 | 83 | 95 | 99 | 101 | 101 | 98 | 103 |
| Block design | 9 | 7 | 9 | 9 | 10 | 10 | 12 | .... |
| Shipley-Hartford | | | | | | | | |
| Vocabulary | 28 | 25 | 27 | 28 | 29 | 32 | 31 | 31 |
| Concept formation | 22 | 14 | 28 | 22 | 28 | 26 | 28 | 30 |
| IQ | 101 | 86 | 108 | 101 | 110 | 111 | 113 | 116 |
| Wechsler Memory Scale quotient | 106 | 76 | 101 | 106 | 108 | 112 | 112 | 118 |
| Bender-Gestalt | | | | | | | | |
| Tremor | 0 | +2 | 0 | ½ | 0 | 0 | 0 | 0 |
| Recall | 7 | 4½ | 8 | 8½ | 7 | .... | .... | 7 |
| MMPI high scores | 21'35 | '2431 | '245 | 4'381 | '546 | '4358 | '45816 | 4'6893 |

*Treatment started in November 1960.

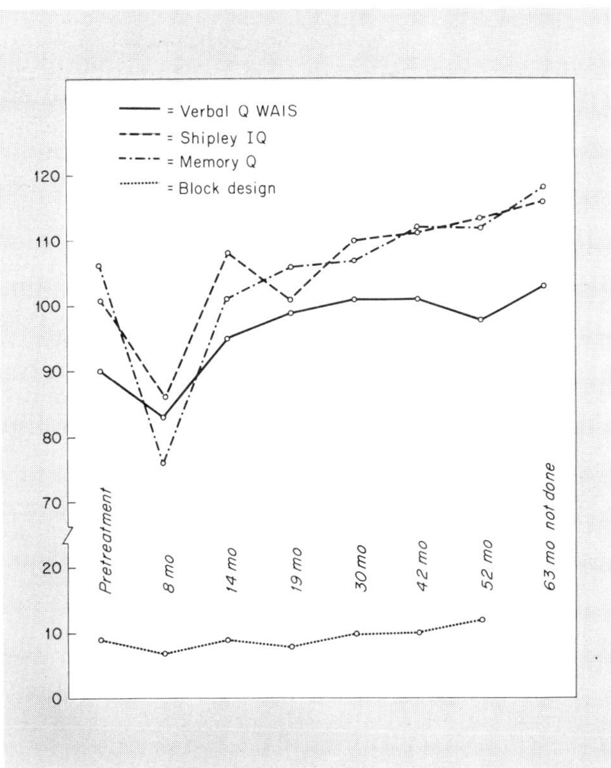


Fig. 2. Results of psychometric tests in case 16.

tarded and quite disturbed when first seen in 1962. Certain aspects of the history, as well as the activities of the patient when hospitalized in our clinical study unit, suggested a psychotic reaction. When last seen, in May 1966, his behavior had improved and he was attending special classes for retarded children. Despite the improvement in his psychosocial adjustment, repeated studies with the Wechsler Intelligence Scale for Children indicated a gradual deterioration with respect to his mental retardation.

### Comment

It is our general impression that the incidence of psychiatric disturbances is higher in patients with Wilson's disease than it is in the average neurologic patient population at the Mayo Clinic. However, these patients were subjected to close observation and psychiatric study over long periods and, thus, many minor psychiatric changes were revealed which otherwise might not have come to our attention.

Thirteen patients had neither a history nor clinical evidence of a psychiatric disorder. In the nine patients with evidence of psychiatric difficulties, there was no common denominator except for the possibility that the symptoms and signs of Wilson's disease contributed somewhat to the psychologic decompensation. We think that these nine patients had personality disturbances which antedated the overt manifestations of Wilson's

**TABLE V**

## RESULTS OF PSYCHOMETRIC TESTS IN CASE 17

| Test | June, 1960 | 8 mos. | 20 mos. | 38 mos. | 73 mos. |
|---|---|---|---|---|---|
| Wechsler (WAIS) | | | | | |
| Information | 11 | 11 | 12 | 12 | 13 |
| Comprehension | 12 | 8 | 10 | 12 | 14 |
| Arithmetic | 13 | 7 | 11 | 11 | 11 |
| Similarities | 10 | 9 | 11 | 11 | 10 |
| Digit span | 9 | 6 | 7 | 7 | 6 |
| Verbal scale IQ | 106 | 89 | 101 | 105 | 107 |
| Block design | 9 | 2 | 9 | 7 | 9 |
| Shipley-Hartford | | | | | |
| Vocabulary | 32 | 29 | 34 | 34 | 35 |
| Concept formation | ---- | 6 | 22 | 20 | 16 |
| IQ | ---- | 81 | 109 | 106 | 102 |
| Wechsler Memory Scale quotient | 106 | 66 | 109 | 113 | 115 |
| Bender-Gestalt | | | | | |
| Tremor | 2 +3 | Unable | ½ | ½ | +1 |
| Recall | 3 | Unable | 6 | 8 | 7 |
| MMPI high scores | 231″ | 5′**23** | 5″21738 | ′1′35**27** | 1″35′6 |

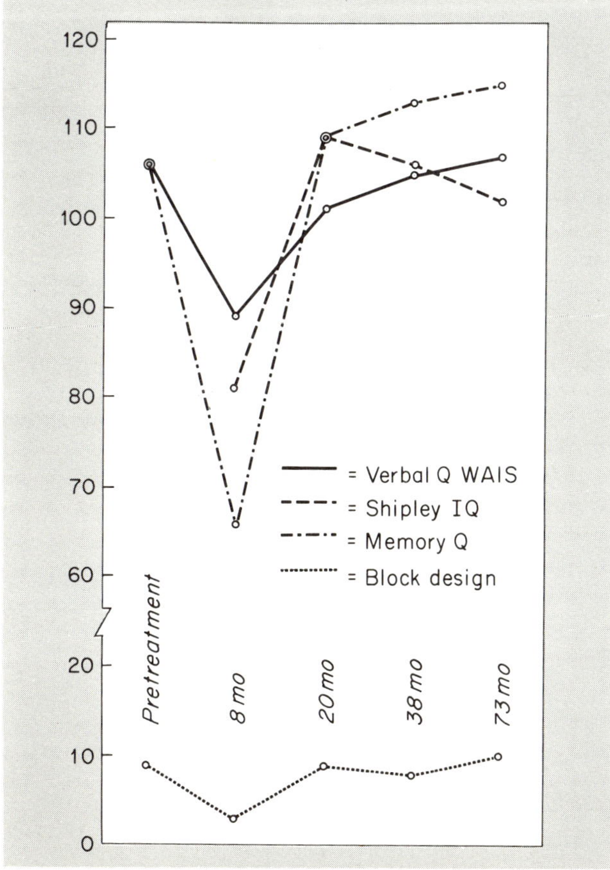


Fig. 3. Results of psychomteric tests in case 17.

disease, although we recognize the possibility that deposition of copper in the brain since infancy could possibly have altered the development of their personality reactions to the psychologic stresses and strains of their lives.

Except for the one patient with mental retardation, the patients did show an improved performance after long-term treatment with penicillamine and a diet low in copper. For example, a patient (case 2) who had a Wechsler Memory Scale quotient of 79 in 1960 had a quotient of 99 in 1966; another patient (case 3) had an IQ of 71 on the Shipley-Hartford tests in 1959 whereas it was 94 in 1966; another patient (case 5) had an IQ of 89 on the Shipley-Hartford tests in 1960, whereas it was 101 in 1965 and a Wechsler Memory Scale quotient of 92 in 1960 and 108 in 1965. In general, the intelligence tests showed slightly improved performance with long-term treatment of the Wilson's disease.

No pattern of scores emerged to suggest any specific or general area of impairment which could be found in common in these patients. Likewise, there was no common denominator in terms of personality pattern or psychologic disturbance. We have noted some tendency for increased emotional lability in a number of our Wilson's disease patients, similar to that seen in patients with multiple sclerosis. This could represent an impairment in cortical function, which is too mild and too subtle to show up on the formal psychometric testing for organic brain disease; despite the name "hepatolenticular degeneration" there is little doubt that copper is deposited in cortical structures as well as in the basal ganglia.

TABLE VI

## RESULTS OF PSYCHOMETRIC TESTS IN CASE 19

| Test | Mar., 1963 | 8 mos. | 13 mos. | 25 mos. | 38 mos. |
|---|---|---|---|---|---|
| Wechsler (WISC) | | | | | |
| Information | 3 | 5 | 3 | 2 | 2 |
| Comprehension | 3 | 2 | 1 | 0 | 2 |
| Arithmetic | 3 | 3 | 2 | 2 | 1 |
| Similarities | 5 | 5 | 2 | 2 | 2 |
| Digit span | 4 | 5 | 5 | 2 | 1 |
| Verbal scale IQ | 60 | 62 | 53 | 50 | 48 |
| Block design | 5 | 7 | 8 | 7 | 5 |
| Bender-Gestalt | | | | | |
| Tremor | .... | 0 | 0 | 0 | 0 |
| Recall | .... | 3 | 5 | 6 | 1.5 |

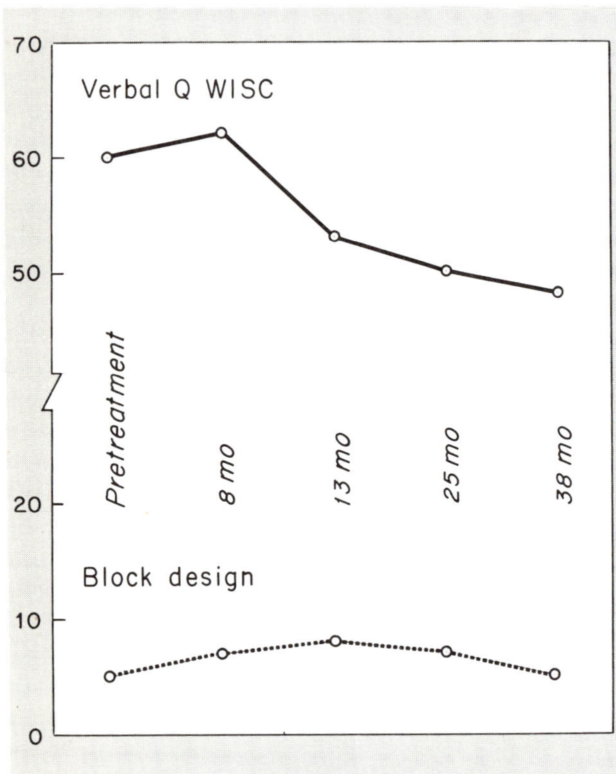


Fig. 4. Results of psychometric tests in case 19.

Finally, it should be pointed out that, with continuous treatment of the Wilson's disease, all of the treated patients except one (case 19) showed improvement on psychometric testing, which paralleled but was much less dramatic than the improvement in the neurologic status.

**Summary**

Twenty-two patients with Wilson's disease have been studied in the years 1952 through 1964. Nine patients had various psychiatric diagnoses; in two of them, there was an organic substrate to the psychiatric diagnosis. Psychometric testing was accomplished in 17 patients; in 13 of these patients, repeated psychometric testing was done periodically over a number of years while these patients were being treated with a low-copper diet and penicillamine. One patient was mentally retarded and four others had IQs at the lower limits of normal or slightly below prior to treatment of the Wilson's disease. In general, the psychometric tests showed slightly improved performance with long-term treatment of the Wilson's disease, except for the one patient with mental retardation.

# Psychiatric Manifestations in Patients with Wilson's Disease*

I. Herbert Scheinberg, M.D.**; Irmin Sternlieb, M.D.†, and Joseph Richman, Ph.D.‡

Thirty of 49 patients with Wilson's disease suffered from significant psychiatric disturbances. In 13 of these patients, psychiatric, neurotic or abnormal behavioral manifestations constituted the first clinical indication of Wilson's disease antedating any overt neurologic or hepatic symptom or sign. Psychiatric disturbances in these patients were detectable in clinical interviews and by objective psychologic tests. Definite improvement, though less dramatic than that of neurologic symptoms and signs, accompanied pharmacologic removal of copper particularly if psychotherapy was also provided.

## Introduction

In Wilson's initial [1] and final [2] publications some description of emotional disturbances in patients appears. Other authors have added many instances of "abnormalities of temperament" [3-8] and of patients in whom psychiatric symptoms preceded any other clinical disorder.[9,10] Some have implied that patients can be classically schizophrenic [11-14] but Beard [15] summarized the literature in 1959 to show convincingly that most were suffering from "nonspecific" disorders. Hall [5] described both intellectual losses and emotional disturbances in patients, adding explicitly that the latter were not schizophrenic. He expressed uncertainty as to whether the somatic disease directly caused the psychic symptoms or whether these were the patients' reactions to their physical disabilities. Knehr and Bearn,[16] who demonstrated impairment of intellect by means of psychologic tests, implied that this might be the result of copper toxicity and that cerebral damage might be detectable and the diagnosis of Wilson's disease made by such tests in patients who had no neurologic symptoms or signs.

In this paper we shall attempt to characterize the psychiatric manifestations in a group of patients with Wilson's disease; to describe the effects of "decopperizing" [17] and psychiatric therapy, and to indicate an implication of this study in the diagnosis and treatment of mentally ill patients with, and without, Wilson's disease.

## Subjects and Methods

Forty-nine patients, in all of whom the diagnosis of Wilson's disease was based on pathognomonic clinical findings or on hypoceruloplasminemia and hypercuprosis of the liver, were the subjects of this study.

Clinical interviews were held with all 49 patients from as frequently as monthly to as rarely as once a year, for periods up to ten years in duration. Clinical psychiatric impressions were compiled from the notes made at the conclusion of each interview.

To 19 of these 49 patients, Rorschach, Wechsler Adult Intelligence Scale (or Wechsler Intelligence Scale for Children), Bender-Gestalt and Figure Drawing tests were given and this battery was administered once or twice more, at intervals of a few years, to nine of these 19 subjects. The tests were interpreted by Doctor Richman independently of the clinical impressions formed by Doctors Scheinberg and Sternlieb.

## Results

From data abstracted from the clinical interview Doctors Scheinberg and Sternlieb tentatively classified the patients' psychiatric symptoms and signs as psychotic, neurotic, or reactive-behavioral. The last category, reactive-behavioral, was used for such emotional disturbances as temper tantrums, excessive irritability, loss of impulse control, fits of rage and destructive behavior. Such symptoms did not seem to be typically neurotic or psychotic, (although they occurred in some instances in patients who were themselves so classified)

*This study was supported in part by grants from the U.S. Public Health Service (AI-1059, TI AM-5384, H.D.-006-74 and 5M01 FR-50) and from the Life Insurance Medical Research Fund (G-65-50).

**Professor of Medicine, Department of Medicine, Albert Einstein College of Medicine and Bronx Municipal Hospital Center, Bronx, New York.

†Associate Professor of Medicine, Department of Medicine, Albert Einstein College of Medicine and Bronx Municipal Hospital Center, Bronx, New York.

‡Assistant Professor of Psychiatry, Department of Psychiatry, Albert Einstein College of Medicine and Bronx Municipal Hospital Center, Bronx, New York.

and appeared to represent in part the reaction and frustration resulting from the patients' physical illness in the manner Hall[5] described 46 years ago.

The psychometric results were categorized in the same three categories by 0, +, or ±. In the 19 patients who had psychologic tests performed, there were 53 pairs of clinical and psychologic evaluations of which 38 were concordant. Although only five patients were concordant for all three of the neurotic, psychotic and reactive-behavioral pairs, in no patient was there discordance for more than one of these three pairs of evaluations. This seemed to be sufficiently good agreement, in such an inherently nonquantitative area, to justify both combining the clinical and psychologic data for further consideration, and "averaging" out the discordances which were present. Sex and age differences did not seem marked, so all patients were considered as one homogeneous group.

**Statistical Results**

Of all of the 49 patients 30, or 61%, had significant psychiatric disturbance, as well as neurologic involvement, at some time.

Thirteen, or 27% of them, had a significant psychiatric manifestation as the first clinical indication of Wilson's disease.

Nine patients were classified as psychotic; six as neurotic; and in 27 reactive-behavioral manifestations were prominent. The total of 42 is due to the fact that several patients exhibited abnormalities in more than one category.

**Clinical Results**

There was a wide variety of psychiatric symptoms and signs including affective changes, such as manic states, euphoria, moodiness, anger, depression, anxiety and apathy—these in almost all 30 patients; and antisocial behavior such as sloppiness, lying and stealing, intellectual deterioration indicated by forgetfulness, and a marked decline in the quality of school work, the latter group in 13 patients. A number of patients exhibited sexual preoccupation—and occupation—sleeplessness, impulsivity, delusions, suicidal attempts, paranoid ideas, alcoholism and concern with death. Nineteen patients were very irritable, many with temper tantrums. Fourteen required psychiatric hospitalization at some time.

**Psychologic Test Results**

As a group, the patients obtained an Average Full Scale I.Q. of 94, with a Verbal I.Q. of 98 and a Performance I.Q. of 90. Individual I.Q. scores ranged from 57 to 135.

From the categorization of personality types, based primarily upon Rorschach patterns and Figure Drawing Styles, it was clear that Wilson's disease occurs in such a variety of personalities that these patients represent a sample from the general population, and not a particular "type."

Twelve out of the 19 tested patients revealed impulse disturbances with a pattern of a buildup, and then explosive discharge, of energy. Such findings, associated with temper tantrums, behavior disturbances, and epileptoid symptoms, constitute much of what could be considered clinically as reactive-behavioral.

The majority of these 19 patients evidenced both cognitive impairment, and emotional or personality disturbances. There were more records with personality

## ABOUT THE SENIOR AUTHOR

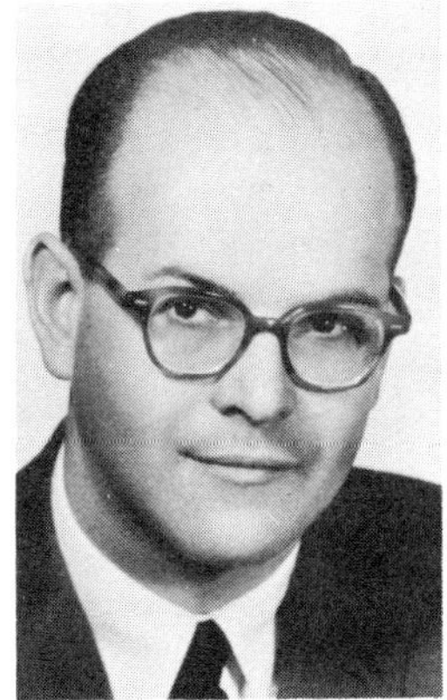

I. Herbert Scheinberg, M.D., Professor of Medicine, Albert Einstein College of Medicine, Yeshiva University; Visiting Physician, Hospital of the Albert Einstein College of Medicine and Visiting Physician, Bronx Municipal Hospital Center of the City of New York, is a Diplomate of the American Board of Internal Medicine, as well as a member of Phi Beta Kappa, Alpha Omega Alpha, American Society for Clinical Investigation, Affiliate Member of the Boston Psychoanalytic Society and Institute, Inc., The Harvey Society and the Association of American Physicians.

He was born in New York City in 1919; awarded an A.B. degree *magna cum laude* from Harvard College in 1940; received his medical degree *cum laude* from Harvard Medical School in 1943 and has held numerous appointments including Research Associate in Chemistry, Massachusetts Institute of Technology; Research Associate in Pediatrics; Instructor, and then Associate in Medicine, Harvard Medical School; Assistant Professor of Medicine, College of Physicians and Surgeons, Columbia University, New York City and Visiting Professor, Department of Physics, University of California, San Diego, at LaJolla, California.

Dr. Scheinberg has been awarded the R. Thornton Wilson Prize, Eastern Psychiatric Research Association of New York City; Research Award of the Association for Research in Nervous and Mental Disease; Ralph E. Miller Lectureship, Dartmouth Medical School; and a Commonwealth Fund Fellowship.

Among other professional appointments are Consultant for the World Health Organization in Geneva, Switzerland; Consultant for the Pan-American Health Organization, World Health Organization; Chairman, National Genetic Alert Program, National Foundation for Neuromuscular Diseases and Member, Scientific Advisory Board of Blood Research Institute, Inc. and the Commission on Plasma Fractionation.

disturbances than cognitive ones; between the two not one patient escaped completely unscathed. Thus, five patients, all of whom were under 20 years of age, appeared fairly intact cognitively. But, four out of the five revealed severe personality disturbances, three with psychotic breaks in thinking or reality testing, and one with severe anxiety and depression. The fifth patient had a history of behavior disturbances.

The most prevalent and indeed almost universal type of personality disturbance was in the area of impulse control, and this appeared both structurally and dynamically related to motor disturbance. In an effort to control their movements patients developed both compulsive compensations and an excessive holding in, or overcontrol, of drives. The result was a buildup of tensions with a sudden release or discharge.

### Results of Treatment

All 49 patients have been treated, with varying intensity, with a decopperizing regimen which, since 1957, has been based on the administration of penicillamine.[17] In 25 of the 30 patients with both significant neurologic and psychiatric disorders, treatment was accompanied by marked and often dramatic improvement in neurologic signs and symptoms, often to the point where incapacitated patients returned to virtually normal lives. Fourteen of these 25 showed also definite improvement in their psychiatric disturbance as judged by clinical or test evaluations or both; four showed equivocal psychiatric improvement. Although neurologic betterment was greater, both in numbers of patients and in the extent of individual improvement, than was the psychiatric improvement, the latter was definite.

One final result seemed quite surprising. Despite the prevalence of psychiatric symptoms and signs in adolescent, as well as adult patients, these were absent in children. Six of our patients were less than 12 years old when treatment was begun and in none of these six was any definite emotional or intellectual disturbance seen.

### Discussion

Consideration of the pathogenesis of the psychiatric effects of Wilson's disease raises two distinct possibilities first clearly stated by Hall.[5] First, the disorders seem characteristic of those in patients with many neurologic disturbances. Depression and euphoria, in particular, have been recognized as typical of patients with organic brain syndromes. There are, however, no specific studies in the literature on such conditions as Parkinsonism, multiple sclerosis or Huntington's chorea, from which one might learn to what degree the psychiatric manifestations observed in patients with Wilson's disease are like those seen in other organic neurologic diseases, and whether these primarily represent reactions to a disabling and life-threatening illness.

On the other hand, it is possible that the psychiatric disorders in Wilson's disease are the direct and fairly specific results of copper toxicity on intellectual, emotional and integrative centers in the brain. The patients certainly and definitely improved as copper was removed from them so it is likely that copper toxicity plays at least some direct role in the causation of their mental disorder. It seems most probable to us that both of these factors—reactions and toxicity—are etiologic.

There can be no doubt from the results presented above, as well as from the earlier material in the literature, that significant emotional and intellectual disturbances occur in a very high proportion of patients with Wilson's disease—over 50% in our group. Furthermore, about a third of our patients first came to the attention of a physician because of such psychiatric disturbances. Because of the therapeutic effectiveness of a decopperizing regimen in this disorder,[17] diagnostic tests for Wilson's disease[18] should be applied to all mentally ill patients who seek medical care.

## REFERENCES


1. Wilson, S. A. K.: Progressive lenticular degeneration: a familial nervous disease associated with cirrhosis of the liver. *Brain,* **34:**295, 1912.
2. Wilson, S. A. K.: Progressive lenticular degeneration. *Neurology* **11:** Williams and Wilkins, Baltimore, 1838 pages, 1940.
3. Boudin, G. and Pépin, B.: Dégénérescence Hépato-Lenticulaire, Masson et Cie., Eds., Paris, 250 pages, 1959.
4. Cumings, J. N.: Heavy metals and the brain. Chas. C Thomas, Springfield, Ill. 1959.
5. Hall, H. C.: La Dégénérescence Hépato-Lenticulaire, Maladie de Wilson – Pseudo-Sclérose, Masson et Cie., Paris, 1 vol. 1921.
6. Steinmann, I.: Genealogische Ermittlungen in 4 Familien mit Westphal-Wilsonscher Pseudosklerose; neurologische und psychische Besonderheiten im klinischen Bild bei 4 erkrankten Geschwisterpaaren. *Arch. Psychiat. Nervenkr.* **105:**514, 1936.
7. Koch, G.: Kasuistischer Beitrag zur Erblichkeit der Westphal-Wilsonschen Pseudosklerose, *Arch. Psychiat. Nervenkr.* **112:**101, 1940.
8. Franklin, E. and Bauman, A.: Liver dysfunction in hepatolenticular degeneration. *Amer. J. Med.* **15:**450, 1953.
9. Konovalov, N. V.: Hepatocerebral dystrophy. *Medgiz,* Moscow, pp. 384-389, 1960.
10. Schwyn, H.: Über zwei Fälle von Wilsonscher Krankheit bei einem Geschwisterpaar. *Schweiz. Arch. Neurol. Psychiat.* **40:**221, 1937.
11. Lisak, A.: Ein Fall von Wilson Pseudosklerose mit katatonen Symptomenkomplex. *Schweiz. med. Wschr.* **19:**161, 1938.
12. Gysin, W. M. and Cooke, E. T.: Unusual mental symptoms in a case of hepatolenticular degeneration, *Dis. nerv. Syst.* **11:**3, 1950.
13. Schmidt, M.: Etudes sur la Pathogénèse de la Dégénérescence Hépato-Lenticulaire, *Acta psychiat. (Kbh.)* **5:**163, 1930.
14. Denny-Brown, D.: Hepatolenticular degeneration (Wilson's disease), *New Engl. J. Med.,* **270:**1149, 1964.
15. Beard, A. W.: The association of hepatolenticular degeneration with schizophrenia, *Acta psychiat. scand.* **34:**411, 1959.
16. Knehr, C. A. and Bearn, A. G.: Psychological impairment in Wilson's disease, *J. nerv. ment. Dis.* **124:**251, 1956.
17. Sternlieb, I. and Scheinberg, I. H.: Pencillamine therapy for hepatolenticular degeneration, *J. Amer. med. Ass.,* **189:**748, 1964.
18. Scheinberg, I. H. and Sternlieb, I.: Wilson's disease, *Ann. Rev. Med.* **16:**119, 1965.

# Morphogenesis of Liver Cirrhosis in Wilson's Disease

Toshio Shikata, M.D.*

The development of liver cirrhosis was studied at various stages of Wilson's disease. Attempts to reproduce changes in rats similar to those found in patients with Wilson's disease were made under various experimental conditions. Copper alone produced liver fibrosis or monolobular cirrhosis, but combinations of copper and a low protein diet or the production of albuminuria by antikidney serum were necessary for the production of postnecrotic cirrhosis. It appeared that deficiency of SH-amino acids secondary to amino-aciduria or albuminuria could be implicated in the development of these lesions.

## Clinical

In a study of autopsy and biopsy material from 19 patients with Wilson's disease we distinguished three stages of morphologic changes in the liver.[1,4] Nine of these patients suffered from the abdominal type of the disease or were asymptomatic.

During the first stage, periportal fibrosis or monolobular cirrhosis was observed. During the second stage, submassive necrosis with parenchymal regeneration was evident. In this stage some cases died of active postnecrotic cirrhosis. During the third stage, multilobular cirrhosis, that is, arrested postnecrotic cirrhosis, was conspicuous. The first stage was found in patients younger than five and the third stage in patients older than ten years of age. Neither abdominal nor nervous symptoms were found in patients during the first stage. Among the siblings of a patient with Wilson's disease, an asymptomatic patient was only detectable by estimation of serum ceruloplasmin. Abdominal symptoms might appear at the second stage, and nervous symptoms became evident at the third stage. At the last stage, the classical features of Wilson's disease finally were well represented.

During the first stage, fine fibrous tissue was increased in amount in the periportal zone of the hepatic lobule, whereas the central zone appeared almost intact. The most advanced feature of this stage was monolobular cirrhosis (Fig. 1). Fine periportal fibrous tissue connected with each other and surrounded the ordinary liver lobules. There were scattered necrotic cells of acidophilic type. Fatty changes or vacuolated nuclei were not constant findings. Copper stains showed few copper granules in the liver cells, although markedly increased hepatic copper content was found chemically.

In the second stage, liver biopsy tissue revealed submassive necrosis of the liver cells (Fig. 2), irregular fibrosis and parenchymal regeneration. In some patients who died of hepatic insufficiency, without showing any nervous symptoms, between the ages of six to nine, liver cell destruction was more conspicuous. Diffuse degeneration and necrosis of liver cells with regenerative nodules in various sizes were prominent features, characteristic of active postnecrotic cirrhosis (Fig. 3).

### ABOUT THE AUTHOR

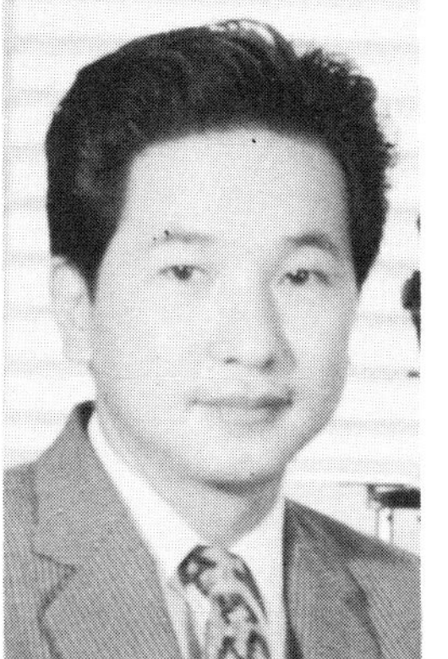

Toshio Shikata, M.D., born in Japan in 1928, is Instructor of Pathology at the University of Toyko, Faculty of Medicine. He received his degree in medicine from the same institution and until 1962 was a member of its Department of Pathology. In 1962 Dr. Shikata came to the United States to become a member of the Department of Experimental Pathology at the City of Hope Medical Center in Duarte, California. In 1964, he returned to the University of Tokyo, Faculty of Medicine.

*Instructor, Department of Pathology, Faculty of Medicine, University of Tokyo, Tokyo, Japan.

Copper granules were demonstrated at the periphery of regenerative nodules, whereas no copper was found in degenerated liver cells. At this stage, degenerative astroglia of Alzheimer II type was seen in the brain.

In the third stage, the liver showed typical coarse nodular cirrhosis. Large multilobular pseudolobules and fine fibrous tissue were characteristic. Transition between active postnecrotic cirrhosis and multilobular arrested postnecrotic cirrhosis was found.

We have summarized these observations and our concept of the morphogenesis of cirrhosis in Wilson's disease in Figure 4.

It has been assumed that chronic copper intoxication, related to failure of ceruloplasmin production, is the etiologic cause for the cirrhosis.[3] However, experimental administration of copper did not result in reproducible pathologic results in experimental animals.[2,6] Long-term feeding of copper sulfate to rabbits produced portal fibrosis or monolobular cirrhosis, which resembled the first stage of Wilson's disease (Fig. 5). This procedure also produced glial changes of Alzheimer type II in the brain which preceded the appearance of morphologic changes in the liver. However, copper administration produces neither submassive necrosis nor postnecrotic cirrhosis. Apparently some additional factor or factors are needed for this to occur.

The abdominal type of Wilson's disease, observed in patients six to nine years of age, was complicated by amino-aciduria. Some of these patients who exhibited albuminuria were often misdiagnosed as suffering from nephritis before hepatic symptoms became obvious. Apparently kidney dysfunction, such as amino-aciduria and albuminuria, is related to the development of severe liver damage. Loss of cystine and serine and albuminuria results in deficiency of SH-amino acids. In fact, copper deposition and degeneration of convoluted tubules in the kidney were more prominent in the second stage.

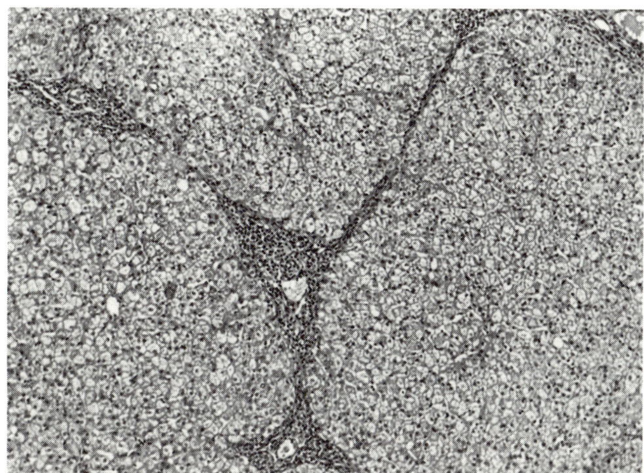

Fig. 1. Monolobular cirrhosis in the first stage of Wilson's disease. Ordinary liver lobule is surrounded by thin fibrous bands, which extend from portal tracts. Centroacinal areas are intact. Haematoxylin-eosin, x33.

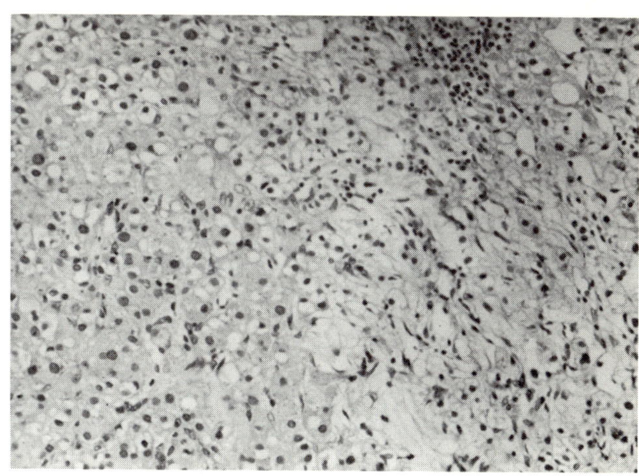

Fig. 2. Submassive necrosis in the second stage. Biopsy specimen. Necrotic area with mild lymphocytic reaction is seen. Haematoxylin-eosin, x72.

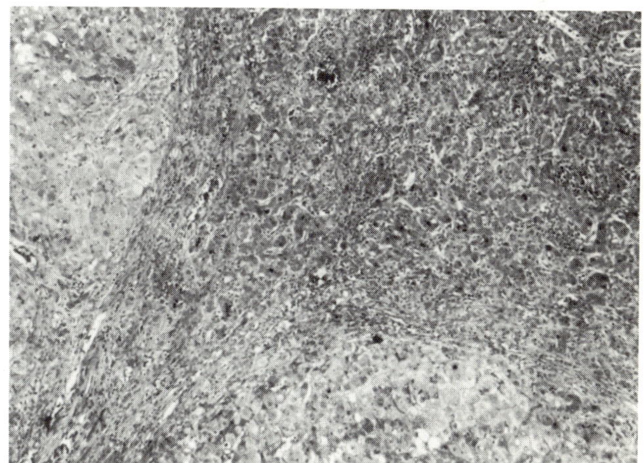

Fig. 3. Active postnecrotic cirrhosis in the second stage. Autopsy specimen. Large regenerative nodules and degenerative liver cells in the broad stroma are evident. Haematoxylin-eosin, x14.

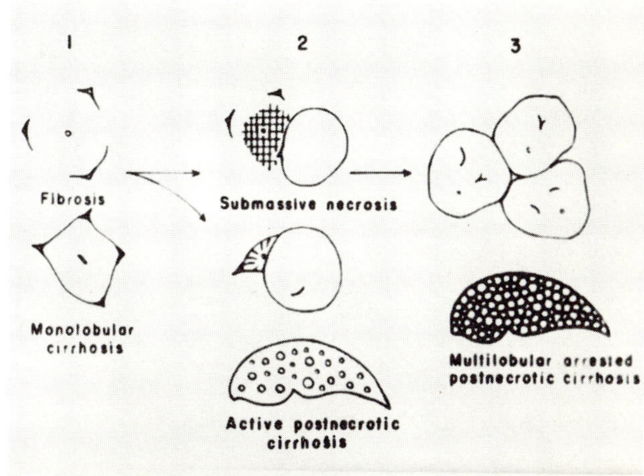


Fig. 4. Schema of morphogenesis of cirrhosis in Wilson's disease.

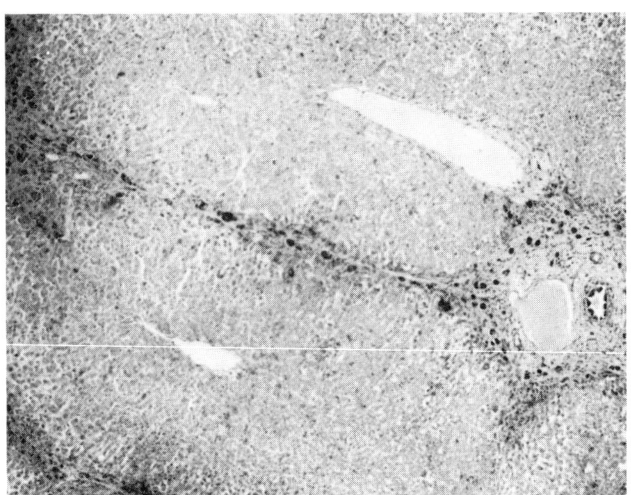

Fig. 5. Monolobular cirrhosis in a rabbit fed 0.5% copper sulfate for twelve months. Haematoxylin-eosin, x14.

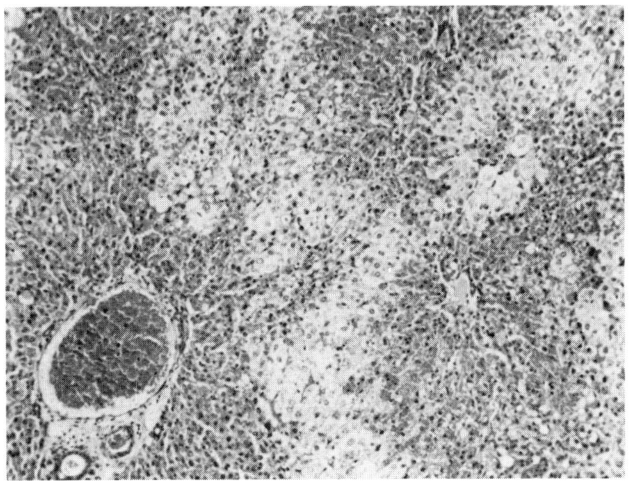

Fig. 6. Massive liver necrosis in a rat fed a low protein diet for one month followed by an injection of copper-albumin complex. Haematoxylin-eosin, x36.

## Experimental

Based on the above observations the following experiments were performed. Rats were fed a low protein diet, as well as injected with antikidney serum, to produce albuminuria. Copper salts were administered parenterally. We also examined whether the effects of low-protein diet could be reversed by adding methionine, vitamin E and selenium to the diet. Procedures and results of the experiments were as follows:

In the first experiment, rats weighing about 100 grams were fed a low protein diet containing 8% casein for one month. The animals were then given a single injection of copper-albumin complex containing 0.6 mg of copper. This procedure produced massive liver necrosis in eight of ten animals (Fig. 6). When 5 mill methionine and 2 mill trytophane were added to the low-protein diet massive necrosis did not occur. Addition of 0.5 mill vitamin E had less of a protective effect. Addition of sodium selenite in 0.15 per million did not show any significant effect. In contrast, oral administration of copper sulfate together with 0.25% ethionine caused massive hepatic necrosis in some rats within three months.

In the second experiment, rats weighing about 100 grams, were injected with antirat-kidney rabbit serum. Ten days later, a single injection of copper-albumin complex, containing 0.6 mg of copper was given. This resulted in massive or submassive necrosis in the liver and postnecrotic cirrhosis developed in some animals in this group (Fig. 7). Finally, the combination of the effect of copper toxicity on kidneys and liver was studied. A single injection of copper-albumin complex alone did not cause significant changes in the liver, but resulted in marked tubular degeneration in the kidneys with the earliest changes appearing in the mitochondria. In the proximal convoluted tubules, these organelles were enlarged and vacuolated (Fig. 8). Destruction of microvilli followed later. After this series of observations, other rats weighing about 100 grams were given a single injection of 0.6 mg of copper-albumin complex

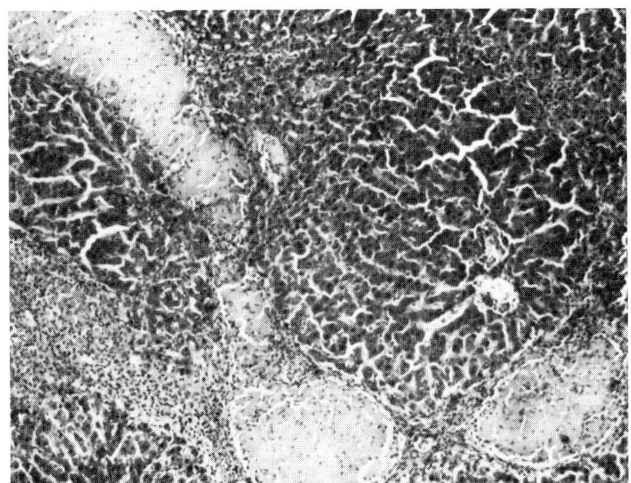

Fig. 7. Postnecrotic cirrhosis in a rat which received antikidney serum and copper. Haematoxylin-eosin, x36.

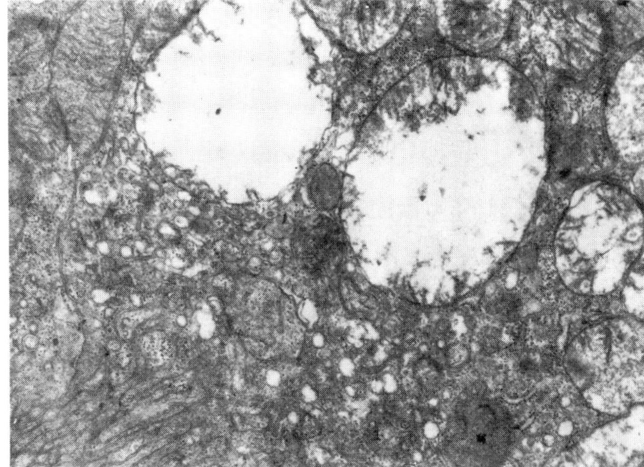

Fig. 8. Enlargement and vacuolization of mitochondria in the epithelium of a proximal convoluted tubule of a rat after a single injection of copper-albumin complex.

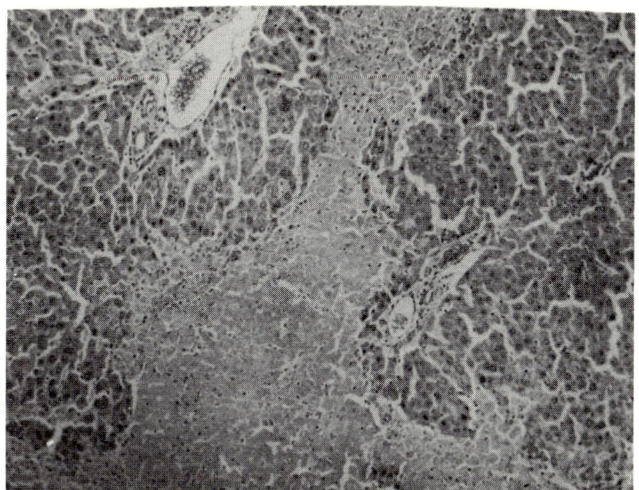

Fig. 9. Submassive necrosis of the liver in a rat (see text). Haematoxylin-eosin, x36.

and 0.3% copper sulfate in drinking water for a week, followed by another injection of copper-albumin complex. This combined procedure produced submassive necrosis of the liver (Fig. 9) which was similar to that of the liver of a patient in the second stage of Wilson's disease.

**Summary**

These studies suggest that copper alone may produce liver fibrosis or monolobular cirrhosis in the first stage of Wilson's disease. In the second stage, renal dysfunction due to copper deposition in the proximal convoluted tubules results in amino-aciduria or albuminuria and consequent secondary SH-amino acid deficiency. The combined effect of SH-amino acid deficiency and toxicity of copper results in submassive or massive necrosis. In the third stage, parenchymal regeneration leads to multilobular postnecrotic cirrhosis.

## *REFERENCES*

1. Anderson, P. J. and Popper, H.: Changes in hepatic structure in Wilson's disease. *Amer. J. Path.* **36:**483, 1960.
2. Mallory, F. B. and Parker, F. J.: Experimental copper poisoning. *Amer. J. Path.* **7:**351, 1931.
3. Scheinberg, I. H.: Copper metabolism, *Fed. Proc.* **20:**179, 1960.
4. Shikata, T.; Arima, M. and Mukai, N.: Morphological changes of abdominal-Wilson. Morphogenesis of Wilson's liver cirrhosis. *Nihonrinsho* **20:**1607, 1962. (in Japanese)
5. Vogel, F. S.: Nephrotoxic properties of copper under experimental condition in mice. *Amer. J. Path.* **36:**699, 1960.
6. Wolff, S. M.: Copper deposition in the rat. *Arch. Path.* **69:**217, 1960.

# Characterization of the Ultrastructural Changes of Hepatocytes in Wilson's Disease

IRMIN STERNLIEB, M.D.*

Biopsy specimens of liver from ten patients with Wilson's disease, ranging in age from three and a half to 36 years, were studied under the electron microscope. Five were asymptomatic patients, but only two of them were untreated; the remaining patients suffered from overt Wilson's disease. In these specimens the abnormalities observed, none of which seemed to be specific for this disorder, were: glycogen nuclei; enlarged, misshapen mitochondria; lipid containing cytoplasmic vacuoles; autophagic vacuoles; separation of lateral cell membranes with formation of intercellular spaces; increased amounts of collagen fibrils in Disse's space and presence of lipocytes.

From studies of biopsy and autopsy specimens of livers of patients with Wilson's disease a composite picture of the sequential changes in hepatic histopathology has been drawn.[1,2] The virtually normal appearing parenchymal cells – occasionally containing glycogen nuclei in the earliest stages – give way to fatty infiltration, accumulation of lipofuscin pigment, necrosis, mesenchymal infiltration, fibrosis, and an ultimate picture typical of postnecrotic cirrhosis. In all of these stages there is a disappointing lack of specificity of any of the morphologic changes. It seemed possible, however, that specific lesions which might lead to a better understanding of the mechanism by which copper, the fundamental etiologic factor in this disease, exerts its toxic effect on hepatocytes, could be detected at the ultrastructural level.

## Materials and Methods

Ten liver biopsy specimens were obtained by the Menghini technic from unanesthetized patients ranging in age from three and a half to 36 years and at various stages of Wilson's disease. Five patients were asymptomatic and were diagnosed biochemically[3]; the other five patients exhibited characteristic clinical manifestations. Two patients in each group had not been treated at the time the liver biopsy was performed. Technics of fixation, embedding and sectioning were identical to those used previously.[4,5] All specimens were examined in an RCA EMU-3C electron microscope at an acceleration potential of 100 Kv.

*Associate Professor of Medicine, Albert Einstein College of Medicine and Bronx Municipal Hospital Center, Bronx, New York.

## Results

In most specimens, from all stages, there is a notable lack of pathologic findings. Many hepatocytes exhibit typically normal appearances, displaying straight, parallel membranes on the lateral surfaces (Fig. 1). Close to biliary canaliculi, junctional complexes reinforce attachments of adjacent cell membranes, and microvilli and lumina of the canaliculi appear unremarkable (Fig. 1). Occasionally, lateral cell membranes exhibit microvilli projecting into spaces forming pericellular canals (Fig. 2). *(Text continues on page 97)*

### ABBREVIATIONS

| | | | |
|---|---|---|---|
| B | Bile canaliculus | Lc | Lipocyte |
| C | Cellular membrane | Li | Lipid |
| D | Junctional complex | G | Glycogen |
| Db | Dense body | Go | Golgi apparatus |
| DS | Disse's space | M | Mitochondrion |
| E | Sinusoidal endothelium | mb | Microbody |
| | | N | Nucleus |
| Er | Endoplasmic reticulum (sEr, smooth; rEr, rough) | n | Nucleolus |
| | | P | Platelets |
| | | R | Ribosomes |
| F | Reticulin fibrils | S | Sinusoid |
| L | Lipofuscin | V | Microvilli |

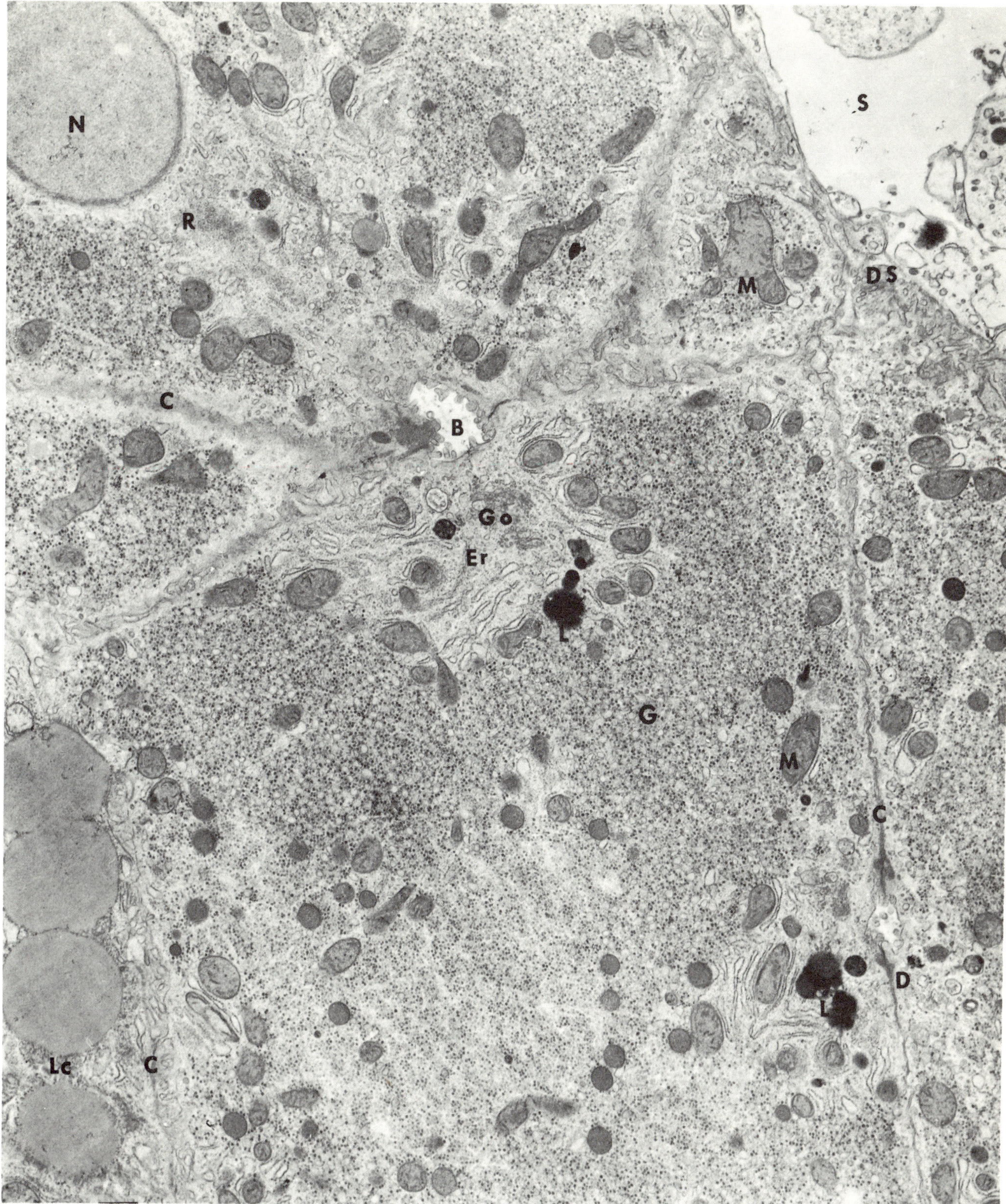


Fig. 1. Low power electron micrograph of biopsy specimen of liver from an 11-year-old girl with a history of a hemolytic episode, hepatic insufficiency and Kayser-Fleischer rings as her only manifestations of Wilson's disease, treated for one year with D-penicillamine. Light microscopy revealed presence of postnecrotic cirrhosis. Group of hepatocytes surrounding bile canaliculus (B) with sinusoid (S) in right upper corner and lipocyte (Lc) in left lower corner. Note "normal" appearance of hepatocytes with straight cellular membranes (C) and rare, misshapen mitochondria (M), abundance of glycogen (G), polarization of stacks of rough endoplasmin reticulum (Er), Golgi apparatus (Go) and lipofuscin pigment bodies (L) towards canalicular poles of cells. Osmium fixation; Epon; lead citrate stain: x 7,200.

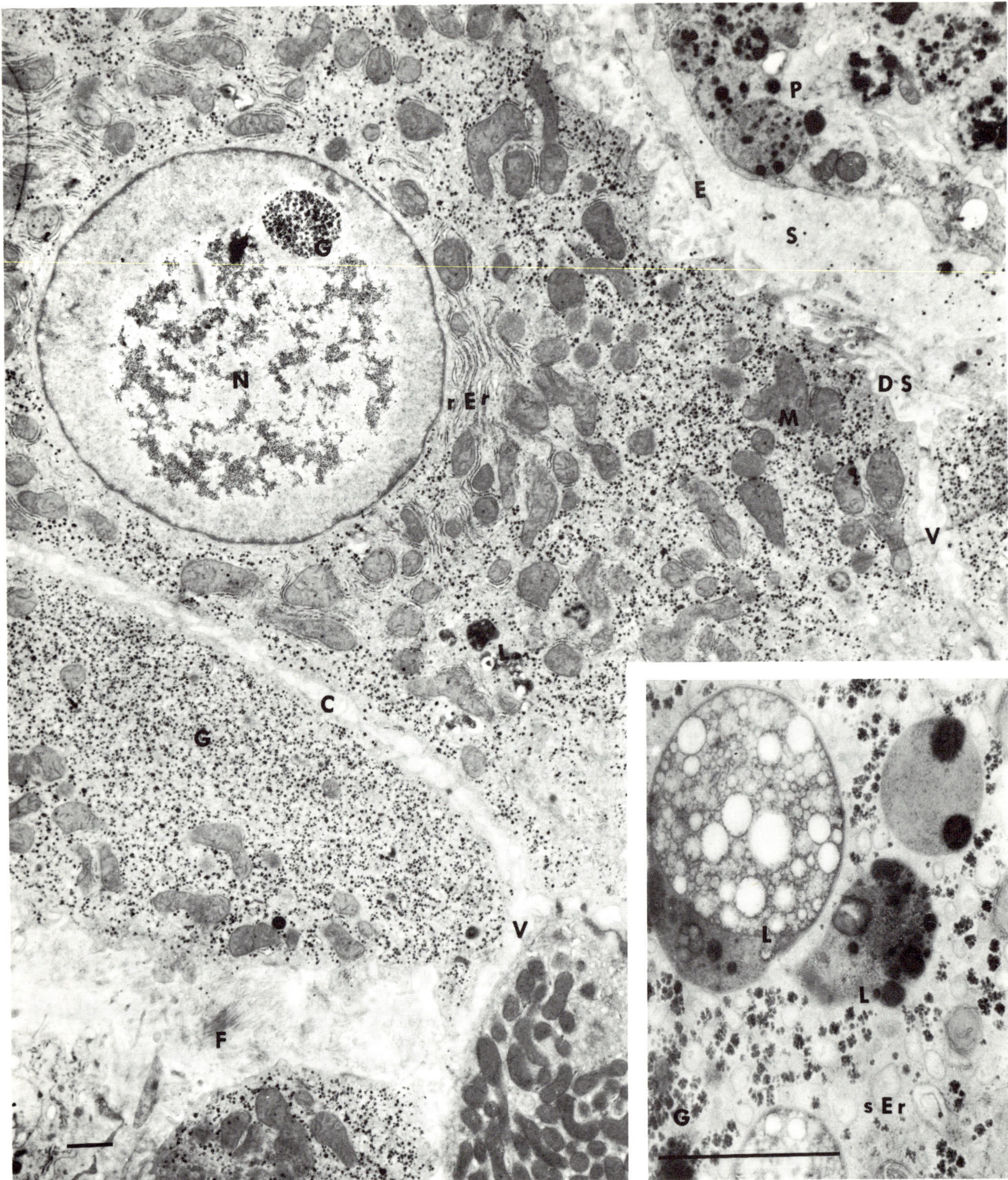


Fig. 2. Low power electron micrograph of biopsy specimen of liver from a 20-year-old man with mostly neurologic and psychiatric manifestations which had become more pronounced after splenectomy. Cirrhosis found at laparotomy and on light microscopy. Patient treated for one year with D-penicillamine. Hepatocytes with microvilli (V) projecting from lateral membranes (C) into spaces separating cells. Note cluster of glycogen rosettes (G) in nucleus (N); bundles of reticulin fibrils (F) in one of the intercellular spaces and cell, probably of mesenchymal origin, insinuating in between hepatocytes at the bottom of picture. x 7,700. Insert: higher magnification of segment of hepatocyte showing glycogen rosettes (G) and heterogeneity of lipofuscin granules (L) x 32,000. Glutaraldehyde and osmium tetroxide fixation; Epon; lead citrate stain.

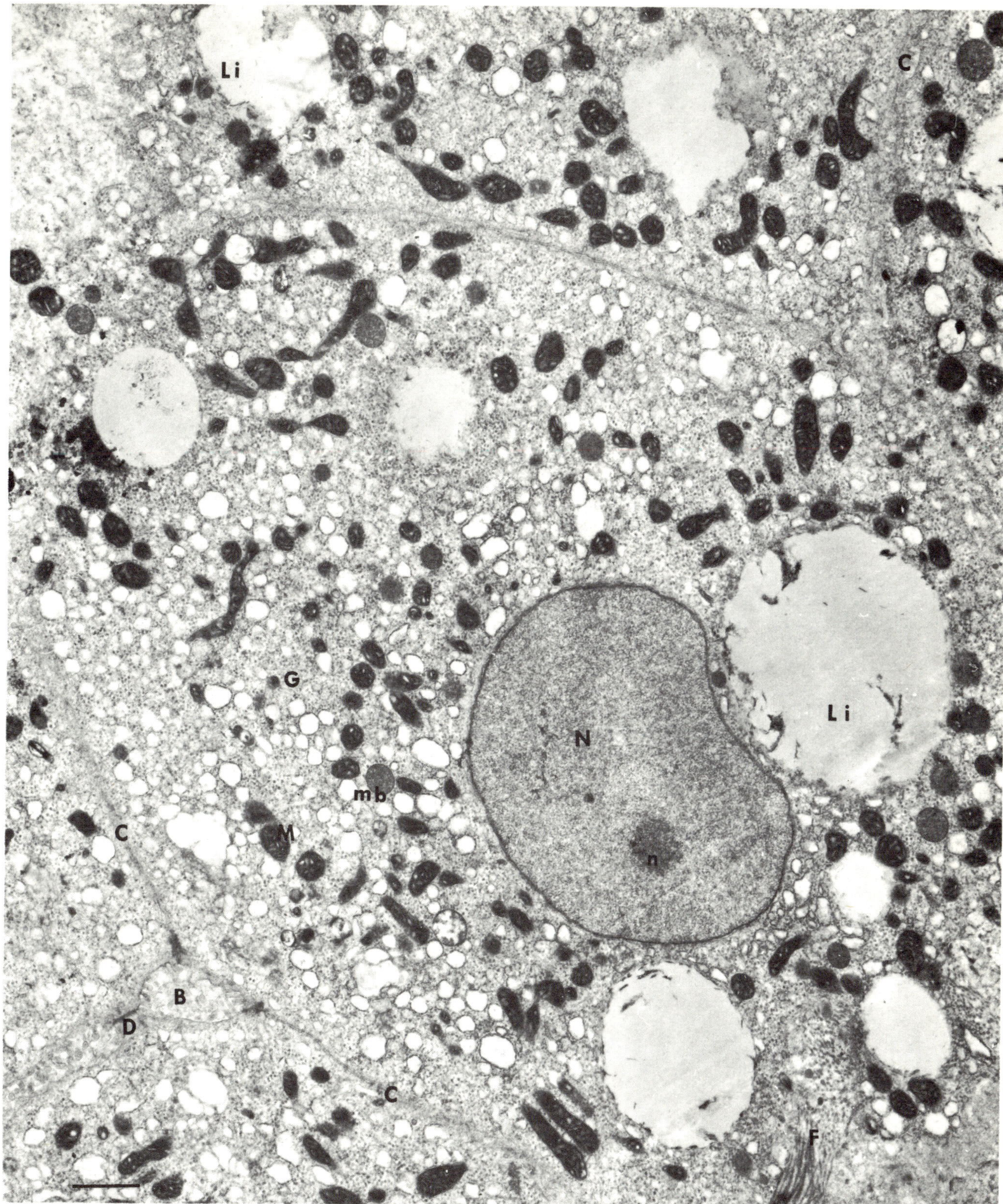


Fig. 3. Electron micrograph of liver biopsy specimen of a ten-year-old asymptomatic patient with no detectable ceruloplasmin in serum and a hepatic copper concentration of 1389 mcg/g dry tissue, before start of therapy. Group of hepatocytes containing several fatty cysts (Li), one of them indenting the nucleus (N). Note straight membranes bordering cells, except for indistinct border on the left with suggestion of spillage of cellular contents, and more markedly vacuolated endoplasmic reticulum than in Figures 1 and 2. Glutaraldehyde and osmium tetroxide fixation; Araldite; uranyl acetate and lead citrate stain; x 11,500.

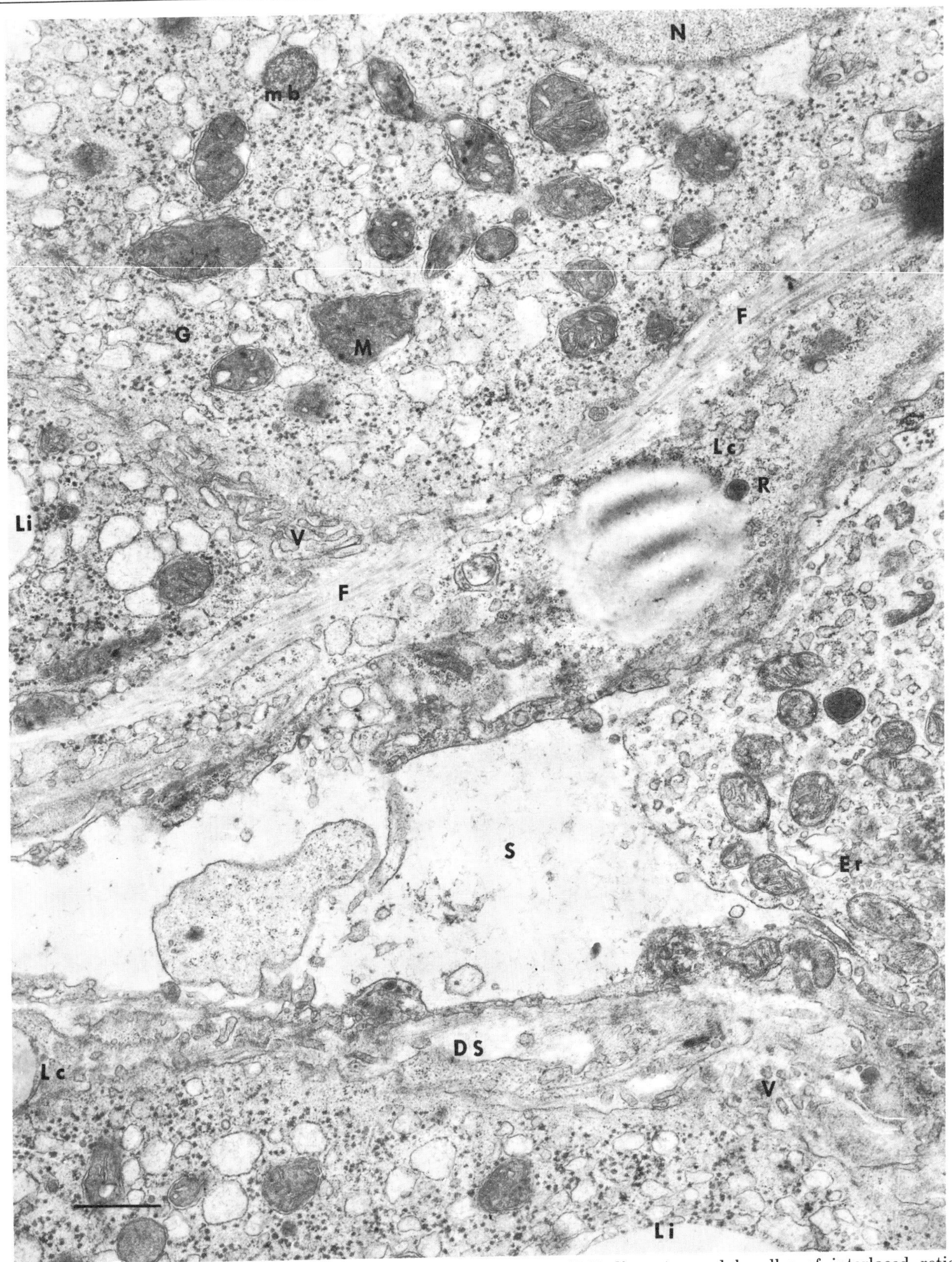


Fig. 4. Same patient as in Figure 3. Electron micrograph showing part of sinusoid (S) surrounded by four hepatocytes with lipid containing vacuoles (Li) and mitochondria (M) with dense matrices and distorted cristae. In Disse's space (DS) lipocytes and bundles of interlaced reticulin fibrils (F) are seen. Osmium tetroxide fixation; Araldite; uranyl acetate and lead citrate stain: x 16,200.

The cytoplasm of many hepatocytes contains stacks of rough endoplasmic reticulum, vacuolated smooth endoplasmic reticulum, Golgi saccules, microbodies, glycogen rosettes, ribosomes, polyribosomes and microtubules – all without any unusual features.

Most nuclei contain a prominent nucleolus and appear round and unremarkable, but a few lipid or glycogen inclusions can be identified (Fig. 2). In tangential sections at high magnifications, perinuclear filaments and microtubules seem to envelop the nuclei.[5]

Mitochondria, normal in size, shape and distribution, occasionally appear enlarged and misshapen (Fig. 1).

A pathologic change which, paradoxically, is more commonly seen in biopsy specimens from young patients is the accumulation of small lipid-containing vacuoles.[6] In early stages, they are few and close to the sinusoidal border of cells; later in the disease process, lipid vacuoles enlarge, coalesce, displace other structures, and even indent the nucleus (Fig. 3). In cells with such vacuoles, the cytoplasm exhibits signs of degeneration: saccules of smooth endoplasmic reticulum appear with larger vacuolation than normal (Fig. 3); myelin figures form; the cristae of mitochondria are distorted and their matrices appear denser than normal (Fig. 4); and clusters of alternating "dark" and "light" cells can be seen. Of course, not all these changes appear in all cells or even in all areas of the same specimen.

Almost all cells contain, in the usual peribiliary localization accumulations of lipofuscin granules, quite heterogenous, surrounded by a membrane and ranging from 0.3 to 3 $\mu$ in diameter (Figs. 1 and 2). Depending on whether lipid has been extracted during fixation, or not, these granules contain vacuoles or electron-dense osmiophilic organelles. Various evolutionary stages of lipofuscin granules and many with copper deposits, demonstrable by electron probe microanalysis[7] and histochemically by Timm's method,[8] can be observed. Autophagic vacuoles and round organelles containing concentric whorles of membranes are also encountered.

Sinusoidal borders are generally normal, with numerous slender microvilli (Figs. 1, 2, 4), but in cells loaded with lipids, cytoplasmic blebs may be seen with apparent breaks in the continuity of sinusoidal membranes and spillage of cytoplasmic contents into the lumen (Fig. 3). It is difficult to evaluate this finding as really pathologic because a mechanical artefact may have a similar appearance. Although endothelial and Kupffer cells do not appear unusual near some sinusoids, mesenchymal cells, "lipocytes" in Disse's space, discontinuous basement membranes and prominent bundles of reticulin fibrils are seen (Fig. 4). Mesenchymal cells, including fibroblasts and "oval cells," are also found in between hepatocytes (Fig. 2).

Biliary ductules, their epithelium and surrounding basement membrane, which have been described in detail elsewhere,[4] appear unremarkable.

**Discussion**

Several ultrastructural abnormalities have been found in these preparations: microvilli on contiguous membranes of hepatocytes; prominent lipofuscin granules; mesenchymal reaction; lipocytes and excessive collagen deposition in Disse's space; glycogen inclusions in nuclei and steatosis unrelated to the usual nutritional factors. But all these, as well as those noted in earlier reports,[9-12] are seen in a variety of other hepatic disorders,[13-17] so that none can be considered characteristic of Wilson's disease. Although this is disappointing, it is consoling to speculate on the basis of the nonspecificity of the lesions seen, that Wilson's disease may serve as a human "experimental" model for the study of many other forms of liver injury. It is also worth noting that we have demonstrated ultrastructural lesions in our youngest patient at a stage when the light microscope could not detect any definite abnormalities.[6]

**ACKNOWLEDGEMENTS**

This work was started during the tenure of a Special Fellowship from the United States Public Health Service (1-F3-AM-7235-01) at the Laboratoire de Synthèse Atomique et d'Optique Protonique in Ivry-sur-Seine, France and was supported in part by grants from the

## ABOUT THE AUTHOR

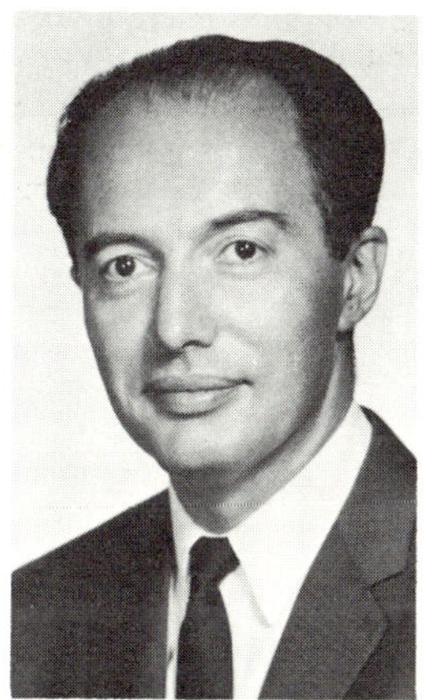

Irmin Sternlieb, M.D., Associate Professor of Medicine at Albert Einstein College of Medicine, Associate Attending Physician at Bronx Municipal Hospital and at the Hospital of the Albert Einstein College of Medicine, and Assistant Visiting Physician at Lincoln Hospital, all of the Bronx, is a Diplomate of the American Board of Internal Medicine and the Subspecialty Board of Gastroenterology.

He was born in Rumania in 1923 and received his B.Sc. and M.D. Degrees from the University of Geneva, Switzerland. He has held numerous appointments in well known hospitals in the New York area, and received a Special Fellowship from the National Institute of Health, U. S. Public Health Service, for research in electron-microscopy at Laboratoire de Synthese Atomique et d'Optique Prontonique, Ivry-sur-Seine, France.

Dr. Sternlieb is a member of the American Society for Clinical Investigation, American Federation for Clinical Research, American Gastroenterological Association, American Association for the Study of Liver Diseases, American Society for Gastrointestinal Endoscopy, Harvey Society, and Societe Francaise de Microscopie Electronique.

National Institutes of Health (AI-1059, TI AM-5384, HD-006-74, 5MO1 FR-50) and by the Life Insurance Medical Research Fund (G-62-58).

I am grateful to Dr. Alex B. Novikoff and Dr. Pierre Favard for permission to use the facilities of their laboratories.

## ADDENDUM

Since this manuscript was submitted for publication a more detailed study of mitochondrial changes in hepatocytes of patients with Wilson's disease has revealed a high incidence of associated mitochondrial and fatty changes, particularly in specimens from young patients (*Gastroenterology,* Abstract, **54**; 169, 1968).

## REFERENCES

1. Scheinberg, I. H. and Sternlieb, I.: The liver in Wilson's disease. *Gastroenterology,* **37:**550-564, 1959.
2. Anderson, P. J. and Popper, H.: Changes in hepatic structure in Wilson's disease. *Amer. J. Path.* **36:**483-497, 1960.
3. Sternlieb, I. and Scheinberg, I. H.: The diagnosis of Wilson's disease in asymptomatic patients. *J. Amer. med. Ass.* **183:** 747-750, 1963.
4. Sternlieb, I.: Electron microscopic study of intrahepatic biliary ductules. *J. Microscopie* (Paris), **4:**71-80, 1965.
5. Sternlieb, I.: Perinuclear filaments and microtubules in human hepatocytes and biliary epithelial cells. *J. Microscopie* (Paris), **4:**551-558, 1965.
6. Jérôme, H. and Sternlieb, I.: La détection préclinique de la maladie de Wilson. *Arch. franc. Pédiat.* (Paris) **23:**669-677, 1966.
7. Goldfischer, S. and Moskal, J.: Electron probe microanalysis of liver in Wilson's disease. Simultaneous assay for copper and for lead deposited by acid phosphatase activity in lysosomes. *Amer. J. Path.* **48:**305-315, 1966.
8. Goldfischer, S.: The localization of copper in the pericanalicular granules (lysosomes) of liver in Wilson's disease (hepatolenticular degeneration). *Amer. J. Path.* **46:**977-983, 1965.
9. Schaffner, F.; Sternlieb, I.; Barka, T. and Popper, H.: Hepatocellular changes in Wilson's disease. Histochemical and electron microscopic studies. *Amer. J. Path.* **41:**315-327, 1962.
10. Angulo, A. G.; Trevino, N.; Perches, A. and Zavala, B. J.: Wilson's disease, an electron microscope study. *Bol. Inst. Estud. méd. biol.* (Mex.), **23:**155-168, 1965.
11. Navarro, F. and Oliva, H.: Microscopia electronica del higado en el sindrome posthepatitis y en la cirrosis de Wilson. *Rev. esp. Enferm. Apar. dig.* (Madrid), **24:**3-10, 1965.
12. Julien, C.; Caroli, J.; Pépin, B; Boudin, G.; Valla, A.; Morin, P. and Pousset, J. L.: Cirrhose splénomégalique chez un homme de 26 ans: Dégénérescence hépato-lenticulaire à expression splanchnique pure. *Bull. Soc. Méd. Paris,* **116:** 847-858, 1965.
13. Novikoff, A. B. and Essner, E.: The liver cell; some new approaches to its study. *Amer. J. Med.,* **29:**102-131, 1960.
14. Popper, H.; Paronetto, F.; Schaffner, F. and Perez, V.: Studies on hepatic fibrosis. *Lab. Invest.,* **10:**265-290, 1961.
15. Phillips, M. J. and Steiner, J. W.: Electron miscroscopical studies on the liver cells in hyperplastic nodules of human cirrhosis. *Rev. int. Hépat.* (Paris), **16:**307-321, 1966.
16. Schnack, H.; Stockinger, L. and Wewalka, F.: Die Bindegewebszellen des Disse'schen Raumes in der menschlichen Leber bei Normalfällen und pathologischen Zuständen. *Wien. Klin. Wschr.* **78:**715-724, 1966.
17. Bronfenmayer, S.; Schaffner, F. and Popper, H.: Fat-storing cells (lipocytes) in human liver. *Arch. Path.* **82:**447-453, 1966.

# Hemolytic Anemia in Wilson's Disease

Sheila Sherlock, M.D.*; Neil McIntyre, M.D.**; Hugh M. Clink, M.B.***; A. Jonathan Levi, M.B.† and John N. Cumings, M.D.‡

Three patients with Wilson's disease were studied. Each presented evidence of acute hemolytic episodes during which large amounts of copper were excreted in the urine. Hematologic investigations and copper studies are discussed.

Jaundice is a common presentation of Wilson's disease and may precede the neurologic features by many years. Infectious hepatitis is commonly invoked to explain this initial episode and Wilson's disease is rarely considered at that time. Subsequent neurologic symptoms may lead to a correct diagnosis for such features as jaundice and ascites are attributed in retrospect to the cirrhosis of Wilson's disease. Following this initial episode no further features suggesting hepatic involvement may appear despite neurologic abnormalities of many years duration. It seems possible that some of these episodes of jaundice might be hemolytic in nature. This has already been suggested in 1934 by Sjövall and Wallgren,[1] in 1947 by Brinton[2] and in 1954 by Cartwright and coworkers,[3] in 1959 by Scheinberg and Sternlieb[4] and by Grüter,[5] in 1962 by Walshe[6] and in 1965 by Carr-Saunders and Laurance.[7] In most of these cases the diagnosis of Wilson's disease was made after the hemolytic episode had subsided. The present three patients are described in whom hemolysis appeared or continued after the diagnosis of hepatolenticular degeneration had been made. Hematologic investigations and copper studies are discussed.

### Case 1

In August 1964 this child of 12 developed a hemolytic jaundice marked by abdominal pain, dark urine and normal colored stools. Transient ascites was controlled with diuretics. Jaundice faded and hemoglobin rose. In February 1965 recurrence of jaundice and ascites led to transfer to the Royal Free Hospital where a diagnosis of Wilson's disease was made by finding Kayser-Fleischer rings and hepatosplenomegaly. An erythrocyte survival was started and during this time the hemoglobin level fell and the reticulocyte count rose to 18%. Serum bilirubin also increased and alkaline phosphatase values fell. Chromium-51 erythrocyte survival was seven days; whole blood loss in the stools was insignificant.

During the hemolytic episode the serum copper was in the normal range, well above the level found in Wilson's disease. Urinary copper was also well above that seen later even when penicillamine was being given. The serum ceruloplasmin value was reduced.

*Professor of Medicine, Department of Medicine, Royal Free Hospital, London, England.

**Lecturer in Medicine, Department of Medicine, Royal Free Hospital, London, England.

***Lecturer in Hematology, Department of Hematology, Royal Free Hospital, London, England.

†Formerly Lecturer in Medicine, Department of Medicine, Royal Free Hospital, London, England.

‡Professor of Chemical Pathology, Institute of Neurology, London, England.

### ABOUT THE SENIOR AUTHOR

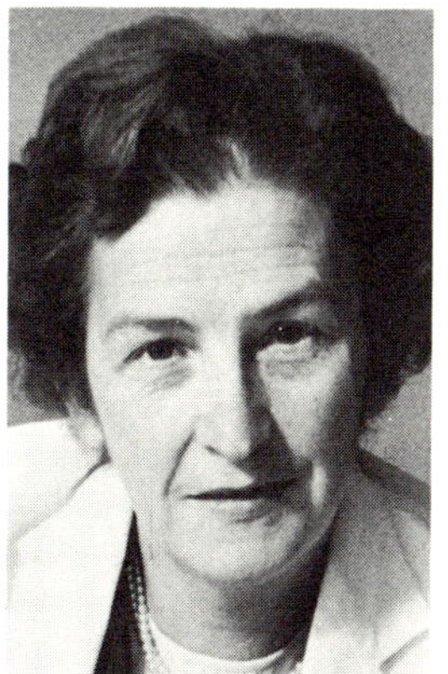

Dr. Sheila Sherlock is Professor of Medicine and Chairman of the Department of Medicine at the Royal Free Hospital School of Medicine (University of London). She received her M.D. from the University of Edinburgh and subsequently trained in Edinburgh and in the Department of Physiological Chemistry, Yale University. For many years she was on the staff of the Royal Postgraduate Medical School, University of London. Her interests are in liver structure and function.

### Case 2

In 1954, this ten-year-old girl had an episode of jaundice with a high proportion of serum unconjugated bilirubin and without bilirubin being detected in the urine. This could have been a hemolytic episode. Later that year Wilson's disease was diagnosed on the basis of finding Kayser-Fleischer rings, hepatosplenomegaly, a serum copper level of 45 μg/100 ml and ceruloplasmin (copper oxidase) of 31 microliter oxygen milliliter per hour. Penicillamine treatment was started. By 1960 Kayser-Fleischer rings had disappeared, liver biopsy showed no histochemical copper and the penicillamine was reduced. In 1965 readmission was necessitated by fever, pallor and jaundice. The hemoglobin was 9.7 g/100 ml; there was 6% reticulocytes and serum alkaline phosphatase was low. During this admission red cell survival was measured and was only four days. The reticulocyte count rose to 24%. At this stage the serum copper was well above that usually found in Wilson's disease. During the hemolytic episode urinary copper excretion was exceedingly high even without penicillamine therapy and reached 6590 μg/24 hours when penicillamine was given. A further mild hemolytic episode was associated with a further increase in urinary copper.

### Case 3

In October, 1965 this nine-year-old boy complained of lower abdominal pain and pallor was noted. A diagnosis of cirrhosis was made on the basis of ascites and hepatosplenomegaly and when Kayser-Fleischer rings were seen, Wilson's disease was confirmed. Hemolysis was marked by a reticulocyte count of 15% and by a reduced cell survival of nine days. The half-life of the transfused cells by the Ashby technic was also very low, (eight days compared with a normal of 50-60 days). Some blood was being lost in the stools but this was too small to account for the reduced red cell life. During hemolysis the serum copper was well above that usually found in Wilson's disease. Erythrocyte copper was also low; ceruloplasmin levels were also low; urinary copper levels were much higher than those usually found in untreated Wilson's disease.

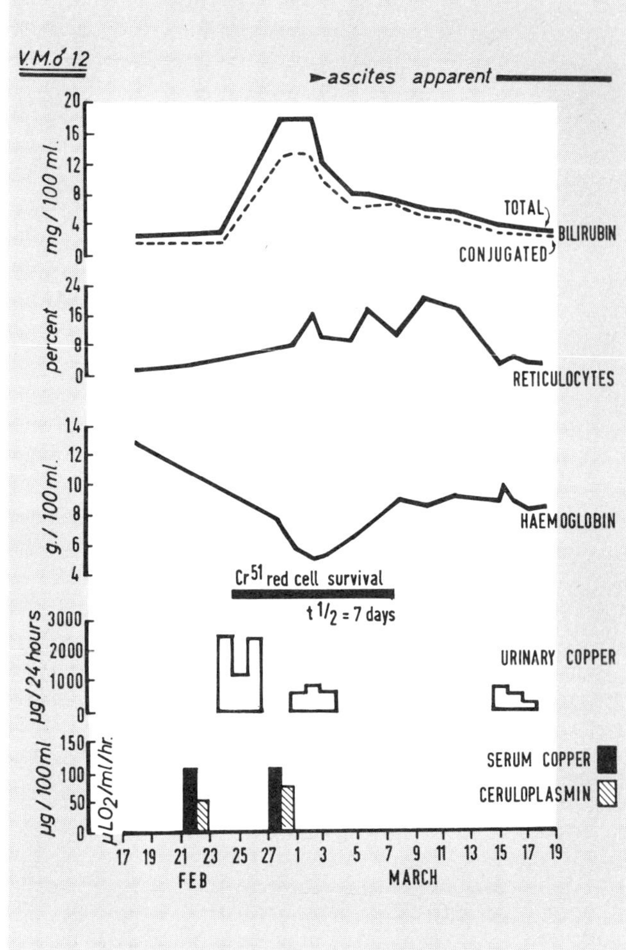


Fig. 1. Hemolytic crisis in Case 1 marked by a rise in total (especially conjugated) serum bilirubin level followed by reticulocytosis and associated with a fall in hemoglobin. The $^{51}$Cr red cell survival was reduced. During the crisis urinary copper was increased, and serum copper was higher than that usually found in Wilson's disease. Ascites developed.

### Discussion

These patients clearly suffered from Wilson's disease. Kayser-Fleischer rings were present, serum ceruloplasmin values were low in two, urinary copper increased in all three, and in two patients liver copper values at autopsy were raised.

Hemolysis was unequivocal; anemia of sudden onset was associated with reticulocytosis and exacerbation of jaundice. Radio chromium half-life of erythrocytes was markedly raised. In two patients, methemalbumin was found in the plasma and haptoglobin levels were low.

In patient three the half-life of transfused red cells was reduced, suggesting that a plasma factor was involved. Cartwright and his colleagues[3] first suggested a relationship between the hemolytic anemia of Wilson's disease and the naturally occurring enzootic jaundice of sheep. In this condition large amounts of hepatic copper accumulate until, for unknown reasons, a large proportion is released into the blood stream. Extensive hemolysis ensues with jaundice and often death from renal impairment associated with hemoglobinuria. The animal may survive the initial attack and suffer several further episodes. Similar conditions have been described in sheep and to a lesser extent in cattle during chronic ingestion of excess copper either accidental or experimental. Rabbits and rats also accumulate copper in the liver but the hemolytic crisis is not a feature of chronic copper poisoning in these animals.[8] In all three patients urinary copper was strikingly elevated above the range usually found in untreated Wilson's disease. In two cases it fell considerably following the initial hemolysis despite the use of penicillamine. These observations suggested that a flux of copper occurred during the period of hemolysis which was not due to hemolysis *per se*. Urinary copper excretion was not strikingly increased during a hemolytic episode in three subjects without Wilson's disease. Furthermore, a calculation of the volume of red cells which would have to have been broken down daily to provide the amount

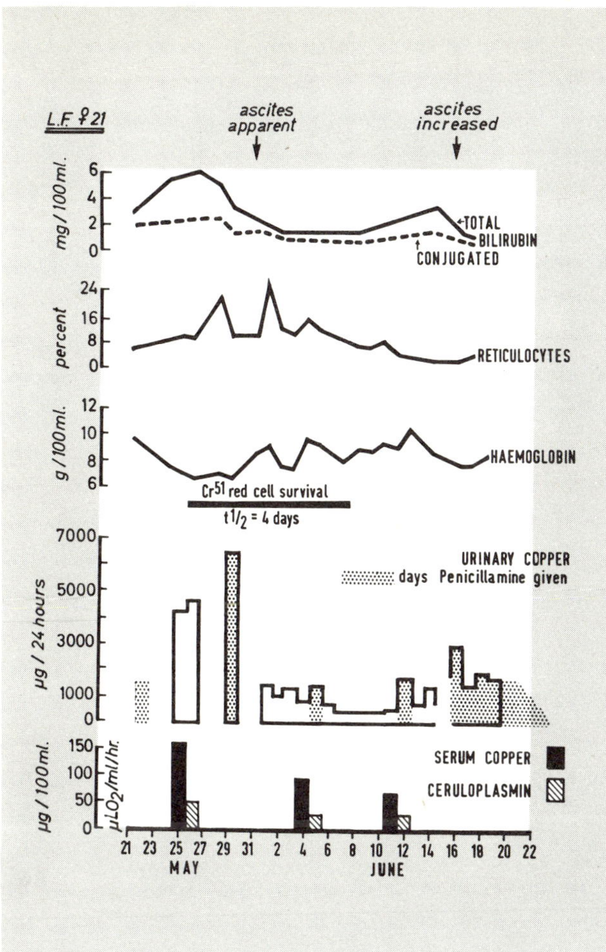


Fig. 2. Hemolytic crisis in Case 2 on admission, marked by a rise in serum (mainly unconjugated) bilirubin and followed by reticulocytosis. The hemoglobin fell and red cell survival was reduced. Urinary copper was very high even without the administration of penicillamine. Serum copper was higher than that usually found in Wilson's disease. Ascites developed. The second episode of hemolysis, which was noted in June, was marked by a slight rise in serum bilirubin and a fall in hemoglobin.

of urinary copper passed by patient three in whom red cell copper was measured during hemolysis, gives results incompatible with his red cell survival figures. The excess copper was probably released from the tissues into the blood. Plasma copper levels were in fact higher than those which would be expected in Wilson's disease and in patients one and three were even above the upper limit of normal. Levels might have been even higher earlier in the episode, as in the experimental hemolysis induced in sheep by chronic copper poisoning, the maximum blood copper level was found at, or within 24 hours of, the appearance of clinical manifestations and thereafter the levels fell quite rapidly. The free copper in the blood was not measured but in patients one and two the plasma copper levels were disproportionately high in relation to the ceruloplasmin level. The high free copper level in the ascitic fluid in patient three also suggests the free copper in the blood was raised. In human acute copper poisoning the severity of the hemolysis correlates better with the copper content of the whole blood than with the serum value. The rise in serum ionic copper is very transient suggesting that the copper moved rapidly into the red blood cells. This is in accord with the experimental results of Gubler *et al*[9] who gave large doses of copper to dogs and demonstrated a very rapid transfer of ionic copper from the plasma into the red cells. In one animal, two hours after the ingestion of copper sulfate, 89% of the blood copper was found in the erythrocytes and only 11% in the plasma. In only one of our patients was the red cell copper measured during an episode of hemolysis, and on two separate occasions it was well above normal. Patients with Wilson's disease normally have no elevation of red cell copper values. Patient two had a normal value when not hemolyzing.

Lambin *et al*[10] showed that ionic copper in low concentration could cause hemolysis of red cells and they suggested that the copper was bound superficially to red cells, probably as a copper protein complex. Their results were confirmed causing hemolysis in a concentration of 75 $\mu$/100 ml in chicken, rabbit and human erythrocytes (Goldberg *et al*).[11] The exact mechanism is not understood. Stein showed that the copper is bound by a N-terminal histidine molecule in the red cell membrane and speculated that this was part of the facilitated transfer system for glycerol. Copper is known to inhibit the transfer of glycerol into erythrocytes. Copper might lower the level of reduced glutathione in the erythrocytes. Todd and Thompson found very low levels of erythrocyte glutathione at the onset of hemolysis in sheep and speculated that this was directly related to the hemolytic process.[12] In the light of these veterinary and experimental studies the hemolytic anemia found in Wilson's disease appears to be of similar type to that found in sheep and cattle chronically intoxicated with copper. Large tissue stores of copper are known to exist in hepatolenticular degeneration, particularly in the liver, and the very high urinary copper excretion at the time of hemolysis in our patients supports the hypothesis that there is a sudden release of copper into the blood with subsequent hemolysis.

In patients one and three the hemolytic episode was initially confused with hepatocellular failure. All three developed ascites at this time which added to the difficulties in diagnosis. Knowledge that hemolytic jaundice is often a presenting feature may lead to an earlier diagnosis and treatment of Wilson's disease and recognition in siblings. Early diagnosis of hemolysis may also permit further study of the hemolytic process at a time when such study is likely to be rewarding.

## Summary

Three patients with Wilson's disease presented evidence of acute hemolytic episodes. During these attacks large amounts of copper were excreted in the urine. The mechanism of production of the hemolysis has been considered. The sudden release of copper from the tissues into the blood with resulting hemolysis of red cells, a mechanism analogous to that of enzootic jaundice in sheep, is considered to be the most likely explanation.

## REFERENCES


1. Sjövall, E. and Wallgren, A.: Some aspects of hepatolenticular degeneration and its pathogenesis. *Acta psychiat.* **9**:435, 1934.
2. Brinton, D.: Wilson's disease. *Proc. roy. Soc. Med.* **40:**556, 1947.
3. Cartwright, G. E.; Hodges, R. E.; Gubler, C. J.; Mahoney, J. P.; Daum, K.; Wintrobe, M. M. and Bean, W. B.: Studies on copper metabolism. XIII Hepatolenticular degeneration. *J. clin. Invest.* **33:**1487, 1954.
4. Scheinberg, I. H. and Sternlieb, I.: Liver in Wilson's disease. *Gastroenterology* **37:**550, 1959.
5. Grüter, W.: Hämolytische Krisen als Frumanifestation der Wilsonschen Krankheit. *Dtsch. Z. Nervenheilk.* **179:**410, 1959.
6. Walshe, J. M.: Wilson's disease: presenting symptoms. *Arch. Dis. Childh.* **37:**253, 1962.
7. Carr-Saunders, E. and Laurance, B. M.: Wilson's disease presenting as acute haemolytic anaemia. *Proc. roy. Soc. Med.* **58:**614, 1965.
8. Marston, H. R.: Cobalt, copper and molybdenum in nutrition of animals and plants. *Physiol. Rev.* **32:**66, 1952.
9. Gubler, C. J.; Lahey, M. E.; Cartwright, G. E. and Wintrobe, M. M.: Studies on copper metabolism. IX. Transportation of copper in blood. *J. clin. Invest.* **32:**405, 1953.
10. Lambin, S.; Bazin, S. and Salas, A.: Action des sels de cuivre sur les erythrocytes. *Ann. Inst. Pasteur,* **81:**572, 1951.
11. Goldberg, A.; Williams, C. B.; Jones, R. S.; Yanagita, M.; Cartwright, G. E. and Wintrobe, M. M.: Studies on copper metabolism. XXII. Haemolytic anaemia in chickens induced by administration of copper. *J. Lab. clin. Med.,* **48:**442, 1956.
12. Todd, J. R. and Thompson, R. H.: Studies on chronic copper poisoning. II. Biochemical studies on blood of sheep during haemolytic crisis. *Brit. vet. J.* **119:**161, 1963.

# Comments

Hans Popper, M.D.*

It has been customary to describe characteristic histologic features in liver disease as an indication of a specific etiology. This holds true for both conventional and electron microscopy. But with additional experience, with either technic, it became clear that one such feature, or even a combination of features, is not specific for any one etiology. For instance, the histologic picture that originally was considered specific for viral hepatitis is also produced by certain drugs. And, of particular relevance to the subject of this symposium, our group was misled in concluding that abundant ballooned hepatic nuclei containing glycogen are — in the absence of diabetes mellitus — a strongly suggestive indication of Wilson's disease. We subsequently learned that such nuclei very frequently occur, even in the livers of normal adolescents. They may, therefore, be a reflection of the age of the patient rather than of Wilson's disease. Although they very frequently are seen in this disorder, we wish to correct the previous implication of ours that they are rather specific.[1] Incidentally, another example of a nonspecific finding is excess of pigment in youth, without wasting, which is not diagnostic for Wilson's disease.

Doctor Shikata's discussion[2] of the evolution of the hepatic lesion in Wilson's disease, a possible role of the kidney in this evolution and a type of cirrhosis rich in copper but different from Wilson's disease, analogous to cirrhosis rich in iron yet different from hemochromatosis, is very interesting. He postulates that the injured kidney may produce hepatic necrosis by inducing protein deficiency as a consequence of aminoaciduria or albuminuria. He has shown that a low protein diet may lead to necrosis progressing to perilobular fibrosis, both of which can be prevented by methionine administration. Protein deficiency may indeed be a causal factor in the hepatic lesion in Wilson's disease, but, since a kidney lesion or a deficient diet complicated the hypoproteinemia of Doctor Shikata's animals, it may be interesting to attempt to produce necrosis in copper-laden animals by simple plasmapheresis which represents a less complicated protein deficiency.

We have seen the acute form of Wilson's disease with submassive necrosis, develop very rapidly — in a few weeks — comparable to the so-called florid cirrhosis of alcoholics. We have in our file five cases of this acute type of Wilson's disease which we designate as a subacute hepatitis. The histologic picture, though somewhat unusual, is again not specific, resembling subacute alcoholic hepatitis and postnecrotic cirrhosis. Extensive, primary collapse of normal parenchyma, with previously intact lobular architecture, and secondary collapse of previously nodular cirrhotic parenchyma can both be seen. In addition bile stasis was usually conspicuous, but the following distinctive findings were encountered: 1) large pigmented liver cells with fine vacuolization; 2) giant liver cells, containing fat and exhibiting several nuclei; 3) liver cells in pseudoductular arrangement (biliary hepatocytes) without surrounding inflammatory reaction; 4) many segmented leukocytes around liver cells and around proliferated bile ductules; and 5) irregular perinuclear cytoplasmic clumps with an off-color in hematoxylin-eosin sections and a blue color in Mallory's aniline blue stains, showing all the characteristics of the alcoholic hyaline of Mallory. The last two features, particularly, are seen in subacute hepatitis and in florid cirrhosis of alcoholics.

We have not examined this lesion in Wilson's disease under the electron microscope as yet, but in the similar alcoholic lesion mitochondrial injury with prominent giant mitochondria can be demonstrated by fine structural technics. In analogy, one may assume that in this subacute hepatitis of Wilson's disease mitochondrial injury is an important feature and this is in keeping with various experimental observations, particularly of Scheuer and Barka in our laboratory, that copper administration leads to mitochondrial damage.[3]

*Professor and Chairman, Department of Pathology, Mount Sinai Medical School, New York, N. Y.

### *REFERENCES*

1. Anderson, P. and Popper, H.: Changes in hepatic structure in Wilson's disease. *Amer. J. Path.* **36:**483-497, 1960.

2. Shikata, T.: Morphogenesis of liver cirrhosis in Wilson's disease In Birth Defects: Orig. Art. Series, *Wilson's Disease,* The National Foundation, New York, Vol. IV, No. 2, 88-91, April, 1968.

3. Barka, T.; Scheuer, P. J.; Schaffner, F. and Popper, H.: Structural changes of liver cells in copper intoxication. *Arch. Pathol.* **78:**331-349, 1964.

# Renal Lesions in Wilson's Disease

Yawara Yoshitoshi, M.D.*; Toshitsugu Oda, M.D.**; Yoshiji Yamane, M.D.**; Mitsumasa Nagase, M.D.**; Kazuo Mori, M.D.** and Toshio Shikata, M.D.***

There were marked morphologic changes found in the proximal convoluted tubules of the kidneys in seven of 18 autopsied patients with Wilson's disease. Functional and morphologic changes similar to those observed in patients, were produced in rats given various combinations of copper, glutathione and penicillamine.

Since amino-aciduria in Wilson's disease was demonstrated by Uzman and Denny-Brown[1] in 1948, there have been several reports on the renal involvement in this disease; renal glycosuria,[2,3,4] phosphaturia[2,4] and slight proteinuria,[2,3] have been ascribed to renal dysfunction caused chiefly by pathologic involvement of proximal convoluted tubules. However, the morphologic changes in the kidneys have been in dispute. Descriptions of glomerular lesions are conflicting and inconclusive.[5] The increased content of copper in the kidney,[3] localized histochemically in the proximal tubules,[6] may account for the tubular dysfunction observed in this disease.

The purpose of the present paper is 1) to study the morphologic changes in the kidneys of patients with Wilson's disease at autopsy and 2) to attempt to reproduce such changes experimentally by copper-induced intoxication in the rat.

**Materials and Methods**

*1. Autopsy material*

Eighteen cases with Wilson's disease autopsied in the Department of Pathology, University of Tokyo, during 1957-1965 were studied. Ten patients suffered from the cerebral type (seven males and three females) seven from the abdominal type (four males and three females) and one was asymptomatic. The age at death ranged from seven to 33 in the cerebral type, six to 12 in the abdominal type and five in the asymptomatic type.

Five patients with fulminant hepatitis and postnecrotic cirrhosis were studied as controls.

*Professor, First Department of Internal Medicine, University of Tokyo, Tokyo, Japan.

**University of Tokyo Faculty of Medicine, Tokyo, Japan.

***Instructor, Department of Pathology, Faculty of Medicine, University of Tokyo, Tokyo, Japan.

The histologic examinations were carried out with the aid of the following stains: hematoxylin and eosin for routine use, Mallory's method for demonstration of fibrous tissue, PAS for identification of the basement membrane, and Sudan III for fat. Histochemical demonstration of copper was done by the method of Okamoto and Utamura[7] using p-dimethyl aminobenzylidine rhodamine.

In one patient treated with a sulfhydryl compound (glutathione), copper content of liver, kidney and brain was determined chemically with sodium diethyldithiocarbamate.[8]

ABOUT THE SENIOR AUTHOR

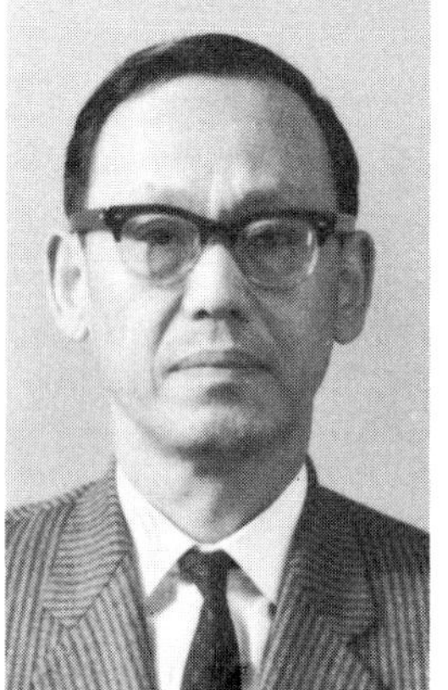

Dr. Yawara Yoshitoshi was born in 1913 and was awarded his M.D. degree in 1938 and D.M.S. degree in 1946, both from the University of Tokyo, Faculty of Medicine. In 1958 he was Associate Professor and since 1962, has been Professor, First Department of Internal Medicine, University of Tokyo.

Dr. Yoshitoshi is a member of the Japanese Society of Internal Medicine, Japanese Society of Nephrology, Japanese Society of Hepatology and the Japanese Society of Clinical Biochemistry and Metabolism.

*2. Experimental copper intoxication of rats*

Male Wistar rats, weighing about 200 g were divided into three groups, which were treated for three months as follows: 1) 0.1% solution of copper acetate put into water given *ad libitum,* 2) 4 mg/100 g body weight of glutathione daily injected intraperitoneally in addition to 1) and 3) 4 mg/100 g body weight of penicillamine orally given daily in addition to 1).

In another series of experiments, rats were similarly divided into three groups and each was treated for 40 days with 1) 0.2% solution of copper acetate given *ad libitum* and 0.2% solution of copper acetate daily injected subcutaneously, 2) glutathione 10 mg/100 g body weight intraperitoneally daily administered in addition to 1), and 3) probenecid 8 mg/100 g body weight per day, orally, in addition to 2). Total amino-nitrogen and amino acids were measured in 24-hour collections of urine obtained prior to and during the experiments.

Tissues for histologic examination were processed like the human autopsy material. Additional specimens were fixed with osmium tetroxide and embedded in Epon for electron microscopic examination.

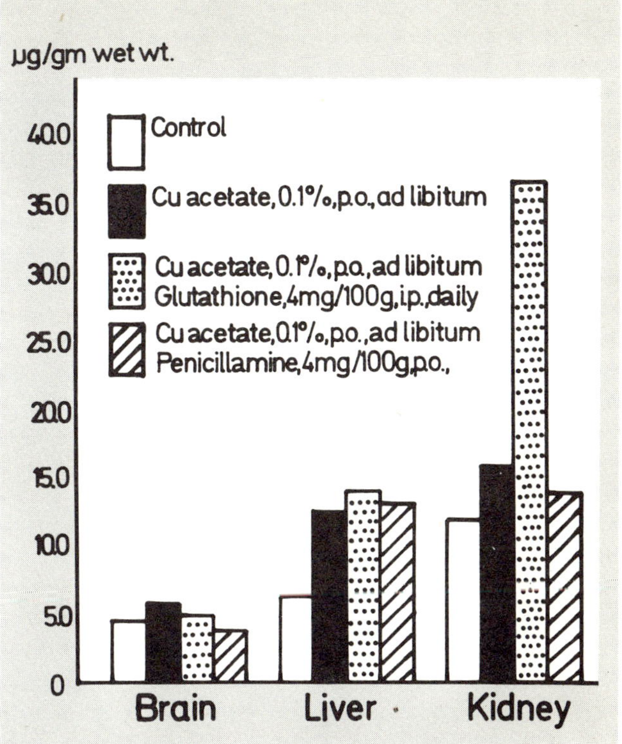


Fig. 1. Copper content of three organs following 3 months' administration of copper acetate with and without sulfhydryl compounds to rats.

## Results

*1. Autopsy material from patients with Wilson's disease*

Marked fat deposition in the proximal convoluted tubules was demonstrated with Sudan III staining, fatty

**TABLE I**

**FREE AMINO ACID PATTERNS IN URINE[1]**

| | Control | GSH[2] | GSH+Pr[3] | Cu[4] | Cu+GSH[5] | Cu+GSH+Pr[6] |
|---|---|---|---|---|---|---|
| No. of Rats | 6 | 4 | 4 | 4 | 4 | 4 |
| Asp | 1.1 | 2.1 | 0.9 | 0.9 | 4.6 | 3.2 |
| Glu | 7.6 | 12.3 | 3.5 | 2.8 | 12.6 | 23.4 |
| Thr | 1.5 | 3.6 | 1.6 | 0.5 | 1.1 | 2.7 |
| Ser | 0.4 | 3.5 | 1.6 | 2.4 | 3.9 | 5.2 |
| Glu•$NH_2$ | 1.1 | 19.3 | 7.1 | 1.9 | 3.6 | 12.5 |
| Pro | trace | trace | trace | trace | trace | trace |
| Asp•$NH_2$ | 0.6 | 0.7 | 0.4 | 22.4 | 21.2 | 32.3 |
| Ala | 5.2 | 12.4 | 7.3 | 2.1 | 5.3 | 1.2 |
| Gly | 5.0 | 14.8 | 17.5 | 15.2 | 12.5 | 21.5 |
| Cys | 3.4 | 4.5 | 1.7 | 11.0 | 4.9 | 6.3 |
| Val, Met[7] Leu, Ileu | 0.6 | 1.3 | 1.3 | 0.8 | 0.6 | 1.3 |
| Phe | 1.8 | 3.3 | 2.0 | 1.4 | 2.2 | 1.9 |
| Lys | 1.6 | 4.0 | 1.9 | 1.1 | 1.6 | 2.2 |
| His | 2.7 | 6.4 | 2.2 | 3.3 | 6.6 | 8.7 |
| Tyr | 0.6 | 4.6 | 1.2 | 2.0 | 1.0 | 1.3 |
| Total $\alpha$-Amino-Nitrogen (mg/day) | 1.10 | 1.47 | 2.25 | 1.51 | 1.60 | 2.39 |

1. Values ($\mu$ moles/day) are the mean of 4 to 6 rats.
2. Glutathione, 10mg/100g i.p., single dose.
3. GSH + Probenecid, 8mg/100mg p.o., single dose.
4. Cu — acetate, 0.1% p.o., 3 months.
5. Cu + Glutathione, 10mg/100g i.p., daily.
6. Cu + GSH + Probenecid, 8mg/100 g p.o., daily.
7. The values of these amino acids estimated as Valine.

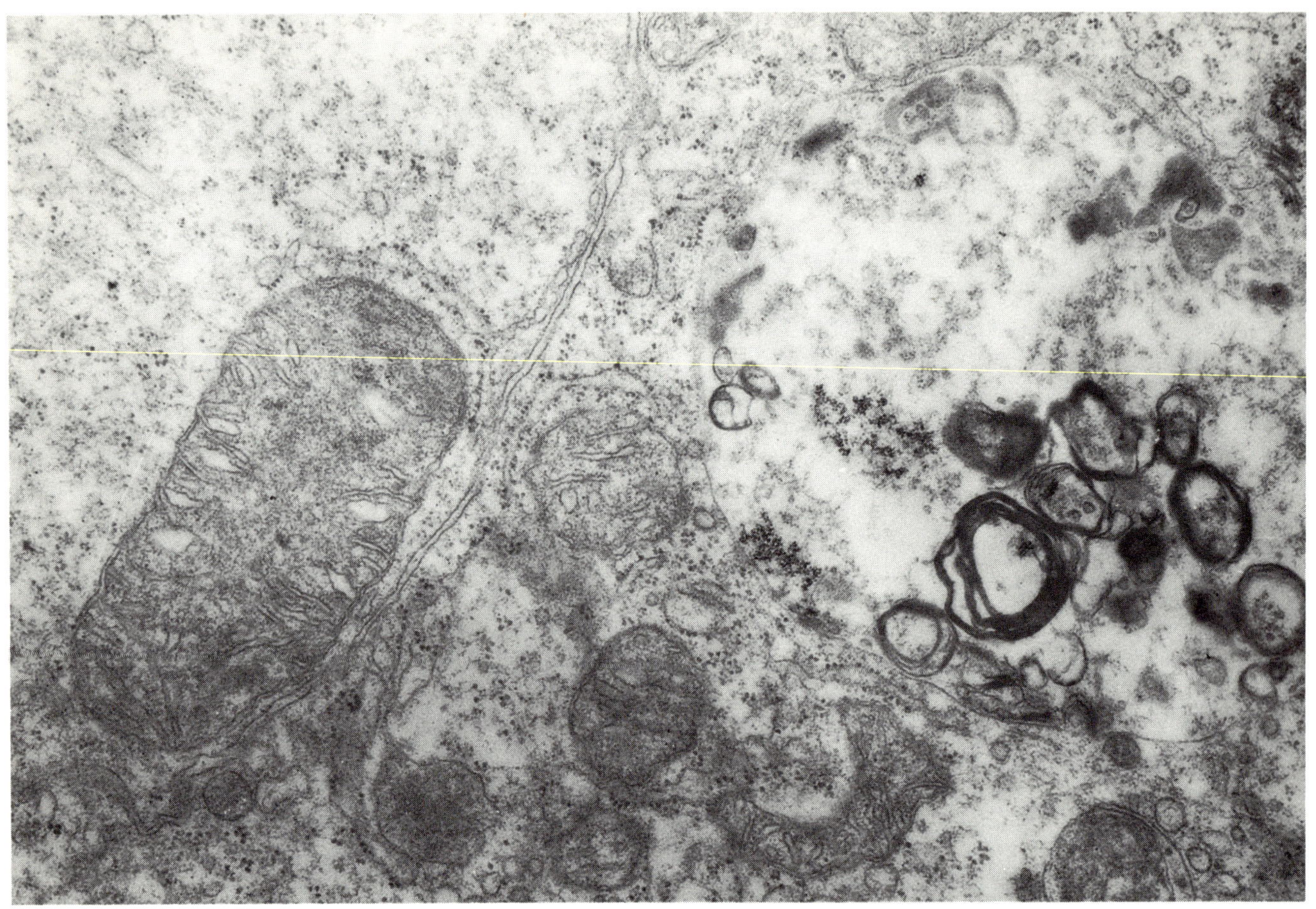

Fig. 2. Renal proximal tubular cells of rat following administration of copper, showing lamellar, lipid structures in lysosomes. Osmium tetroxide in phosphate buffer (pH 7.4) fixation; Epon; uranyl acetate and lead nitrate x 10,500; Japan Electronoptics, Type C.

droplets being visible even on hematoxylin and eosin staining in the cases of the abdominal type. In addition, some of the proximal tubules showed hydropic changes, while none were seen in the distal tubules. No abnormalities were found in the cases of the cerebral type, except in one patient, treated with glutathione, whose proximal tubules showed slight fatty and hydropic changes. Glomerular capillaries and mesangial cells were not thickened and no hypercellularity was noted in the glomeruli. The copper content of the kidney in this case was markedly increased (251.5 mcg/g wet weight) while that in the liver was only moderately increased (49.1 mcg/g wet weight).

Histochemical study revealed copper granules in the cytoplasm and occasionally in the nuclei of the proximal epithelial cells, but none in the glomeruli.

Similar changes to those observed in the abdominal type of Wilson's disease were seen in the kidneys of patients with fulminant hepatitis or postnecrotic cirrhosis though they appeared less pronounced. In addition, however, the control kidneys contained bilirubin casts or droplets within the epithelial cells, which suggested presence of bilirubin which could have caused these changes.

*2. Experiments with rats*

The kidneys of rats treated with both copper and glutathione for three months contained more copper than those of the other groups to which copper alone or copper and penicillamine were given (Fig. 1); these findings are similar to the result observed in the patient treated with glutathione.

Electron microscopic study of the kidneys revealed loss of cristae and vacuolization of mitochondria, and lamellar structures of lipoid in the proximal tubular cells (Figs. 2, 3).

In the experiment designed to investigate the effect of probenecid, renal copper content was about twice that of animals treated with glutathione.

In the short-term experiment lasting for 40 days, copper content of kidneys in the glutathione-treated group of rats was not as high as that in the long-term experiment (Fig. 4).

Paper chromatography of rat urine revealed slightly increased total amino-nitrogen in rats given copper alone and in those receiving copper and glutathione. Probenecid increased the excretion of amino-nitrogen,

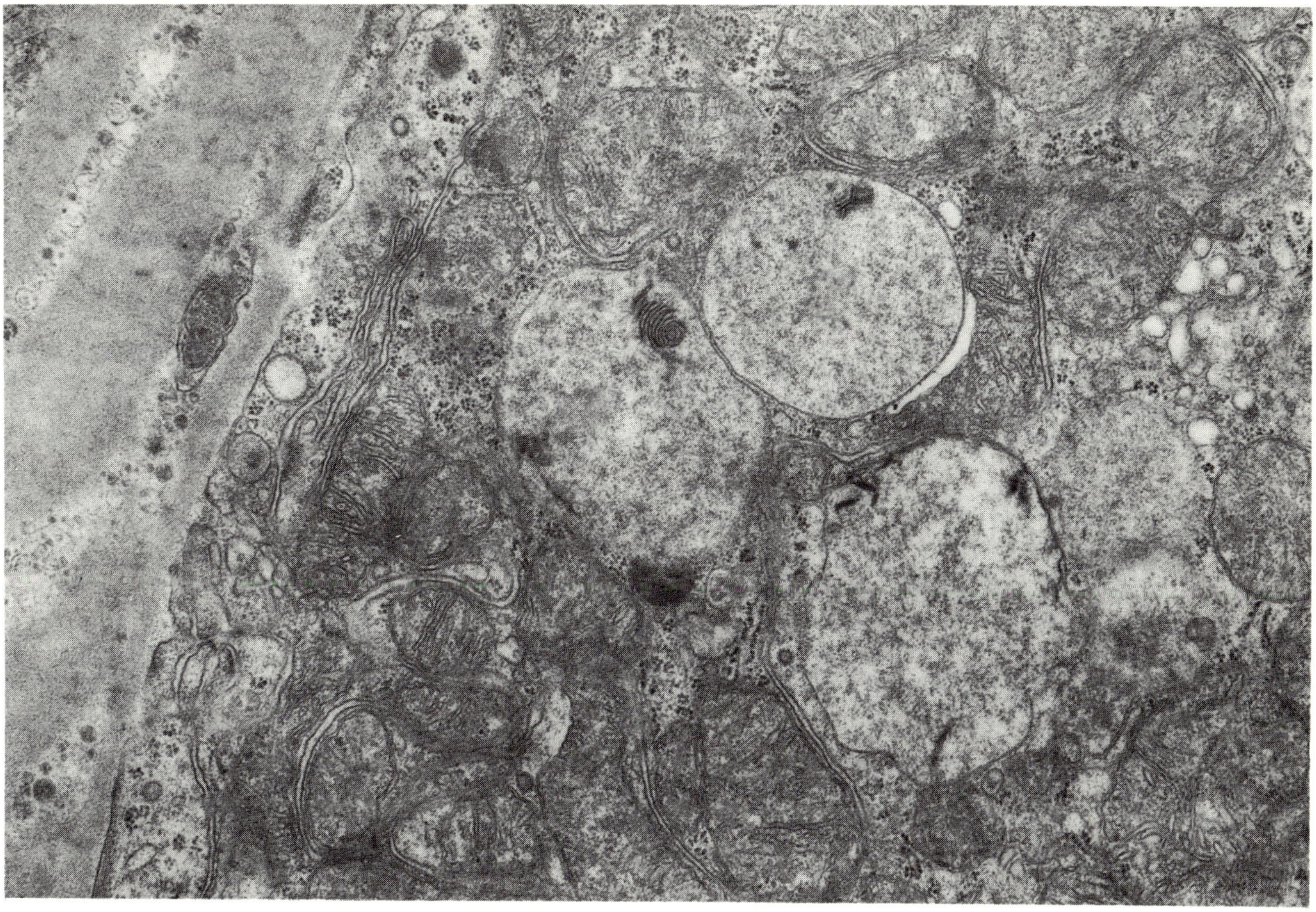

Fig. 3. Renal proximal tubular cell of rat following administration of copper, showing loss of cristae and vacuolization of mitochondria (x 10,500).

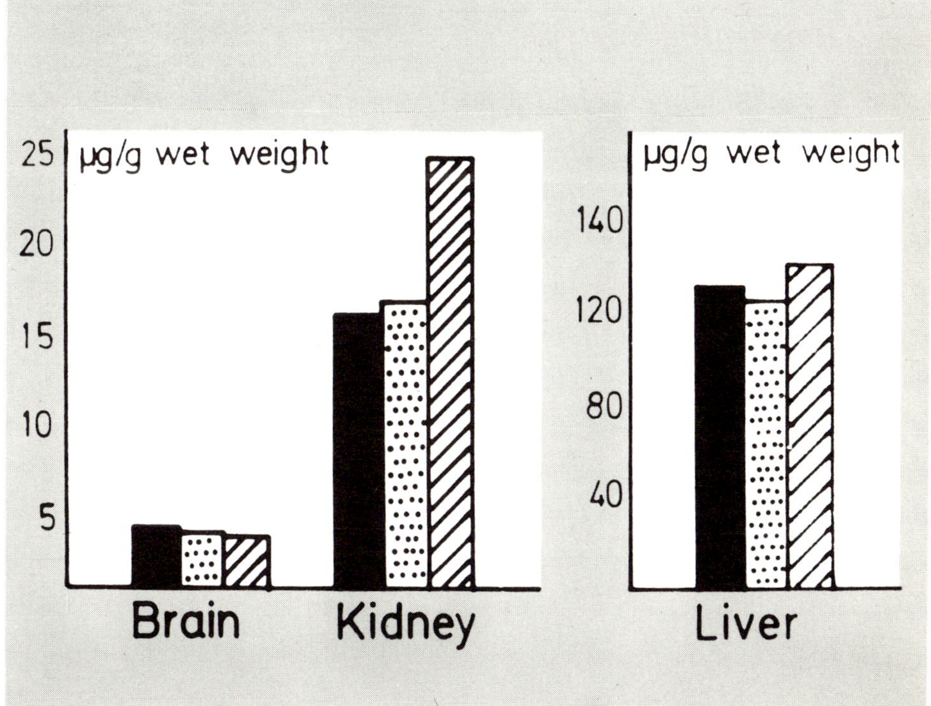


Fig. 4. Copper content of three organs following administration of copper acetate, sulfhydryl compounds and probenecid to rats. Solid bars, copper acetate, 0.2% p.o. and 1mg/100g s.c. daily for 40 days; stippled bars, copper acetate and glutathione, 10mg/100g i.p., daily; striped bars, copper acetate, glutathione and probenecid, 8mg/100g, daily.

presumably due to a diminished reabsorption by the renal tubules. Excretion of asparagine, glycine and cysteine was increased in rats given copper (Table I).

### Discussion

Other abnormalities of renal function have become apparent after amino-aciduria was discovered in patients suffering from Wilson's disease.[1] Diminished renal blood flow and lowered glomerular filtration rate have been reported,[2] as well as renal glycosuria. Some of these abnormalities resemble chronic heavy metal intoxication of renal tubules with dysfunction. Dallenbach[9] demonstrated diminished secretion of phenol red and absorption of trypan blue by epithelial cells of proximal renal tubules following chronic lead intoxication. Wolff[6] related the tubular dysfunction observed in Wilson's disease to the deposition of copper. It is therefore of interest that cystinuria, which is frequently encountered in this disease was also observed in the animals poisoned with copper.

A comparison of the effects of two sulfhydryl containing compounds, glutathione and penicillamine, was attempted. There was less copper excreted into the urine following administration of the former although surprisingly, the kidneys of glutathione treated rats contained more copper than those of the other groups, both chemically and histochemically. These findings suggest that copper chelated with glutathione may be trapped in the proximal renal tubules. Because of its inhibitory effect on tubular reabsorption, probenecid was administered in addition to copper and glutathione with the expectation that copper excretion would increase. Surprisingly, however, copper deposits in the kidneys were increased further. Since these observations are inconclusive, further investigation of the role of glutathione is required.

Light microscopy revealed lesions in the proximal renal tubules including deposition of fat and copper and hydropic degeneration. Similar hydropic degeneration was present in the kidneys of patients with fulminant hepatitis, presumably secondary to accumulation of bilirubin. From these observations, it is likely to assume that copper, when present in excess in the cells, by combining with sulfhydryl containing enzymes of mitochondria, may damage the oxidation-reduction system, resulting in dysfunction of proximal tubules. This hypothesis, however, is not yet proven.

### Summary

We investigated 1) the role of copper in the renal lesions of Wilson's disease and 2) the effect of SH-compounds on copper excretion. Histologic study of kidneys from 18 autopsy cases with Wilson's disease showed marked deposition of fat and hydropic changes in proximal convoluted tubules in cases of abdominal type while in patients with the cerebral type none of these abnormalities were encountered. Copper deposits in the proximal tubules were seen in one case with the cerebral type, treated with glutathione.

In parallel experiments the effects of copper, penicillamine and glutathione on the kidneys of rats were studied. Long-term oral administration of copper and glutathione produced lesions similar to those seen in the proximal renal tubules of patients. Copper deposition was not decreased by administration of probenecid. Excretion of total amino-nitrogen, asparagine, glycine and cysteine in the urine of copper-intoxicated rats was increased.

## REFERENCES

1. Uzman, L. and Denny-Brown, D.: Aminoaciduria in hepatolenticular degeneration (Wilson's disease). *Amer. J. med. Sci.* **215:**599, 1948.
2. Bearn, A. G.; Yü, T. F. and Gutman, A. B.: Renal function in Wilson's disease. *J. clin. Invest.* **36:**1107, 1957.
3. Bickel, H.; Neale, G. C. and Hall, G.: A clinical and biochemical study of hepatolenticular degeneration (Wilson's disease). *Quart. J. Med.* **26:**527, 1957.
4. Morgan, H. G.; Stewart, W. K.; Lome, K. G.; Stomers, J. M. and Johnstone, J. H.: Wilson's disease and the Fanconi syndrome. *Quart. J. Med.* **31:**361, 1962.
5. Reynolds, E. S.; Tannen, R. L. and Tyler, H. R.: The renal lesion in Wilson's disease. *Amer. J. Med.* **40:**518, 1966.
6. Wolff, S. M.: Renal lesions in Wilson's disease. *Lancet* **i:**843, 1964.
7. Okamoto, K. and Utamura, M.: Biologische Untersuchungen des Kupfers. *Acta Sch. med. Univ. Kyoto* **20:**573, 1937.
8. Lahey, M. D.; Gubler, C. J.; Chase, M. S.; Cartwright, G. E. and Wintrobe, M. M.: Studies on copper metabolism. II. Hematologic manifestations of copper deficiency in swine. *Blood* **7:**1053, 1952.
9. Dallenbach, F. D.: Phenolrotausscheidung und Trypanblauausscheidung bei der Blei-Nephropathie der Ratte. *Arch. path. Anat.* **338:**91, 1964.

# Calcium Studies in Wilson's Disease*

Venard R. Kinney, M.D.**; Raymond V. Randall, M.D.***; John W. Rosevear, M.D., Ph.D.†; W. Newlon Tauxe, M.D.‡ and Norman P. Goldstein, M.D.§

Forty-eight studies were performed on ten patients. Calcium-balance studies were performed with individual periods being delineated by a carmine marker. Radiocalcium absorptive studies were performed using calcium-47. In patients with hypercalciuria, oral radiotracer studies revealed hyperabsorption. D-penicillamine did not affect the intestinal efficiency of calcium absorption. The urinary calcium of patients with hypercalciuria was diminished in response to a low calcium diet. Concurrent balance and radiotracer studies revealed absorption efficiencies which correlated to a significant degree, although they were not quantitatively equal.

Abnormalities of calcium homeostasis thus far reported in patients with Wilson's disease (hepatolenticular degeneration) include hypercalciuria,[1] nephrolithiasis,[1] osteomalacia,[2] and osteoporosis.[3] Some of these abnormalities may be explained by the renal tubular dysfunction which is demonstrable in some patients with Wilson's disease,[2] but a definite relationship between the renal abnormalities and hypercalciuria has not been established. Although both osteoporosis and hypercalciuria have been mentioned in the literature, the reported data are not sufficient to implicate the increased renal excretion of calcium as a definite etiologic factor in the bone disorder. Of the 15 patients with Wilson's disease whom we have studied,[4] nine have had hypercalciuria. One of the nine patients had a solitary renal stone and another had bilateral nephrocalcinosis and a history of renal stones. One of the patients without hypercalciuria also had a renal stone. None of the patients had evidence of skeletal demineralization on roentgenographic survey.

The purpose of the present investigation was to evaluate whether increased intestinal absorption of calcium is a significant causative factor of hypercalciuria.

Because fecal material contains both unabsorbed dietary calcium and endogenous calcium of gastrointestinal origin, conventional balance studies measure not the intestinal absorptive efficiency for calcium but the net result of both of these processes. As we have previously described,[5] a radioisotopic tracer study (with $^{47}Ca$) reflects actual intestinal absorptive efficiency for calcium. Ten of the previously mentioned 15 patients with Wilson's disease were evaluated by means of the oral radiocalcium method to determine absorptive efficiency. One of these ten patients had a stone in the left kidney.

## Methods

The diagnosis of Wilson's disease in each of the ten patients was established by the usual clinical and neurologic manifestations and by the presence of Kayser-Fleischer rings and hypercupriuria. Six of the patients had clinical or laboratory evidence of the hepatic disease, although none had evidence of significant hepatic insufficiency during the present studies. Each patient had been treated with D-penicillamine; however, determinations to evaluate hypercalciuria were done before treatment with penicillamine had been started or at a time when it was temporarily suspended. Fifty-two studies were performed on these ten patients during a three-

*This investigation was supported in part by Research Grants AM-6908 and NB-3655 from the National Institutes of Health, Public Health Service.

**Consultant, Section of Medicine, Mayo Clinic; Instructor in Medicine, Mayo Graduate School of Medicine (University of Minnesota), Rochester, Minnesota.

***Consultant, Section of Medicine, Mayo Clinic; Associate Professor of Medicine, Mayo Graduate School of Medicine (University of Minnesota), Rochester, Minnesota.

†Consultant, Section of Biochemistry, Mayo Clinic; Assistant Professor of Biochemistry, Mayo Graduate School of Medicine (University of Minnesota), Rochester, Minnesota.

‡Consultant, Section of Clinical Pathology, Mayo Clinic; Associate Professor of Clinical Pathology, Mayo Graduate School of Medicine (University of Minnesota), Rochester, Minnesota.

§Consultant, Section of Neurology, Mayo Clinic; Professor of Neurology, Mayo Graduate School of Medicine (University of Minnesota), Rochester, Minnesota.

year period. Nine of these patients had 43 oral radiocalcium studies performed while they were in a hospital metabolic unit and were consuming diets similar to those followed at home (containing the same amounts of calcium or isocaloric diets containing different amounts of calcium). One patient had four studies performed while he was consuming his regular diet and one additional study performed while he was in the metabolic unit. Studies were performed without additional medication and also while the patients were taking D-penicillamine. Calcium balance periods were from two weeks to two months, with individual periods being delineated by carmine markers. Four of the ten patients also were studied by whole-body counting after intravenous administration of radiocalcium tracer to provide an independent measurement of fecal and urinary losses of radiocalcium.

## ABOUT THE SENIOR AUTHOR

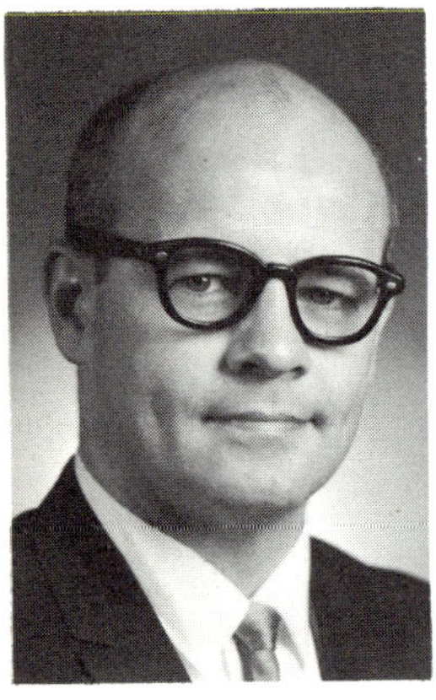

Dr. Venard R. Kinney, a consultant in medicine at the Mayo Clinic, Rochester, Minnesota, from 1962 to 1967, and instructor in Medicine in the Mayo Graduate School of Medicine of the University of Minnesota at Rochester from 1963 until June, 1967, was born in Yonkers, New York, in 1931. He received the degree of bachelor of science *summa cum laude* in chemistry from Iona College in 1953, and the degree of doctor of medicine from New York Medical College in 1957.

Dr. Kinney came to Rochester, Minnesota, on October 1, 1958, as a fellow in medicine of the Mayo Graduate School of Medicine. In 1959, with his colleagues, he was the recipient of a grant for research in physiology from the National Institutes of Health. In 1961 he received the Herschel V. Jones Award for superior ability in medical science as a fellow of the Mayo Graduate School of Medicine. He was appointed an assistant to the staff of the Mayo Clinic in medicine (gastroenterology) on January 1, 1962, and to the staff of the Mayo Clinic as a consultant in medicine on April 1 of that year. In 1962, also, he received the degree of doctor of philosophy in medicine from the University of Minnesota; the title of his dissertation was "The Mechanism of Chloride Absorption in the Ileum of Dogs." In 1963 he became an instructor in medicine in the Mayo Graduate School of Medicine.

Dr. Kinney has maintained a special interest in the metabolism of electrolytes, and particularly in the absorption of calcium from the intestine. He has contributed to the literature of his specialty.

Dr. Kinney became a diplomate of the National Board of Medical Examiners in 1958. He is an associate of the American College of Physicians and a member of the American Medical Association, the Minnesota State Medical Association, the Zumbro Valley Medical Society, the Society of the Sigma Xi, the Phi Chi professional medical fraternity, the Galen Society, the DaVinci Society, the Tara Knights and the Alumni Association of the Mayo Graduate School of Medicine.

*Procedures.*—The tracer dose of 3 to 6 $\mu c$ of $^{47}CaCl_2$ was given orally after the patient had fasted overnight, and fasting was continued for four additional hours. The $^{47}Ca$ was added to a solution containing 100 mg of calcium carrier as the chloride. When the intravenous method was employed, 1 to 3 $\mu c$ of high-specific-activity $^{47}Ca$ was administered as calcium chloride.* The procedure for measuring the radiocalcium content of each individual stool and each 24-hour urine sample is detailed in our previous report.[5] Whole-body counting was performed in a chamber (six and one-half feet wide, seven and one-half feet high and eight feet long) made of six-inch steel, lined with lead one-eighth-inch thick.

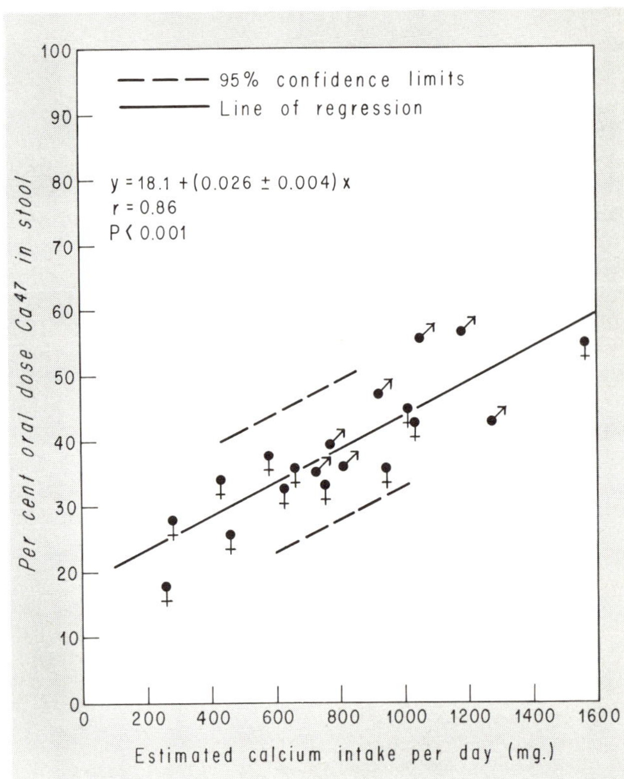


Fig. 1. Fecal excretion of orally administered $^{47}Ca$ plotted against daily calcium intake for 19 control subjects. (Reproduced from Kinney, V. R.; Tauxe, W. N. and Dearing, W. H.: Isotopic tracer studies of intestinal calcium absorption. *J. Lab. clin. Med.* **66**:187-203, 1965. By permission of the publisher, the C. V. Mosby Company.)

*Supplied by the Oak Ridge National Laboratory (Oak Ridge, Tenn.) as $^{47}CaCl_2$ with less than 1% $^{45}Ca$ contamination (specific activity, 130 to 180 mc/gm).

TABLE I

## Summary of Calcium Absorption and Urinary Excretion Data in 10 Patients with Wilson's Disease

| Patient | Sex | Age (yr.) | Calcium absorption* | Urine Ca (mg/24 hr.) | Hypercalciuria |
|---|---|---|---|---|---|
| 1 | M | 15 | N (0/5) | 69-87 | — |
| 2 | F | 44 | N (0/4) | 107-124 | — |
| 3 | M | 22 | H (2/6) | 246-235 | + |
| 4 | M | 33 | H (1/2) | 347 | + |
| 5 | M | 42 | N (2/4) | 239 → 185 | +† |
| 6 | M | 17 | N (0/3) | 357 → 153 | + |
| 7 | M | 34 | H (1/7) | 231 → 159 | + |
| 8 | M | 31 | H (4/5) | 289 → 211 | + |
| 9 | F | 34 | H (4/6) | 288 → 108 | + |
| 10 | F | 30 | H (6/8) | 242 → 134<br>118 → 189 | + |

*N = normal absorption by radiocalcium study; H = hyperabsorption.
In parentheses are shown number of abnormal tests/number of tests performed.
†This patient had a renal stone.

Eight plastic scintillation detectors were arranged in two banks, four above and four below the patient. Each detector consisted of an 18- by 18- by six-inch NE-102 plastic scintillator viewed by four EMI 9530 B multiplier phototubes.[6]

To determine if hypercalciuria existed, the daily urinary excretion of calcium was measured in each patient over a three-day period during which the patient consumed a diet designed to contain 105 mg of calcium/24 hr. (Chemical analysis of the diet showed that its content of calcium varied from 97 to 115 mg/24 hr.) Each patient was allowed to drink deionized water (calcium-free, by analysis) as desired. We consider a urinary excretion of calcium greater than 170 mg/24 hr to be hypercalciuria under these conditions.

*Chemical methods.*—The serum calcium was determined by permanganate titration of calcium oxalate precipitated from serum[7] or by the complexometric titration method of Jones and McGuckin[8]; urinary calcium was measured by the method of Holth.[7] Calcium content of the diet and stool was determined by the method of Clark and Collip.[9]

### Results

*Controls.*—The percentage of oral tracer recovered in the stool of 19 control subjects previously reported[5] is shown in Figure 1. There is a statistically significant correlation between percentage of recovery and estimated dietary calcium intake. There is no correlation with age, height, or weight.

*Wilson's disease.*—The results of the 48 oral radiocalcium tracer studies in the patients with Wilson's disease are shown in Figure 2. Each symbol indicates an individual patient studied while being maintained on diets of different calcium content. Two patients who have always had normal calcium excretion had a total of nine studies and all indicated normal calcium absorptive efficiency. Two patients who have had hypercalciuria demonstrated hyperabsorption during three of eight tests (Table I).

During the period of observation, which ranged from 18 to 36 months, the six remaining patients improved with reference to their hypercalciuria; five of these patients reverted to normal urinary calcium excretion and

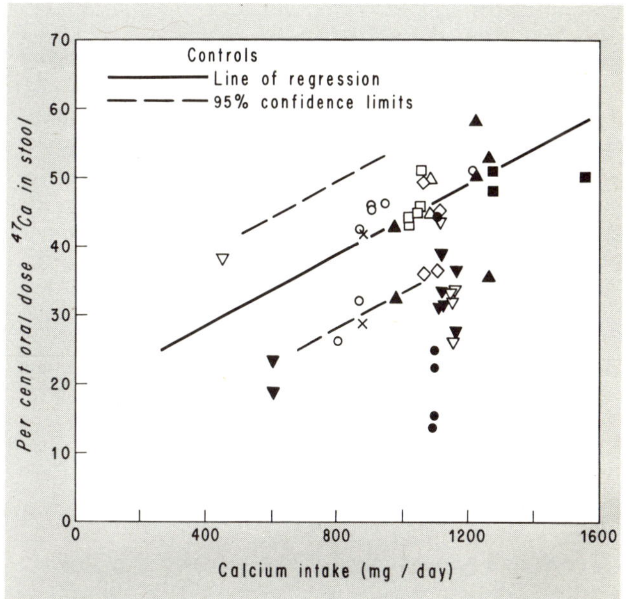


Fig. 2. Fecal excretion of orally administered $^{47}Ca$ plotted against daily calcium intake: results of 48 tests on nine patients with Wilson's disease.

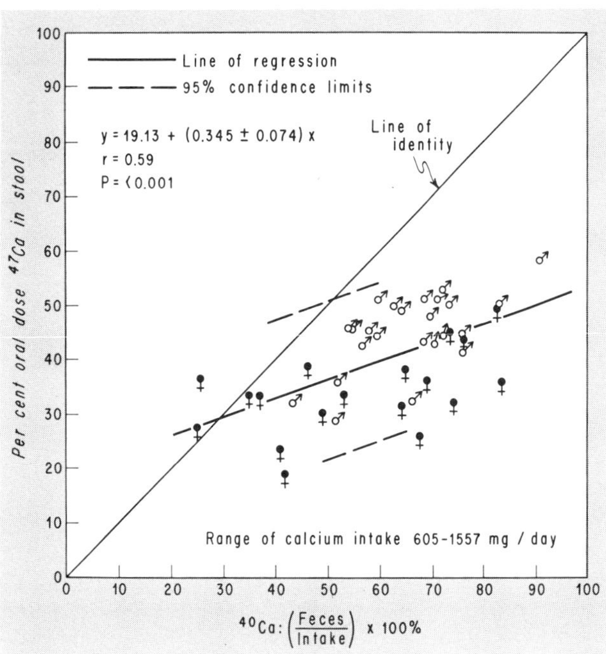


Fig. 3. Correlation between conventional calcium balance studies and $^{47}$Ca studies.

one patient, to a lesser degree of hypercalciuria. In five patients of this group, the first abnormality to return to normal was calcium absorption, and then the urinary calcium excretion subsequently became normal. In one patient, the converse was observed. One of the five patients whose urinary calcium excretion returned to normal has again demonstrated hypercalciuria after hyperabsorption was indicated in the absorption test.

Comparison of studies performed while the patients were taking penicillamine and when this medication had been discontinued indicated that there was no effect of penicillamine on calcium absorptive efficiency. All of the patients studied had normal serum calcium values.

*Concurrent radiocalcium and conventional balance studies.*—In 42 studies there was a significant correlation between the recovery of fecal radiocalcium (as percentage of dose) and the fecal calcium content (as percentage of dietary intake) during concurrent balance periods ($r = 0.59$, $P < 0.001$) (Fig. 3). The percentage of the $^{47}$Ca recovered in the stool was generally less than the percentage of dietary (stable) calcium present in the stool, which is a reflection of the fact that fecal calcium contains both unabsorbed dietary calcium and endogenous calcium. Correction for this latter factor results in a closer agreement between the two observations.

*Whole-body retention.*—Whole-body retention after the intravenous administration of $^{47}$Ca in four patients is shown in Figure 4. Agreement between the directly measured value and the predicted body retention on the basis of cumulative fecal and urinary losses was very close. The greatest difference between the predicted and observed values was 2.7% at the end of an eight-day period. These observations validate the methods employed for determining radiocalcium excretion and show that there is no significant loss of calcium through the skin.

## Discussion

The demonstration that hyperabsorption of calcium occurs in patients with Wilson's disease who have hypercalciuria does not clarify which abnormality is primary. Variations in urinary excretion of calcium in response to changes in dietary intake of calcium is a temporary phenomenon; on a long-term basis, the gastrointestinal tract is the major site that adjusts to alterations of calcium intake.[10] Long-term studies in normal males reveal the urinary excretion of calcium to vary slightly with dietary calcium intakes ranging from 400 to 1,000 mg/day.[10] When hypercalciuria occurs, the absorptive efficiency of the intestinal tract increases; however, the absolute amount of calcium absorbed is limited by the amount of calcium in the daily dietary intake. Thus, in patients with an habitual diet of low calcium content, a negative balance would exist with a consequent decrease in calcium content of bone. If hypercalciuria in patients with Wilson's disease is the result of a renal abnormality, then this physiologic sequence would be a possible explanation for the demineralization noted in some patients with Wilson's disease. The renal tubular resorptive defects for amino acids and uric acid typical of patients with Wilson's disease were present in the ten patients in the present series, but none had any evidence to indicate renal tubular acidosis.[4] It is still plausible to consider that an independent renal tubular abnormality of calcium resorption may occur. Although hypercalciuria existed in the majority of the patients we have studied, none had any evidence of skeletal demineralization, suggesting that their intestinal absorption of calcium had compensated for the loss or that, if negative calcium balance did exist, the time interval had not been sufficient to produce roentgenographic evidence of osteoporosis.

Osteoporosis has been reported in patients with liver disease even when clinical icterus and steatorrhea was not clinically significant.[11] This may be another possible explanation for the skeletal abnormalities noted in patients with Wilson's disease.

Because increased absorption of one divalent cation, copper, is known to occur in Wilson's disease, hyperabsorption of another divalent cation, calcium, may occur. The results of the present study suggest but do not prove, that hyperabsorption of calcium may be the primary abnormality. In five of the six patients whose urinary excretion of calcium became normal or decreased significantly, normal calcium absorption was evident before the hypercalciuria diminished. If the hyperabsorption were a consequence of the hypercalciuria, then a reverse sequence of events would have been expected.

## Summary

Forty-eight radiocalcium absorption tests (oral method) were performed in ten patients with Wilson's disease. Two patients who had normal urinary excretion of

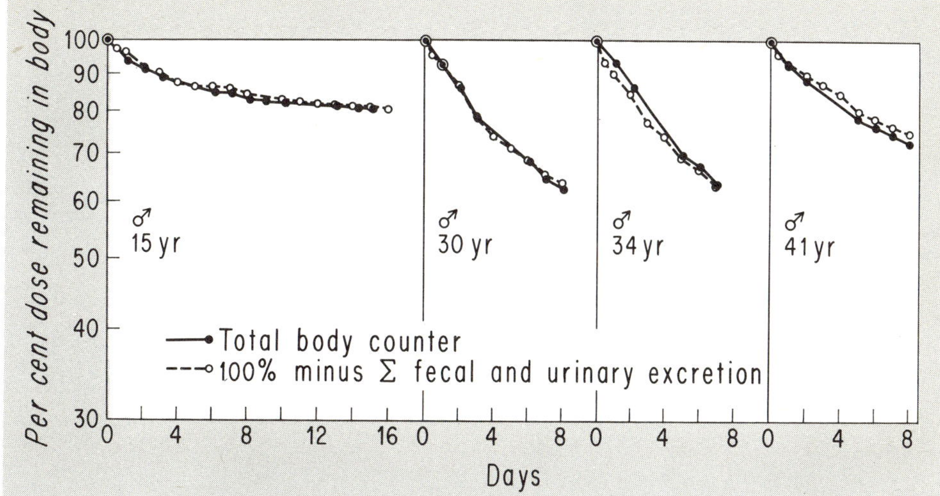


Fig. 4. Whole-body retention of $^{47}Ca$ after intravenous administration in four patients with Wilson's disease. *Solid line* = direct estimate by whole-body counting. *Broken line* = calculated as 100% minus sum of fecal and urinary excretion.

calcium had normal absorption during a total of nine studies. Two patients with hypercalciuria demonstrated hyperabsorption on three of eight tests. Of the six remaining patients, five became normocalciuric and one had a significant decrease of the hypercalciuria during the three-year period of observation. In five of these six patients, calcium absorption was the first parameter to return to normal, suggesting that the gastrointestinal abnormality was the primary feature with the hypercalciuria secondary to it.

Concurrent calcium balance and radiocalcium studies revealed significant correlation between the two different measurements of absorptive efficiency, although the absolute values were not equal.

Monitoring of radiocalcium retention by a whole-body counter verified the reliability of the excretory measurements and showed that there are no significant losses of calcium except by urinary and fecal excretion.

## REFERENCES


1. Litin, R. B.; Randall, R. V.; Goldstein, N. P.; Power, M. H. and Diessner, G. R.: Hypercalciuria in hepatolenticular degeneration (Wilson's disease). *Amer. J. med. Sci.* **238:**614-620, 1959.
2. Morgan, H. G.; Stewart, W. K.; Lowe, K. G.; Stowers, J. M. and Johnstone, J. H.: Wilson's disease and the Fanconi syndrome. *Quart. J. Med.* **31:**361-384, 1962.
3. Rosenoer, V. M. and Michell, R. C.: Skeletal changes in Wilson's disease (hepato-lenticular degeneration). *Brit. J. Radiol.* **32:**805-809, 1959.
4. Randall, R. V.; Goldstein, N. P.; Gross, J. B. and Rosevear, J. W.: Hypercalciuria in hepatolenticular degeneration (Wilson's disease). *Amer. J. med. Sci.* **252:**715-720, 1966.
5. Kinney, V. R.; Tauxe, W. N. and Dearing, W. H.: Isotopic tracer studies of intestinal calcium absorption. *J. Lab. clin. Med.* **66:**187-203, 1965.
6. Tauxe, W. N. and Orvis, A. L.: The Mayo Clinic whole-body counter. *Mayo Clin. Proc.* **41:**18-23, 1966.
7. Holth, T.: Separation of calcium from magnesium by oxalate method: a critical study. *Anal. Chem.* **21:**1221-1226, 1949.
8. Jones, J. D. and McGuckin, W. F.: Complexometric titration of calcium and magnesium by a semiautomated procedure. *Clin. Chem.* **10:**767-780, 1964.
9. Clark, E. P. and Collip, J. B.: A study of the Tisdall method for the determination of blood serum calcium with a suggested modification. *J. biol. Chem.* **63:**461-464, 1925.
10. Malm, O. J.: Calcium requirement and adaptation in adult men. *Scand. J. clin. Lab. Invest.* **10** (suppl. 36):1-280, 1958.
11. Summerskill, W. H. J. and Kelly, P. J.: Osteoporosis with fractures in anicteric cirrhosis: observations supplemented by microradiographic evaluation of bone. *Proc. Mayo Clin.* **38:**162-174, 1963.

# Diagnosis and Treatment Studies of Patients in Asymptomatic Stage of Wilson's Disease*

JUN-BI TU, M.D., D.M.Sc.**; R. QUENTIN BLACKWELL, Ph.D.***; JAMES W. FRESH, M.D., CDR, MC† and RAYMOND H. WATTEN, M.D., Capt., MC‡

Detection of asymptomatic cases among siblings of Wilson's disease patients allows early therapy and more favorable prognosis. Useful screening tests for this purpose include determinations of urinary copper, plasma ceruloplasmin, and serum transaminase. Any screening abnormalities should be confirmed with other work such as liver biopsies, radio-copper studies, and copper balances. Penicillamine-induced cupriuresis improves the screening effectiveness of urinary copper studies and copper balance studies provide valuable support both in establishing final diagnosis during the asymptomatic stage and in monitoring therapy.

## Introduction

Wilson's disease is recognized as a genetically determined degenerative disease which requires an environmental factor, copper, for its development; therefore, the rate of degeneration depends in part on the amount of dietary copper available. The asymptomatic stage of Wilson's disease has become the subject of attention recently because it is now recognized as the stage of the disease most susceptible to therapeutic control[1-8] and as the time of the best prognosis. Hence it is of obvious importance to locate the asymptomatic patient at the earliest possible age in order to begin preventive therapy. However, the incidence of Wilson's disease is relatively low and proposals for mass population screening to locate susceptible individuals have not yet gained wide support; therefore, the screening of members of families with known occurrence of the disease presently is the only practical means to locate the asymptomatic patient.[5]

In the course of studies on the clinical and biochemical features of several Chinese families with Wilson's disease in Taiwan, three young asymptomatic female patients have been identified in three separate families. One patient has been receiving intensive treatment for four years; the other two patients were treated only after the development of initial clinical manifestations. This paper summarizes our experience in the diagnosis and treatment of these three patients.

## Diagnosis

The diagnostic procedure is composed of the initial screening procedures and the methods for further investigation of the suspected homozygotes for the disease. All of the high risk members of a known family should be screened, particularly the siblings of known patients in whom the chance for homozygosity is one in four.[9] Individuals with normal results from the screening tests are considered unlikely to be homozygous for the disease; those showing one or more abnormal results require further investigation.

Based on reports of other investigators and our own experience, three tests appear most useful for screening. They include a) 24 hour urinary copper determinations before and during oral penicillamine administration; b)

*This work was accomplished under the Bureau of Medicine and Surgery Work Unit MR005.09-0040. The study was funded in part under U.S. Public Law 480, Section 104(c) and in part by the Bureau of Medicine and Surgery, Department of the Navy, Washington, D.C. The opinions and assertions contained herein are those of the authors and are not to be construed as official or reflecting the views of the U.S. Navy Department or the U.S. Naval Service at large.

**Research Associate, Department of Biochemistry, U.S. Naval Medical Research Unit No. 2, Taipei, Taiwan, Republic of China. Present address: Kingston General Hospital, Kingston, Ontario, Canada.

***Head, Department of Biochemistry, U.S. Naval Medical Research Unit No. 2, Taipei, Taiwan, Republic of China.

†Head, Department of Pathology, U.S. Naval Medical Research Unit No. 2, Taipei, Taiwan, Republic of China.

‡Commanding Officer, U.S. Naval Medical Research Unit No. 2, Taipei, Taiwan, Republic of China.

plasma ceruloplasmin or copper oxidase determination and c) determination of the serum transaminases, SGOT and SGPT.

Among the three proposed screening procedures, urinary copper determination was found to be the most useful diagnostic criterion. As illustrated in Table I, hypercupriuria appears to be the most regular abnormality found both in patients with asymptomatic and those with advanced Wilson's disease. Normal urinary excretion of copper has never been reported in patients with advanced Wilson's disease including those with normal concentration of ceruloplasmin.[10-13] While this is also true for the majority of asymptomatic patients reported,[1-8] Sternlieb *et al* reported three out of eight cases with normal urinary copper levels.[8] However, at least two of those three patients had urinary copper excretion levels above the usual normal values found by other workers.[12, 14, 15]

Penicillamine will induce significantly higher copper excretions in the homozygote for Wilson's disease[14] regardless of the urinary copper excretions before penicillamine. This apparently is true for the asymptomatic as well as for symptomatic patients.

Some of the heterozygotes in our series also showed higher than normal levels of urinary copper without penicillamine although some studies[15, 16] have reported the heterozygote to have normal urinary copper excretion. All 12 heterozygotes studied in our series showed marked increases in urinary copper after oral penicillamine; however their increases were not as great as those of the homozygotes and the two groups were distinguishable. This is particularly important because as many as 20% of the heterozygotes may have subnormal levels of serum ceruloplasmin[16, 17]; this, coupled with an elevated urinary copper excretion without penicillamine, would tend to confuse the distinction between

## ABOUT THE SENIOR AUTHOR

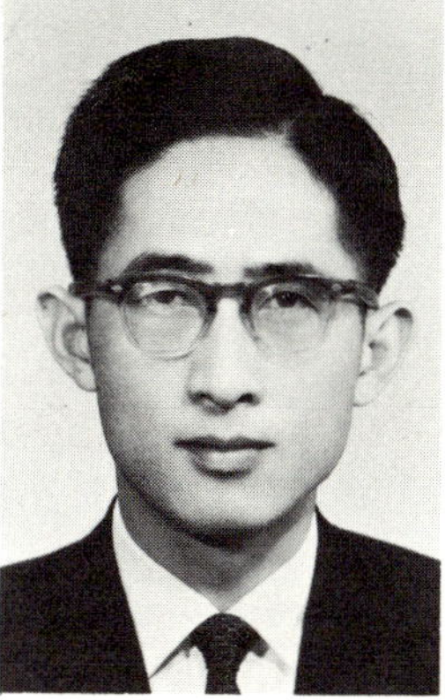

Dr. Tu was born in Fukien, China, received his medical education at the National Taiwan University, Republic of China, and graduated in July 1956.

He served at the Department of Neurology and Psychiatry of the National Taiwan University Hospital as Resident, Instructor, and Visiting Lecturer, respectively, from 1956 to 1966. He joined the Department of Biochemistry of the U. S. Naval Medical Research Unit No. 2 in Taiwan as Research Fellow from 1960 to 1964, and as Research Associate from 1965 to 1966. During the period 1964 to 1965 he worked with Professor Hans Zellweger on the biochemical aspects of Down's Syndrome and Pediatric Neurology at the Pediatric Department, State University of Iowa.

He is most interested in the genetic and biochemical study of mental and neurologic disorders and has been working on Wilson's disease, phenylketonuria, Down's syndrome, gargoylism, and hepatic porphyria since 1960.

In 1964 he was awarded a Doctor of Medical Science degree from the Kyushu University, Japan, for his achievement in the study of Wilson's disease in Taiwan.

In 1966, Dr. Tu moved to Canada where he continues his research career at Queen's University Medical School, Kingston, Ontario.

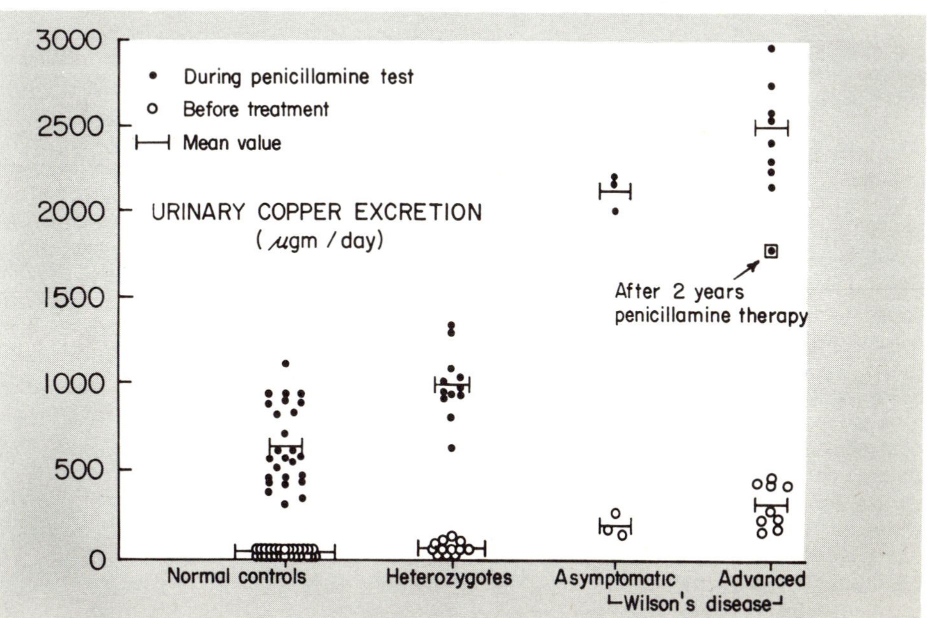


Fig. 1. Results of penicillamine-induced cupriuresis test under various conditions.

TABLE I

RESULTS OF SCREENING TESTS IN ASYMPTOMATIC WILSON'S DISEASE.

| Subjects | | Age and Sex | Urinary Copper μg/24 hr Before Penicillamine | Urinary Copper μg/24 hr During Penicillamine | Copper Oxidase Ravin Units | SGOT Frankel Units | SGPT Frankel Units |
|---|---|---|---|---|---|---|---|
| Asymptomatic Wilson's Disease | | | | | | | |
| Case 1 | | 5F | 140 | 2220 | 0.041 | 116 | 121 |
| Case 2 | | 7F | 120 | 2000 | 0.040 | 35 | 16 |
| Case 3 | | 6F | 250 | 2160 | 0.254 | 120 | 89 |
| Advanced Wilson's Disease | | | | | | | |
| Mean Value | | | 290 | 2330 | 0.035 | | |
| Range | low | | 120 | 2140 | 0.005 | Variable | |
| | high | | 560 | 2960 | 0.087 | | |
| Normal Control Subject | | | | | | | |
| Mean Value | | | 24 | 640 | 0.410 | | |
| Range | low | | 6 | 270 | 0.217 | Below 40 | |
| | high | | 57 | 1160 | 0.686 | | |

the two groups. The oral penicillamine definitely serves to accentuate the differences in the urinary copper excretions of heterozygotes and homozygotes[14] as illustrated in Figure 1.

Low ceruloplasmin levels have been claimed to be the most consistently abnormal finding in Wilson's disease,[9] and the test is widely recommended as a screening test for the asymptomatic patient.[18] However, in recent years a significant number of firmly established cases of Wilson's disease, including Case 3 (Table I), have had normal serum ceruloplasmin concentrations.[4, 5, 10-13] The reason for these differences still remains obscure; periodic follow-up observations on these subjects would be of interest. For example, Figure 2 shows the results of our follow-up study on Case 3. It was found that during the three years of study a striking fall of both plasma copper oxidase and total plasma copper, from the normal range to the characteristic low levels of the disease, took place in this patient. Although the patient was asymptomatic when first examined she gradually deteriorated and showed initial symptoms of the disease at the age of nine when repeated plasma copper oxidase and total plasma copper determinations disclosed low values. Two similar cases were reported in discussions held during the first International Symposium on Wilson's Disease in 1961, in which initially normal levels of ceruloplasmin decreased markedly to very low levels following penicillamine therapy. At that time it was suggested that the fall in serum copper and ceruloplasmin in the patients may have been a result of the decoppering effect of penicillamine.[19] In view of our experience with Case 3 such an explanation appears less likely because our patient did not receive any treatment prior to the change of ceruloplasmin levels. Our results suggest that ceruloplasmin deficiency is a secondary product of the Wilson's disease gene. A recent animal study by Williams *et al*[20] to investigate the relationship of liver damage and serum ceruloplasmin levels indicated that alteration of ceruloplasmin levels is secondary to some phase of liver damage. This supports the position that an asymptomatic sibling of a known patient with Wilson's disease with a normal concentration of ceruloplasmin still may be in danger of being affected with the disease. Therefore, it appears to be extremely important that screening for Wilson's disease should not rely on the results of ceruloplasmin assay alone, but should include additional independent tests.

Although nonspecific, serum transaminase levels generally are elevated at the initial stage of liver diseases including that of Wilson's disease. High serum transaminase levels were found in our asymptomatic patients and have been reported in the literature.[4-6, 21] It is interesting to note that elevated transaminase levels in Case 3 occurred before the diminution of plasma copper oxidase activity (Fig. 2). Because of lack of active treatment, this patient eventually developed Kayser-Fleischer

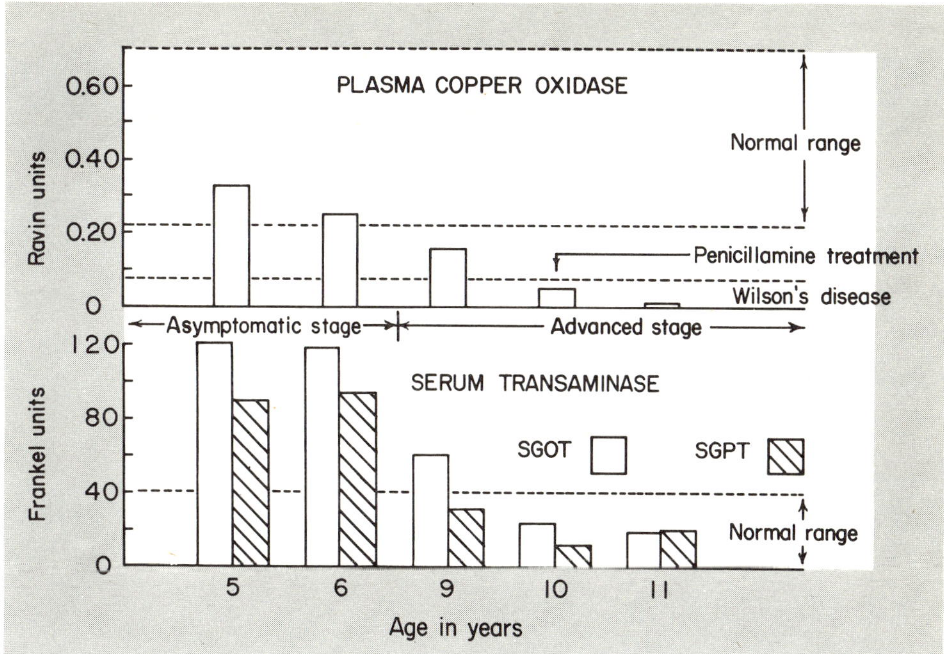


Fig. 2. Results of follow-up study of plasma ceruloplasmin levels in Case 3.

rings, slight mental retardation and progressive slowness of movement. Since two of her elder sisters died with all of the usual clinical and biochemical findings of Wilson's disease,[22] the present sequence of the biochemical changes in the patient seems not to represent an unusual type of the disease. Whether other asymptomatic patients may be subject to the same sequence of biochemical changes remains as a challenging problem for further investigation. Such an investigation not only may lead to a more precise method for the screening test, but also may clarify the basic pathogenesis of the disease.

Numerous conditions in which tissue destruction occurs with attendant release of transaminases and other cellular enzymes into the circulation are known to be characterized by elevations in serum transaminase activities; these include myocardial infarction, hepatitis, and skeletal myopathy. In most cases they should cause no confusion in the diagnosis of asymptomatic Wilson's disease. However, because anicteric hepatitis, a condition which usually is accompanied by a high serum transaminase activity, frequently occurs in some populations,[23] it requires special consideration. This is of particular importance because a few patients with severe icteric hepatitis are known to exhibit ceruloplasmin deficiency in addition to high serum transaminase levels.[24, 25]

In 1962 during a survey on subclinical hepatitis in Taiwan, a separate study of this problem was made. Copper oxidase activity was measured in a group of 72 patients with histologically proven anicteric hepatitis who were selected in a screening survey by the finding of two elevated SGPT values.[23] The results are shown in Figure 3. The mean and standard deviation values were $0.311 \pm 0.031$ which were significantly lower ($p<0.05$)

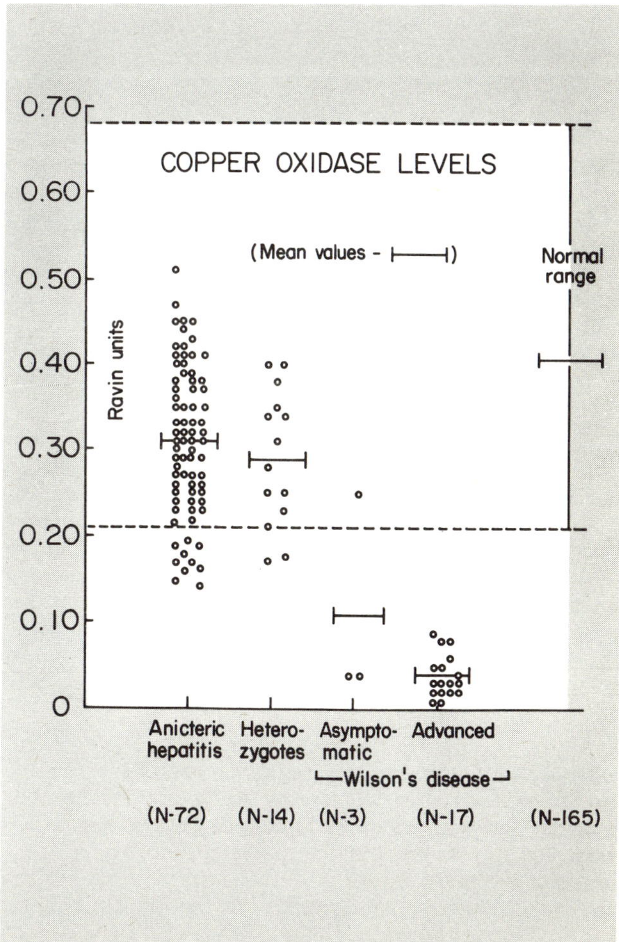


Fig. 3. Measure of copper oxidase activity in a group of 72 patients with anicteric hepatitis.

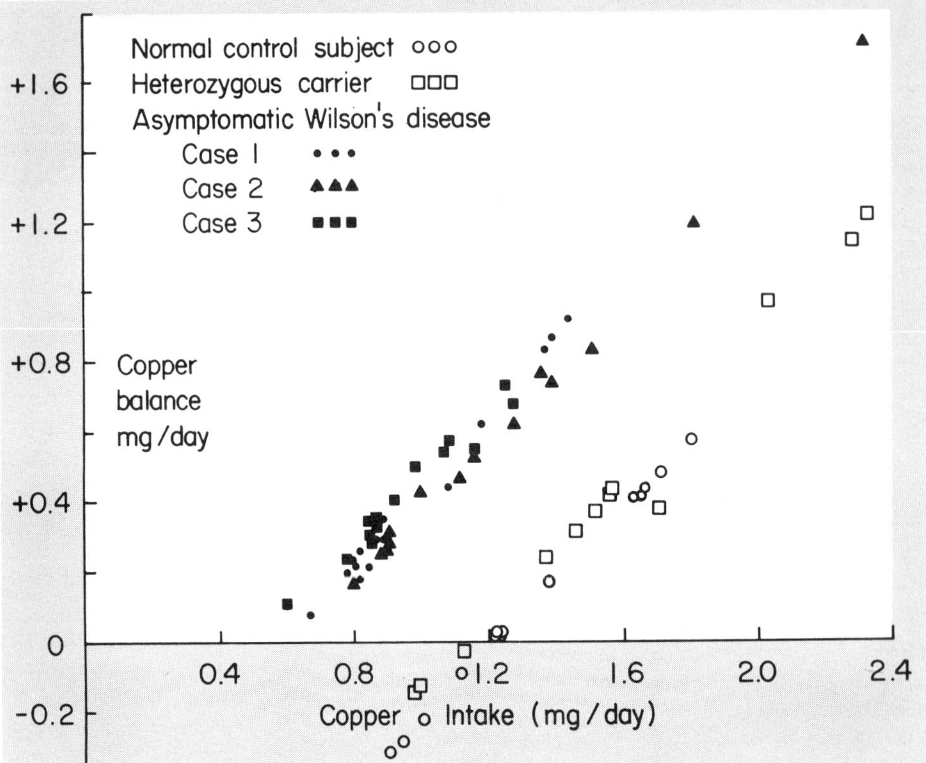


Fig. 4. Results of copper balance determination.

than the corresponding normal control values of 0.410 ± 0.085. Ten cases, (14%) of the anicteric subjects showed a definite subnormal level of copper oxidase activity, but none fell to levels commonly observed in typical Wilson's disease. In addition, the changes did not last more than a few weeks, and there was no hypercupriuria. These findings suggest that changes of copper oxidase activity in anicteric hepatitis are infrequent, and when they occur they are mild and transient in nature; therefore, they are unlikely to cause confusion in the detection of asymptomatic Wilson's disease.

The screening tests discussed above may be hampered during infancy when the serum transaminase values are normally elevated[26] and the serum ceruloplasmin is low.[27] Furthermore, although it has not been thoroughly investigated, it seems likely that urinary copper levels in homozygotes for Wilson's disease would not vary much from those of normal infants.[8] Further work is required to determine those urinary copper levels and the possible effect of penicillamine-induced cupriuresis in infants.

Methods for further examination of subjects with abnormal responses to the screening procedures include a) liver biopsy; b) radiocopper studies and c) copper balance determinations. Other methods also are available; our experience is limited to liver biopsies and copper balance studies.

Liver biopsy changes in asymptomatic patients generally include excessive deposition of copper and varying degrees of parenchymal damage.[28] In the present series, one open wedge liver biopsy was taken in Patient 1 at the age of five before treatment started.[22] The liver copper was found to be 315 μg per gram of wet tissue which is approximately 30 times higher than the mean control value; by contrast the bile copper was 0.5 μg per ml which is about 1⁄13 of the control value.[22] Histologic examination revealed marked damage of the liver with parenchymal cell degeneration, areas of focal necrosis, distortion of lobular architecture, ballooning of nuclei in some hepatic cells, patchy cytoplasmic glygocen deposition, and fatty changes with large and small fat vacuoles.[29] The other two asymptomatic subjects refused liver biopsy examination until recently when Case 3 was studied. By that time, however, she was showing initial signs of the disease and had received penicillamine treatment for seven months. Her liver tissue was found to be moderately fibrotic with a moderate lymphocytic infiltration and slight parenchymal cell degeneration. These changes agree with those found by other investigators and indicate that liver biopsy can provide decisive information to confirm the presence of the disease.[28] However, the histologic changes in liver are nonspecific[8] and may be very mild in the early asymptomatic stage.[30] Furthermore, very high copper content of the liver also has been demonstrated in conditions other than Wilson's disease such as neonatal giant cell hepatitis,[31] primary biliary cirrhosis,[32] and juvenile cirrhosis.[33]

Asymptomatic patients, like the patients with advanced disease, incorporate very little $^{64}$copper into ceruloplasmin; the other radioisotope tests including rate of clearance from blood, and urinary excretion of labeled copper following intravenous administration were reported to be normal.[31] Sternlieb *et al*[17] demonstrated that measurement of incorporation of radiocopper into ceruloplasmin can provide a fairly reliable means of distinguishing the heterozygote from the normal subject but it does not separate them from the homozygote patients. Osborn *et al*[21] found an impaired hepatic uptake of injected radiocopper in eight patients with Wilson's disease, including one asymptomatic subject. There also was an overlap between patients and heterozygotes. Since the differentiation of these two conditions is of great importance in the management of patients with asymptomatic Wilson's disease, the current methods of radiocopper study apparently have limited value in establishment of the diagnosis.

It seems clear that there is no single specific test to detect the asymptomatic Wilson's disease patient; such may continue to be true until the primary genetic defect of the disease is established.[31, 34] The current tests appear to be dealing with the secondary effects of the abnormal genes. Our experience with copper balance studies and the consistent results obtained from them suggest that the abnormality which results in increased accumulation of copper in the tissues must be closer to the genetic defect than the other abnormalities such as serum ceruloplasmin levels. If this assumption is correct, balance determination may provide more reliable information for the diagnosis of Wilson's disease in the extremely early stage. We have proposed a reliable method of daily copper balance determination.[35] Results of such a study are shown in Figure 4 for the three asymptomatic subjects, including Case 3 whose balance determination was made while she was beginning to develop the initial clinical manifestations. It is clear that they exhibited strikingly positive copper balances which are quite similar to that of the advanced patients.[36] The heterozygote, whose results are also shown in the figure, had mild hypoceruloplasminemia and hypercupriuria. That subject demonstrated a slightly higher positive balance than the control subject but was clearly separable from those of the three patients.

Whether hepatic damage associated with higher copper content in conditions other than Wilson's disease would show a distinguishable balance slope remains to be determined.

## Treatment

Beginning in 1951 with the use by Cumings[37] of dimercaprol (BAL) as a copper removing agent in the treatment of Wilson's disease, a number of copper binding agents have been tried. Most investigators agree that oral penicillamine is the most effective one for the purpose.[3, 29, 34] In those patients who do not respond to penicillamine[3,35,38] it appears likely that either irreversible damage occurred prior to treatment or the therapy was not sufficiently intense.[34, 35] The latter possibility exists particularly when copper balance studies are not employed to assess the effect of therapy upon the patient's copper balance status.[29]

Accumulating experience concerning the effectiveness of the therapy of Wilson's disease by copper removal suggests that complete recovery of normal physiologic function in organs and tissues will not occur in those patients who were symptomatic before treatment began.[3, 38] Intensive treatment beginning in the asymptomatic stage would appear to offer a better prognosis.[29] This is illustrated by our experience with Case 1.

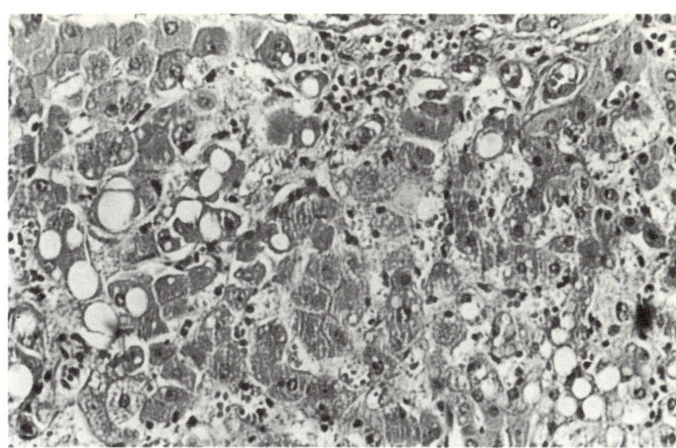

Fig. 5. Liver biopsy of patients. Case 1 shows extensive necrosis of hepatic cells with ballooning of nuclei and fatty metamorphosis. Hematoxylin and eosin, x 340.

The patient was placed on penicillamine therapy and a low copper diet and has continued to remain asymptomatic and in apparent good health for four years. Copper balance studies, electroencephalograms, psychometric tests, liver function tests, and liver biopsies were done before and at intervals after therapy began. Results of the tests show improvement following therapy.

A description of the copper balance determinations in the management of Wilson's disease (including this patient) will be presented in a separate paper.[36] Two sets of copper balance data determined on this patient have been reported previously.[29] The first balance study was made when the patient was five years old and receiving dietotherapy alone. The second study was performed after seven months of oral DL-penicillamine therapy with dosage of one gram per day. The results were closely similar to those found in symptomatic patients; dietotherapy had definite but limited value whereas the combination of low copper diet with penicillamine established a definite negative balance.[29, 35, 36]

The liver biopsy results before therapy are described along with Figure 5. Following therapy, three needle biopsies of the liver were taken; two were obtained about one week apart during the 16th month of treatment (Fig. 6). Both of these specimens were read as normal liver tissue. The third specimen was taken about four years after therapy began. The liver parenchymal cells still appear normal. There was only minimal fibrosis in the portal areas (Fig. 7). In addition, the initial findings of abnormal liver function tests and electroencephalographic changes in this patient were all diminished. The patient has remained cheerful, playful and clinically asymptomatic during the entire four year course. Her mental and physical development appears quite normal. She has been attending regular school since the age of

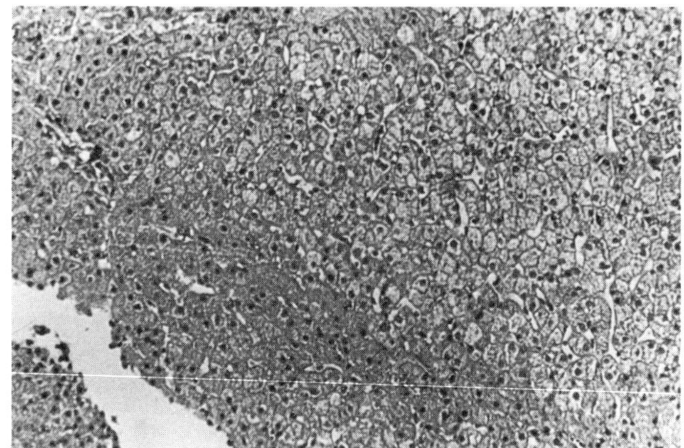

Fig. 6. Normal liver biopsy tissue after 16 months of treatment. Hematoxylin and eosin, x 85.

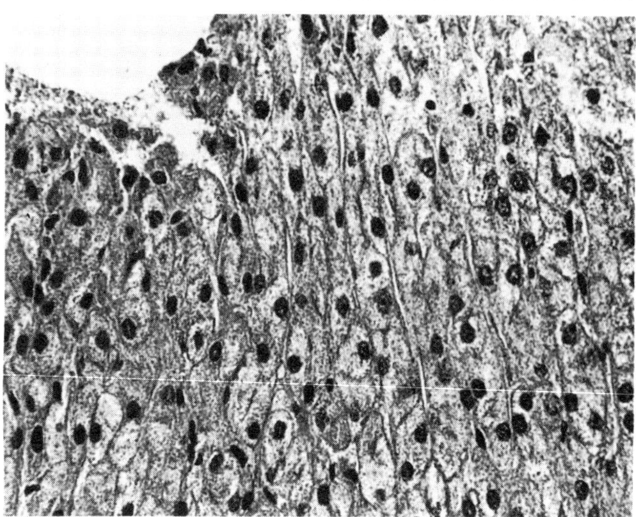

Fig. 7. Normal liver biopsy tissue after four years of treatment. Hematoxylin and eosin, x 340.

seven and shows above average scholastic achievement. Although we cannot predict with certainty at this early point that the present treatment program, continued for life, will prevent development of symptomatic Wilson's disease in this patient, the favorable results after four years are encouraging.

Unfortunately, Cases 2 and 3 were unable to receive drug therapy at the time their condition was diagnosed. Both developed clinical signs and symptoms of the disease approximately two years after their initial examination; age of onset for Case 2 was seven and one-half years and for Case 3, eight years of age. Recently, they both have been placed on oral D-penicillamine, one gram per day; a six-month follow-up observation shows some evidence that the advance of the disease has been retarded in Case 3 but little evidence of benefit is apparent thus far in Case 2.

## Summary

Procedures for screening and diagnosis of patients in the asymptomatic stage of Wilson's disease have been reviewed. It is considered highly desirable that high risk subjects, particularly all siblings of known cases, be screened with at least three tests: urinary copper excretion, plasma ceruloplasmin, and serum transaminases. Any subjects showing one or more abnormal results in these tests should be studied further by liver biopsy, radiocopper studies if convenient, and copper balance determinations.

Particular emphasis has been placed on the use of penicillamine-induced cupriuresis as a screening procedure and the use of the copper balance study as an important aid in diagnosis of Wilson's disease in the asymptomatic stage.

Early diagnosis of the disease and institution of intensive therapy with penicillamine and low-copper diet while the patient is still asymptomatic appears to be a reasonable and desirable goal of the clinician.

## REFERENCES


1. Bickel, H.; Neale, F. C. and Hall, G.: A clinical and biochemical study of hepatolenticular degeneration (Wilson's disease). *Quart. J. Med.* **26:**527-558, 1957.

2. Lygren, T.; Sörensen, E. W. and Bernhardsen, A.: Hepatolenticular degeneration (Wilson's disease): A case diagnosed biochemically before clinical manifestations. *Lancet* **i:**276-277, 1959.

3. Walshe, J. M.: Treatment of Wilson's disease with penicillamine. *Lancet* **i:**188-192, 1960.

4. Arima, M.; Oshima, M.; Shima, N.; Obe, Y. and Suzuki, M.: Wilson's disease in children. *Paediat. Univ. Tokyo* **5:**14-19, 1960.

5. Tu, J. B.; Cooper, W. C.; Blackwell, R. Q. and Hou, T. Y.: Asymptomatic Wilson's disease. *Acta paediat. Sinica* **3:**154-160, 1962.

6. Warren, C. B. M. and Broughton, P. M. G.: Wilson's disease. *Arch. Dis. Childh.* **37:**242-252, 1962.

7. Walshe, J. M.: Wilson's disease: The presenting symptoms. *Arch. Dis. Childh.* **37:**253-256, 1962.

8. Sternlieb, I. and Scheinberg, I. H.: The diagnosis of Wilson's disease in asymptomatic patients, *J. Amer. med. Ass.* **183:**747-751, 1963.

9. Bearn, A. G.: Genetic and biochemical aspects of Wilson's disease. *Amer. J. Med.* **15:**442-449, 1953.

10. Enger, E.: Wilson's disease. Report of a case with normal serum ceruloplasmin level. *Acta med. Scand.* **163:**121-124, 1959.

11. Rosenoer, V. M. and Franglen, G.: Caeruloplasmin in Wilson's disease. *Lancet* **ii:**1163-1164, 1959.

12. Sass-Kortsak, A.; Cherniak, M.; Geiger, D. W. and Slater, R. J.: Observations on ceruloplasmin in Wilson's disease. *J. clin. Invest.* **38:**1672-1682, 1959.

13. Kurtzke, J. F.: Normal ceruloplasmin in Wilson's disease. *Arch. Neurol.* **7:**371-376, 1962.

14. Tu, J. B. and Blackwell, R. Q.: Studies on levels of penicillamine-induced cupriuresis in heterozygotes of Wilson's disease. *Metabolism* **16:**507-513, 1967.

15. Neale, F. C. and Fischer-Williams, M.: Copper metabolism in normal adults and in clinically normal relatives of patients with Wilson's disease. *J. clin. Path.* **11:**441-447, 1958.

16. Cartwright, G. E.; Markowitz, H.; Shields, G. S. and Wintrobe, M. M.: Studies on copper metabolism XXIX, a critical analysis of serum copper and ceruloplasmin concentrations in normal subjects, patients with Wilson's disease, *Amer. J. Med.* **28:**555-563, 1960.

17. Sternlieb, I.; Morell, A. G.; Bauer, C. D.; Combes, B.; De Bobes-Sternberg, S. and Scheinberg, I. H.: Detection of the heterozygous carrier of the Wilson's disease gene. *J. clin. Invest.* **40:**707-715, 1961.

18. Aisen, P.; Schorr, J. B.; Morell, A. G.; Gold, R. Z. and Scheinberg, I. H.: A rapid screening test for deficiency of plasma ceruloplasmin and its value in the diagnosis of Wilson's disease. *Amer. J. Med.* **28:**550-554, 1960.

19. Rosenoer, J. M.: In *Wilson's Disease. Some Current Concepts* Walshe, J. M. and Cumings, J. N. eds), Charles C. Thomas, Springfield, Illinois, pp. 110-112, 1961.

20. Williams, A. O.: Studies on copper, caeruloplasmin and cirrhosis in relation to Wilson's disease. *Brit. J. exp. Path.* **46:**564-568, 1965.

21. Osborn, S. B.; Roberts, C. N. and Walshe, J. M.: Uptake of radiocopper by the liver. A study of patients with Wilson's disease and various control groups. *Clin. Sci.* **24:**13-22, 1963.

22. Tu, J. B.: A genetic, biochemical and clinical study of Wilson's disease among Chinese in Taiwan. *Acta paediat. Sinica* **4:**81-104, 1963.

23. Cooper, W. C.; Gershon, R. K.; Sun, S. -C. and Fresh, J. W.: Anicteric viral hepatitis. A clinicopathological follow-up study in Taiwan. *New Engl. J. Med.* **274:**585-595, 1966.

24. Walshe, J. M. and Briggs, J.: Caeruloplasmin in liver disease: A diagnostic pitfall. *Lancet* **ii:**263-265, 1962.

25. Gault, M. H.; Stein, J. and Arnoff, A.: Serum ceruloplasmin in hepatobiliary and other disorders: Significance of abnormal values. *Gastroenterology* **50:**8-18, 1966.

26. Stanton, R. E. and Joos, H. A.: Glutamic-oxalacetic transaminase of serum in infancy and childhood. *Pediatrics* **24:**362-366, 1959.

27. Scheinberg, I. H.; Harris, R. S.; Morell, A. G. and Dublin, D.: Some aspects of the relation of ceruloplasmin to Wilson's disease. *Neurology* **8:**44-51, 1958.

28. Schaffner, F.; Sternlieb, I.; Barka, T. and Popper, H.: Hepatocellular changes in Wilson's disease: histochemical and electron microscopic studies, *Amer. J. Path.* **41:**315-327, 1962.

29. Tu, J. B.; Cooper, W. C.; Blackwell, R. Q. and Hou, T. Y.: Treatment of hepatolenticular degeneration (Wilson's disease) in the asymptomatic stage, *Neurology* **15:**402-408, 1965.

30. Scheinberg, I. H. and Sternlieb, I.: The liver in Wilson's disease. *Gastroenterology* **37:**550-564, 1959.

31. Sass-Kortsak, A.: Copper metabolism. *Advanc. clin. Chem.* **8:**1-67, 1965.

32. Hunt, A. H.; Parr, R. M.; Taylor, D. M. and Trott, N. G.: Relation between cirrhosis and trace metal content of liver with special reference to primary biliary cirrhosis and copper. *Brit. med. J.* **ii:**1498-1501, 1963.

33. Butt, E. M.; Nusbaum, R. E.; Gilmour, T. C. and DiDio, S. L.: Trace metal patterns in disease states. *Amer. J. clin. Path.* **30:**479-497, 1958.

34. Scheinberg, I. H. and Sternlieb, I.: Wilson's disease. *Ann. Rev. Med.* **16:**119-135, 1965.

35. Tu, J. B.; Blackwell, R. Q. and Watten, R. H.: Copper balance studies during the treatment of patients with Wilson's disease, *Metabolism* **14:**653-666, 1965.

36. Watten, R. H.; Tu, J. B.; Blackwell, R. Q. and Hou, T. Y.: Contributions of copper balance studies to investigation and management of Wilson's disease. In Birth Defects: Original Article Series, *Wilson's Disease.* The National Foundation, New York, Vol. IV, No. 2, pp. 35-40, April, 1968.

37. Cumings, J. N.: The effects of BAL in hepatolenticular degeneration. *Brain* **74:**10-22, 1951.

38. Sternlieb, I. and Scheinberg, I. H.: Penicillamine therapy for hepatolenticular degeneration. *J. Amer. med. Ass.* **189:**748-754, 1964.

# The Detection of Wilson's Disease and the Prevention of the Clinical Manifestations in Apparently Healthy Subjects*

Irmin Sternlieb, M.D.** and I. Herbert Scheinberg, M.D.***

A systematic search for the presence of biochemical abnormalities characteristic of Wilson's disease in siblings and children of known patients has uncovered apparently healthy subjects in whom Wilson's disease is latent. A combination of hypoceruloplasminemia (serum ceruloplasmin concentration of less than 20 mg/100 ml) and increased hepatic copper concentration (more than 250 mcgm/gm dry liver) was the basis for the diagnosis in 28 of 43 subjects. Thirty-six of these patients have regularly followed an "anti-copper" regimen and none of them has developed any symptom of the disease during a total follow-up period of more than 120 patient-years. In contrast all seven untreated patients developed Wilson's disease.

Although the disturbance in copper metabolism which characterizes Wilson's disease is inherited, signs and symptoms have never been reported to occur before four years of age and may not occur until the fifth decade. When an early diagnosis is made it is generally because isolated stigmata of the disease – Kayser-Fleischer rings, mild neurologic abnormalities, hepatomegaly, splenomegaly, or a few spider angiomata – are observed by a physician who is astute enough to suspect Wilson's disease. Even earlier diagnosis is possible, however, in asymptomatic subjects, with none of these signs, in whom the presence of Wilson's disease can be established exclusively by biochemical means.[1-16] It now appears possible to prevent Wilson's disease from manifesting itself in such patients.

From ten years of observation of the states of health of 48 asymptomatic subjects, 40 of whom were treated with a "decopperizing" regimen,[17-18] we have, first, confirmed our earlier conclusion that a decreased serum ceruloplasmin concentration and an increased hepatic copper concentration are almost always necessary, while the latter is sufficient to establish the diagnosis of Wilson's disease in an asymptomatic subject.[7] Second, we have learned that if such a biochemical diagnosis is made, prophylactic therapy is mandatory no matter how healthy the patient appears to be.

## Methods

*Diagnostic:* serum ceruloplasmin concentrations were determined by measuring the oxidase activity of serum towards paraphenylenediamine.[19,20] Quantitative methods[20,21] were used in 28, and semiquantitative methods[19] in the remaining 20 patients.

Hepatic copper concentrations of surgical or needle biopsy specimens were determined by wet ashing and measurement of color developed with dicyclohexanone-oxalyldihydrazone[22] or biquinoline,[23] in 23 of 33 samples obtained. No details of the analytic method used in ten samples were available, and hepatic copper concentrations were not determined at all in the remaining 15 patients. In seven of the last the diagnosis of Wilson's disease was established by the demonstration of hypercupriuria, abnormal liver function or morphology, and a characteristic result of a test of incorporation of $^{64}Cu$ into ceruloplasmin; and, in one, by abnormal liver histology and the same $^{64}Cu$ test.[15] In the remaining seven patients of this group the diagnosis was based on hypoceruloplasminemia and no further tests were obtained initially. Five of these subjects were not treated and classical Wilson's disease developed[1,4,8]; in the other two who were aceruloplasminemic siblings of a patient with manifest Wilson's disease, therapy was instituted

*Supported in part by grants from the U.S. Public Health Service (A1-1059, TI AM-5384, HD-006-74, and 5 MO1 Fr-50) and from the Life Insurance Medical Research Fund (G-62-58).

**Associate Professor, Department of Medicine, Albert Einstein College of Medicine and Bronx Municipal Hospital Center, Bronx, New York.

***Professor, Department of Medicine, Albert Einstein College of Medicine and Bronx Municipal Hospital Center, Bronx, New York.

without any additional tests and hepatic biopsy is planned in the near future.

Thirty-four liver biopsy specimens were examined histologically. A variety of other determinations discussed below, was carried out in some patients.

*Therapeutic:* prophylactic therapy was administered to 40 of the asymptomatic subjects in whom the diagnosis of Wilson's disease was made.[6,7,9-11,13,14,16] The prime component of the regimen was D-penicillamine.[17,18]

*Results of diagnostic tests:* of the 28 patients in whom quantitative measurements of ceruloplasmin was made, 17, or 61%, had no trace of this protein detectable, (a striking contrast with our accumulated group of 161 patients who were ill with Wilson's disease of whom only 27% had no ceruloplasmin). Nineteen of the 20 semi-quantitative determinations of ceruloplasmin concentration were below the lower limit of normal for the method used, and, in the one patient with a concentration above this, the diagnosis of Wilson's disease, based only on hypercupriuria and elevated serum transaminase levels, was confirmed when, without treatment, characteristic clinical manifestations appeared.[5]

The mean of the 33 hepatic copper concentrations was 1008 mcg/g dry liver with a range of 152* to 1828 (normal: 20-45 mcg/g). In 25 symptomatic patients the mean copper concentration of the biopsy specimens was 649 mcg/g with a range of 101-1727 mcg/g.

The 34 biopsy specimens examined histologically showed pathologic changes ranging from fatty infiltration to inflamation and cirrhosis, in all but five children.[7,9-11,13,14,16] In all of the latter, who were 15 months to seven and one-half years of age, glycogen nuclei in hepatocytes constituted the sole, and nonspecific, abnormality.

The following miscellaneous findings are recorded since results of these kinds are of some significance in the diagnosis of Wilson's disease:

**a)** In only 22 of the 34 asymptomatic patients in whom urinary copper excretion was measured was there over 100 mcg of copper found in 24-hour collections (normal: below 50 mcg/24 hours).

**b)** Of 14 specimens stained for copper histochemically,[24,25] nine gave negative results although quantitative determinations, performed in seven of these showed hepatic copper concentrations ranging between 152 and 1823 mcg/g.

**c)** Abnormal amino-aciduria was observed in only four of the 14 patients in whom this was looked for.

**d)** Serum uric acid concentrations were within normal limits in our nine patients.

*Nine months later a repeat biopsy sample from this patient contained 400 mcg/g.

*Results of prophylactic therapy:* in seven of the eight untreated patients characteristic and unequivocal signs of Wilson's disease developed[1,4,5,8] and five of them died within one to six years after the diagnosis was first made.

In none of the 40 treated patients did significant neurologic or hepatic abnormalities develop during more than 135 patient-years. Two patients developed Kayser-Fleischer rings within eight months after therapy was started but there was doubt that one of them had adhered to his regimen during this period. Stuttering appeared in one patient; the spleen became palpable in another; and a fine tremor of one hand appeared in a boy who took penicillamine intermittently.

**Discussion**

Determinations of the serum concentration of ceruloplasmin are being performed increasingly often in relatives of patients with Wilson's disease as well as in healthy children unrelated to such patients. If a value of less than 20 mgm per 100 ml is confirmed, and if the patient can be shown not to have one of the acquired conditions associated with hypoceruloplasminemia,* we believe a biopsy specimen of the liver must be quantitatively analyzed for copper. A value of 250 or more mcgm of copper per gram of dry liver means that it is highly probable that the individual will ultimately sicken and die of Wilson's disease, unless he is treated appropriately. With adequate therapy, the outlook for health and life is excellent.

Heterozygous carriers of one "Wilson's disease" gene never become clinically ill and need no treatment. Yet in the serum of about 20% of heterozygotes the concentration of serum ceruloplasmin is below 20 mg%.[7] Determination of the hepatic copper concentration of a hypoceruloplasminemic subject yields the best criterion by which the physician must decide whether to withhold lifelong and risky treatment from a heterozygote, or to administer lifesaving therapy to an abnormal homozygote. Even with such a procedure, incorrect decisions will occasionally be reached. Thus we made the diagnosis of Wilson's disease in an asymptomatic man of 20 who 1) had no ceruloplasmin in his serum; 2) had hepatic copper concentrations of 261, 183 and 258 mcgm/g dry liver in three biopsy samples taken within a four-year interval; and 3) had a brother of 23 with similar findings and clinical manifestations of Wilson's disease. The younger brother, however, differed from the older in having neither hypercupriuria, nor significant histopathologic changes in his liver, and, in remaining asymptomatic during five years despite his refusal, because of his well-being, to follow the regimen prescribed. Finally, when we realized that his hepatic copper concentration was not increasing with time, although that of an untreated patient does, and that his mother was also aceruloplasminemic and perfectly healthy at age 55,[7] we concluded that he and she were both heterozygous.

*sprue, kwashiorkor, nephrotic syndrome, protein-losing enteropathy, and very rare instances of hepatitis.

Sixty-one percent of the asymptomatic patients discussed in this paper had no detectable ceruloplasmin; in marked contrast only 27% of the symptomatic patients had such a low level of the protein. It seems quite possible that asymptomatic subjects, with only moderate deficiencies of ceruloplasmin, may be overlooked while a symptomatic patient, with the same concentration, would not be. Thus, for example, from our own experience, we failed to investigate further an apparently healthy child with 17 mgm of ceruloplasmin per 100 ml of serum several years ago, in part because his siblings with manifest Wilson's disease exhibited much lower concentrations. Yet within a year hepatomegaly developed in this boy and his incorporation of $^{64}Cu$ into ceruloplasmin was characteristic of patients with Wilson's disease.[26]

One out of the 48 patients reviewed had a normal concentration of serum ceruloplasmin,[5] a finding which has been verified rarely in symptomatic patients with Wilson's disease.[27] In this patient, as in at least some of the earlier cases, liver dysfunction was present and may have elevated a usually depressed level.

Although the interpretation of serum ceruloplasmin concentrations has its limitations and the performance of accurate quantitative measurements of hepatic copper concentration is difficult, these tests are, we believe, essential for reliable diagnosis in an asymptomatic individual. True, in a hypoceruloplasminemic subject the diagnosis may be made if hypercupriuria and definite histologic abnormalities are found, but normal findings in both of the latter do not rule the diagnosis out. Histochemical staining, and searches for amino-aciduria have proved misleading in several instances[28,29] and determinations of serum uric acid concentrations are of no diagnostic help.

These results make it difficult to overestimate the importance of therapy in asymptomatic patients. Of eight asymptomatic patients, untreated because of the unavailability of penicillamine, five have died and two are ill with Wilson's disease. In contrast, all of the 40 asymptomatic patients who have been treated are alive and well.

Because of the rarity of Wilson's disease a study such as this, to be meaningful, could only be collaborative. We have many colleagues to thank for their generous help:

Dr. Masataka Arima, Tokyo; Dr. Lester Baker, Philadelphia; Dr. Jean-Pierre Benhamou, Clichy; Dr. Ira K. Brandt, New Haven; Prof. John N. Cumings, London; Dr. W. Dangerfield, London; Dr. D. K. Dastur, Bombay; Dr. Kazuhiko Fukuda, Sendai; Dr. Norman P. Goldstein, Rochester; Dr. Bechir Hamza, Tunis; Dr. Frank Iber, Baltimore; Prof. Hénri Jérôme, Paris; Prof. J. Lange, Gummersbach; Dr. A. Jonathan Levi, London; Dr. C. Charlton Mabry, Lexington; Dr. Richard W. Reilly, Chicago; Dr. Fred Rosen, Boston; Prof. Sheila Sherlock, London; Dr. Jun-bi Tu, Taipei; Dr. N. H. Wadia, Bombay; Dr. John M. Walshe, Cambridge; Dr. C. B. M. Warren, Chelmsford; Dr. Claus Weiner, Munich; Doz. Dr. Friedrich Wewalka, Vienna.

## REFERENCES


1. Lygren, T.; Sörensen, E. W. and Bernhardsen, A.: Hepatolenticular degeneration (Wilson's Disease). A case diagnosed biochemically before clinical manifestations. *Lancet* **i:**276-277, 1959.

2. Arima, M.; Oshima, M.; Shima, N.; Obe, Y. and Suzuki, M.: Wilson's disease in children. Report of eleven cases with special reference to juvenile cirrhosis. *Paediatria Univ. Tokyo* **5:**14-19, 1960.

3. Lange, J.: Über den klinisch asymptomatischen Morbus Wilson. *Dtsch. med. Wschr.* **87:**541-544, 1962.

4. Giagheddu, M. and Chessa-Perle, E.: Studio dell-attività rame-ossidasica serica in otto famiglie colpite da Malattia di Strümpel-Wilson (Degeneraziona epato-lenticolare). *Sist. nerv.* (Milano) **13:**237-52, 1962.

5. Tu, J. B.; Cooper, W. C.; Blackwell, R. A. and Hou, T. Y.: Asymptomatic Wilson's disease. *Acta Paed. Sin.* **3:**154-160, 1962.

6. Warren, C. B. M. and Broughton, P. M. G.: Wilson's disease. *Arch. Dis. Childh.* **37:**242-252, 1962.

7. Sternlieb, I. and Scheinberg, I. H.: The diagnosis of Wilson's disease in asymptomatic patients. *J. Amer. med. Ass.* **183:**747-750, 1963.

8. Wadia, N. H. and Dastur, D. K.: Wilson's disease in four Indian families (clinical, genetical and biochemical aspects). *Neurology, (Bombay)* **11:**1-18, 1963.

9. Arima, M.; Komiya, K.; Kamoshita, S. and Mukai, N.: Clinical and pathological characteristics in Wilson's disease in cases under ten years of age. *Paed. Univ. Tokyo,* **9:**17-22, 1963.

10. Weiner, C.: Morbus Wilson im Kindesalter. *Münch. med. Wschr.* **106:**387-402, 1964.

11. Tu, J. B.; Cooper, W. C.; Blackwell, R. Q. and Hou, T. Y.: Treatment of hepatolenticular degeneration (Wilson's disease) in the asymptomatic stage. *Neurology,* **15:**402-408, 1965.

12. Fukuda, K.: Clinical and pathological aspects of Wilson's disease in cases of one and the same family. *Tohoku J. exp. Med.,* **85:**55-71, 1965.

13. Sigwald, J.; Raverdy, P.; Jérôme, H.; Raverdy, E.; Ficzlewicz, P.; Boutelier, D. and Peigné, F.: A propos d'une observation de dégénérescence hépatolenticulaire (D.H.L.). Intérét du déspistage systématique des homozygotes cliniquement indemnes. *Rev. neurol.* (Paris) **113:**33-37, 1965.

14. Jérôme, H. and Sternlieb, I.: La détection préclinique de la maladie de Wilson. *Arch. franc. Pédiat.* **23:**669-677, 1966.

15. Tauxe, W. N.; Goldstein, N. P.; Randall, R. V. and Gross, J. B.: Radiocopper studies in patients with Wilson's disease and their relatives. *Amer. J. Med.* **41:**375-380, 1966.

16. Levi, A. J.; Sherlock S.; Scheuer, P. J. and Cumings, J. N.: Presymptomatic Wilson's disease. *Lancet,* **ii:**575-579, 1967.

17. Walshe, J. M.: Wilson's disease, new oral therapy. *Lancet,* **i:**25-26, 1956.

18. Sternlieb, I. and Scheinberg, I. H.: Penicillamine therapy for hepatolenticular degeneration. *J. Amer. med. Ass.* **189:**748-754, 1964.

19. Ravin, H. A.: Rapid test for hepatolenticular degeneration. *Lancet,* **i:**726-727, 1956.

20. Morell, A. G.; Windsor, J.; Sternlieb, I. and Scheinberg, I. H.: Measurement of the concentration of ceruloplasmin in serum by determination of its ovidase activity. In F. W. Sunderman and F. W. Sunderman, Jr., *Laboratory Diagnosis of Liver Diseases.* St. Louis, W. H. Green, Inc., Chapter 16B (in press).

21. Jérôme, H. and Girault, M.: Dosage de la ceruloplasmine par détermination de son activité enzymatique. *Rev. franc. Etud. clin. biol.* (In press).

22. Morell, A. G.; Windsor, J.; Sternlieb, I. and Scheinberg, I. H.: The spectrophotometric determination of microgram quantities of copper in biological materials. In F. W. Sunderman and F. W. Sunderman, Jr., *Laboratory Diagnosis of Liver Diseases.* St. Louis, W. H. Green, Inc., Chapter 16C (in press).

23. Jérôme, H. and Girault, M.: Microméthode spectrophotométrique de dosage du cuivre dans les tissus et les liquides biologiques. *Bull. Soc. Chim. biol.* (In press).

24. Uzman, L. L.: Histochemical localization of copper with rubeanic acid. *Lab. Invest.* **5:**299-305, 1956.

25. Howell, J. S.: Histochemical demonstration of copper in copper-fed rats and in hepatolenticular degeneration. *J. Path. Bact.* **77:**473-484, 1959.

26. Sternlieb, I.; Morell, A. G.; Bauer, C. D.; Combes, B.; de Bobes-Sternberg, S. and Scheinberg, I. H.: Detection of the heterozygous carrier of the Wilson's disease gene. *J. clin. Invest.* **40:**707-715, 1961.

27. Scheinberg, I. H. and Sternlieb, I.: Wilson's disease and the concentration of caeruloplasmin in serum. *Lancet* **i:**1420-1421, 1963.

28. Barbeau, A.; Reilly, R. W.; Marver, H. and Kirsner, J. B.: An early defect in Wilson's disease. *Rev. canad. Biol.* **20:**25-36, 1961.

29. Forssman, O.: Wilson's disease in a Swedish family. *Acta med. scand.* **166:**237-239, 1960.

# Some Observations on the Treatment of Wilson's Disease with Penicillamine

JOHN M. WALSHE, Sc.D., F.R.C.P.*

A review of 11 years of experience with the use of the drug penicillamine, which included treatment of 33 patients with Wilson's disease. It is concluded that all patients with this disease will benefit from treatment with penicillamine once a negative copper balance has been established and maintained.

Until the year 1948 Wilson's disease was a hopeless therapeutic problem with an invariably fatal outcome even though a few cases ran a remarkably chronic course.[2] However, Cumings,[3] realizing the possibilities of Peters'[6] work in Oxford on the design of the BAL molecule for the treatment of arsenical war gas poisoning, suggested that BAL might be of value for mobilizing excess stores of copper from patients with Wilson's disease. Although BAL has undoubtedly helped many patients with Wilson's disease[1] it is far from an ideal therapeutic agent both because of the painful nature of the injection and the frequent toxic reactions. In 1956 I suggested that penicillamine (dimethyl cysteine) by virtue of the relative stability of its thiol group, and hence its ability to mobilize copper when given by mouth, should be of value in the treatment of Wilson's disease.[7] Time has proved the accuracy of this prediction. It is my object to review 11 years experience with the use of this drug and to summarize the results of maintenance treatment on both the biochemical and the clinical course of the illness. This work has been recorded in detail elsewhere.[8]

My first patient was started on penicillamine in December 1955. At that time her dosage was limited by the problems of preparing the penicillamine and packing it into capsules in my laboratory. She received on average 450 mg daily during the first year and this small dose, I believe, explains why it took nearly 12 months before improvement occurred. This young woman, who was originally bedridden, is now leading a normal married life though she has not as yet propagated her abnormal gene.

Since 1955 it has been possible to see a relatively large number of cases of this rare disease so that I can now report findings on an additional 32 patients.

*Reader in Metabolic Disease, Department of Investigate Medicine, University of Cambridge, England.

## The Effect of Penicillamine on Copper Stores

In 26 patients there was a significant fall in the concentration of copper in the serum and also in the basal copper excretion in the urine following continuous treatment with penicillamine for a mean period of two years (Table I). In patients in whom there was a measurable concentration of ceruloplasmin in the serum when first seen, this was observed to fall with treatment (Fig. 1). The basal rate of copper excretion fell from an average of 0.24 $\mu$g/minute before treatment to 0.08 $\mu$g/minute after two years of treatment; there was a corresponding fall in the response to a test dose of penicillamine but the renal clearance remained virtually unchanged (Table II). Studies with radiocopper ($^{64}$Cu) have confirmed that the apparent reduction in the cupruretic response to penicillamine was not associated with drug resistance, and therefore, presumably resulted from depletion of the body stores of excess copper. For instance patient S.T., when first seen was given radiocopper intravenously together with full therapeutic doses of penicillamine. He excreted 35% of the radioisotope in 24 hours. When tested under exactly similar conditions, E.M., who had been taking penicillamine for six years, excreted 38% of the radiocopper. Clearance studies after injec-

### ABOUT THE AUTHOR

Dr. J. M. Walshe is reader in metabolic disease in the Department of Investigative Medicine in the University of Cambridge. He received his training in the study of metabolic disease in Professor Charles Dent's Unit at University College Hospital in London. It was while working on the Harvard Medical Unit at the Boston City Hospital that he first became interested in Wilson's disease and after returning to England he took up the appointment in the Medical School of Cambridge University which permitted him to make Wilson's disease his major interest.

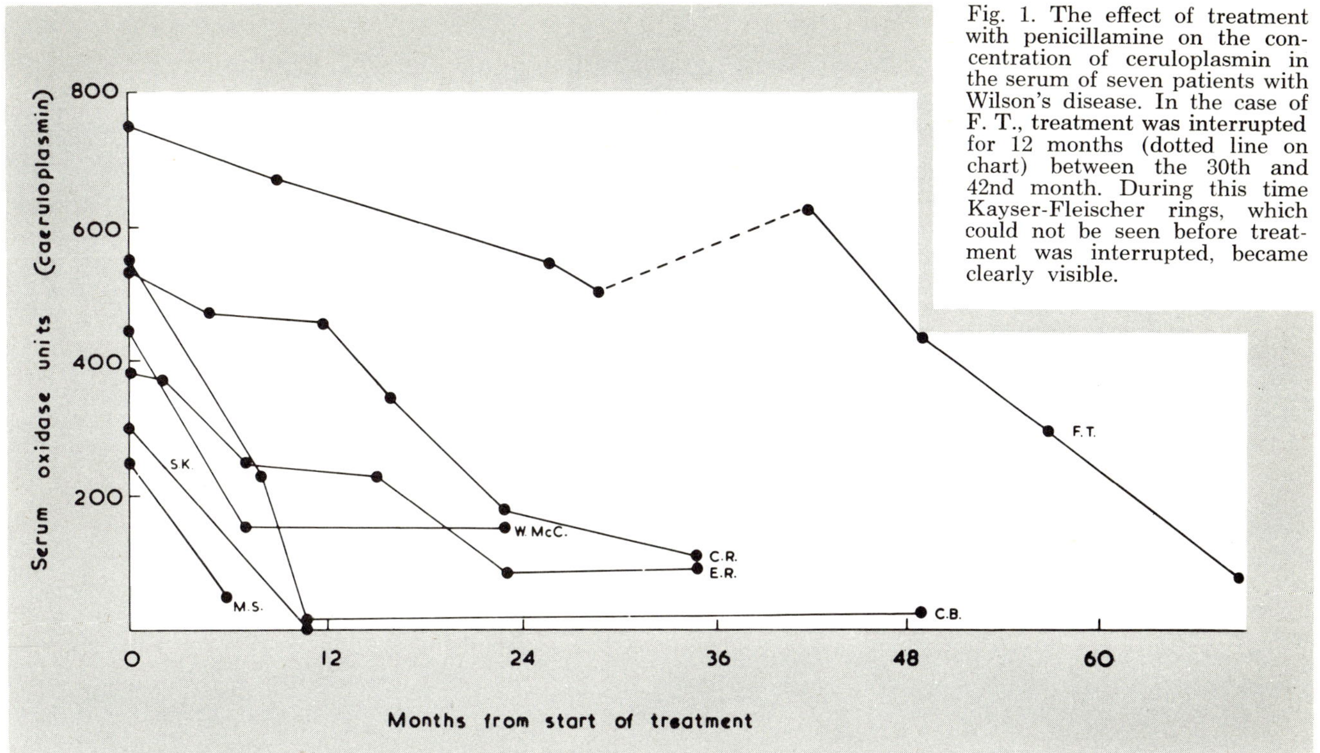


Fig. 1. The effect of treatment with penicillamine on the concentration of ceruloplasmin in the serum of seven patients with Wilson's disease. In the case of F. T., treatment was interrupted for 12 months (dotted line on chart) between the 30th and 42nd month. During this time Kayser-Fleischer rings, which could not be seen before treatment was interrupted, became clearly visible.

tion of $^{67}Cu$ also showed an identity of response between J. Ba. who had been on treatment for five years and D.C. who had only been taking penicillamine for three months.[8] Further evidence of depletion of abnormal copper stores has been seen in the fading or complete disappearance of the Kayser-Fleischer rings. On the other hand, there has been no suggestion of a deficiency of copper for essential metabolic requirements such as cytochrome c oxidase or hemoglobin synthesis, or for the formation of the other copper proteins; the copper content of the hair has remained uninfluenced by treatment.[4]

### Therapeutic Regimen

Most patients received between 900 mg and 1,800 mg D-penicillamine HCl daily. The maximum dose given, calculated as free base, was 48 mg/Kg for a period of one year but most patients received 35 mg/Kg. At the time of writing one patient (H.L.) has taken 3,600 g without toxic effects. BAL was not given and potassium sulfide was given only to a few patients who specifically requested it. Slavish adherence to a low copper diet was not enforced but patients were counseled to eschew certain high copper foods, shell fish, liver, nuts, cocoa and chocolate, mushrooms, dried fruit and whisky (the best whiskies are made in copper stills). Apart from this they have been encouraged to lead as nearly normal lives as possible. Pyridoxine (vitamin B6) has been given only to growing children or to adults living at great distances who could not receive adequate supervision, (indeed evidence of pyridoxine deficiency has been strikingly absent).[5]

### Results of Treatment

These have been encouraging and 27 out of 32 patients have benefited, but five have died. In the early days one died of progressive neurologic disease. Retrospective judgment points to inadequate dosage as the cause of failure; the patient's serum copper concentration actually rose while on treatment and at postmortem examination the tissue concentrations of copper were still markedly elevated.[8] Her maximum dose of penicillamine was 1,200 mg daily for a few weeks; otherwise she received only 900 mg daily. It has been observed over the

**TABLE I**

## Effect of Continuous Penicillamine Therapy on Serum and Urine Copper Levels* in Wilson's Disease (mean of 26 patients).

| | Plasma Copper, μg/100 ml | Urine copper, μg/min. |
|---|---|---|
| Before therapy | 50.0 | 0.24 |
| On therapy | 20.0 | 0.08 |

*Treatment was stopped 48 hours before specimen collection.

TABLE II

**Effect of Continuous Penicillamine Therapy on Endogenous Copper Clearance in Wilson's Disease* (mean of 26 patients).**

| | Urine copper, μg/min. | | Clearance, ml/min. | |
|---|---|---|---|---|
| | Basal | After 600 mg Penicillamine | Basal | After 600 mg Penicillamine |
| Before therapy | 0.24 | 4.13 | 0.50 | 13.2 |
| On therapy | 0.08 | 2.07 | 0.37 | 19.1 |

*Treatment was discontinued 48 hours before clearance studies.

years that clinical response is always preceded by a fall in the serum copper and ceruloplasmin concentrations (Fig. 1) and if this does not occur the dose of penicillamine should be increased. Of the other four patients who died two had severe toxic or sensitivity reactions as soon as penicillamine was given. Adequate treatment could not be established while two were in the terminal stage of the disease and they died very soon after penicillamine was started. These have been discussed in detail elsewhere.[8] Of these five patients two died of neurologic disease, one of hepatic failure, one of hemorrhage from a ruptured esophageal varix and one of mixed hepatic and neurologic disease.

Five patients were diagnosed in the presymptomatic stage of the illness when an elder sibling was found to be affected. All have remained well for periods of up to six years on prophylactic treatment. In all these subjects routine laboratory tests of liver function strongly suggested hepatic involvement, the serum transaminases being a particularly useful test at this stage of the disease (Table III). Abnormalities of the serum proteins were less marked, but one girl of nine years of age had a considerable elevation of gamma globulin. This returned slowly to normal over a period of two years.

Five patients had hepatic disease with fluid retention and jaundice and three had a mixed hepatic and neurologic illness with psychiatric involvement. The serum transaminases were less abnormal in this group, but they too returned to normal with treatment (Table III). Clinically these patients have done well except for the psychiatric disturbances which though improving are still troublesome at the time of writing. Edema and ascites have resorbed so that diuretics and salt restriction are no longer necessary for these patients. One patient in this group, in addition to liver disease, had had a series of severe hemolytic crises which have not recurred since treatment was started two years ago.

Fifteen patients were seen whose symptoms were confined to the nervous system; these patients had only minor abnormalities in laboratory tests of liver function (Table III) even though, in some cases, there was a definite history of jaundice earlier in the illness. The most severely affected patients were totally disabled by tremor or ballistic movements and were entirely dependent on nursing help for feeding and personal toilet. The duration of symptoms varied from around 18 months to 20 years. All patients in this group have improved since starting treatment which has been continued for periods of from one to 11 years. Nine patients are now virtually symptom free. At the start of treatment there may be an initial period of deterioration and real improvement may not be obvious for as long as nine months but most patients show benefit sooner. Several years may elapse before maximum improvement is achieved. Late deterioration has only been seen occasionally when, without my knowledge, the patient's dose of penicillamine has been reduced; such deterioration is always associated with and usually preceded by a rise in the serum copper and basal urine copper excretion. When the penicillamine dose is restored to its initial level the patient will again respond. To reduce the dose is potentially hazardous and should never be undertaken without full biochemical control.

TABLE III

**Effect of Continuous Penicillamine Therapy on Mean Serum Transaminase Values in Patients with Wilson's Disease.**

| | Before therapy | | On therapy | |
|---|---|---|---|---|
| | SGOT. | SGPT. | SGOT. | SGPT. |
| Normal range | $< 40$ | $< 30$ | | |
| Presymptomatic (5)* | 128 | 200 | 29 | 27 |
| Hepatic and mixed cases (8)* | 57 | 58 | 22 | 26 |
| Neurologic (14)* | 36 | 34 | 26 | 27 |

*Figures in brackets denote the number of cases studied.

Serious toxic symptoms have not been seen though some patients have chronic thrombocytopenia. Anemia and iron deficiency have not been recorded[9] and biochemical changes suggesting pyridoxine depletion have been observed in only one of 19 patients studied.[5] Evidence for penicillamine incorporation into protein in place of cysteine has been sought in hydrolysates of protein from liver, red cells, serum and hair, but has not been found in any of these tissues.

### Conclusions

The results of treatment of 33 patients with Wilson's disease have been reviewed. In 28 the response has been good. Five patients died and the reasons for these deaths have been reviewed. In one case treatment was clearly inadequate and in two it was initiated too late to influence the course of the illness. In two cases there were severe reactions to the drug which prevented establishment of adequate dosage.

It is concluded that all patients will benefit from treatment with penicillamine once a negative copper balance has been established and maintained; it seems probable that therapeutic failures reported in the literature are due more to shortcomings on the part of the physician than on the part of the drug.

## REFERENCES


1. Bearn, A. G.: The place of BAL in the therapy of Wilson's disease. *Amer. J. Med.* **21**:134, 1956.
2. Cumings, J. N.: Heavy metals and the brain. Blackwell, Oxford, p. 21, 1959.
3. Cumings, J. N.: The copper and iron content of brain in the normal and in hepatolenticular degeneration. *Brain,* **71**:410-415, 1948.
4. Gibbs, K. and Walshe, J. M.: Penicillamine and pyridoxine requirements in man. *Lancet,* **i**:175-179, 1966.
5. Gibbs, K. and Walshe, J. M.: A study of the copper content of hair in normal families and those with Wilson's disease. *J. Med. Genet.* **2**:181-184, 1965.
6. Peters, R. A.; Stocken, L. A. and Thompson, R. H. S.: British antilewistie BAL. *Nature,* **156**:616-619, 1945.
7. Walshe, J. M.: Penicillamine. A new oral therapy for Wilson's disease. *Amer. J. Med.* **21**:487-495, 1956.
8. Walshe, J. M.: The physiology of copper in man and its relation to Wilson's disease. *Brain,* **90**:149-176, 1967.
9. Walshe, J. M. and Clark, V.: Effect of penicillamine on serum iron. *Arch. Dis. Childh.* **40**:651-653, 1965.

# Long-Term Treatment of Wilson's Disease with D-Penicillamine

JOACHIM LANGE, M.D.*

The results of therapy of 12 patients with manifest Wilson's disease and of six asymptomatic patients are reviewed. Therapy was based principally on the administration of D-penicillamine-HCl in doses of 0.9-1.35 gm daily. Neurologic manifestations responded very well to therapy. Improvement of liver function tests was also noted. Kayser-Fleischer rings disappeared or diminished in four patients. No significant clinical manifestations appeared in the treated, asymptomatic patients.

## Introduction

Since 1956, when Walshe discovered the copper-binding quality of penicillamine,[1] Wilson's disease,[2] has been studied intensively.

The clinical and biochemical criteria of Wilson's disease are by now so distinct that it is possible to diagnose the disease at a very early stage, even before the appearance of any clinical manifestation. This is important for the discovery and prophylactic treatment of apparently healthy homozygous siblings.[3-5]

In cooperation with several colleagues in West Germany** who kindly put their observations at my disposal, we focused our attention on early diagnosis by biochemical methods and therapy, both of which have improved remarkably since 1956. There is no doubt that penicillamine is more effective, easier to apply and more compatible than previously used drugs, e.g. BAL.

We observed 12 patients with manifest Wilson's disease and six asymptomatic siblings. They have been treated from two to seven years with D-penicillamine-HCl (Metalcaptase®, Heyl & Co.) which was administered in a daily dosage of 0.9 to 1.35 g of free base. Potassium sulfide was given in doses of 20 mg during the three main meals. In order to minimize the absorption of dietary copper, patients received a low copper diet and were advised to avoid drinking water high in copper content. Special consideration was also given to the use of copper-free cooking equipment.

In the 12 patients of group 1 (Table I) the disease first manifested at ages varying from seven to 26 years, with a mean of 15.3 years. The interval between the first evidence of symptoms and the onset of treatment with penicillamine ranged from one month to 22 years. Three patients (Nos. 9, 10, 11), diagnosed for five, seven and 12 years, had been treated with BAL earlier, which did not stop progression of the disease. In case No. 9 copper excretion increased slightly, but copper balance remained positive.[6]

Group 1a (Nos. 1-6) consisted of six patients with predominent Parkinson-like symptoms and indications of hepatic dysfunction (Wilson-type). In group 1b (Nos. 7-12) generalized tremors predominated with only minimal signs of liver disease (pseudosclerotic-type). Onset of symptoms in patients of group 1b occurred on the average six years later than in patients of group 1a

### ABOUT THE AUTHOR

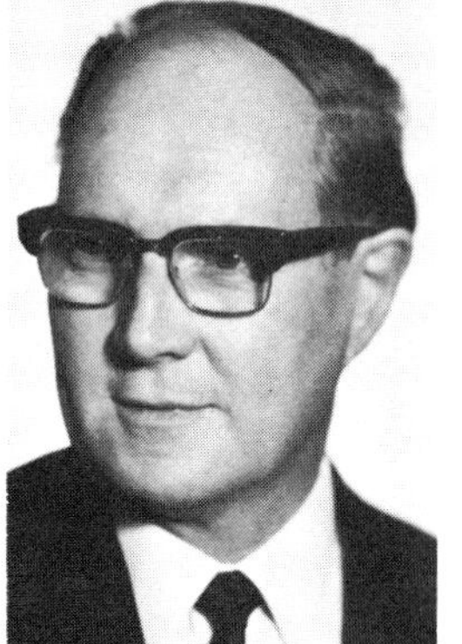

Dr. Joachim Lange, born in Germany in 1919, studied in Freiburg, Jena, Berlin and Hamburg. In 1944 he was appointed assistant to Dr. Med. H. H. Berg in Hamburg-Eppendorf. From 1946 to 1963 he did clinical work at the University of Bonn and was appointed Professor of Internal Medicine there in 1962. Since 1964 he has been Chief of the Department of Medicine at the Städtische Krankenhaus in Gummersbach, Germany.

*Professor of Internal Medicine, University of Bonn, Germany.

**Dr. F. Bläker, Hamburg; Dr. J. Duderstadt, Braunschweig; Dr. W. J. Henry, Berlin; Dr. H. Lange, Berlin-Buckow; Dr. P. Wallauer, Marburg; Dr. C. Weiner, München; Dr. T. Werner, Landau; Prof. Dr. E. Welte, Mönchengladbach.

(19.3 and 13.3 years, respectively). Severity of the disease was greater and rate of progression more rapid in patients of group 1a. Distinction between the two types of Wilson's disease is difficult although this classification seemed to be of prognostic importance as judged by our experience with therapy.

The diagnosis was based on clinical findings, abnormalities of copper metabolism, evidence of liver disturbance and presence of corneal rings in all cases. Mean serum-copper was 53 $\mu$g/100 ml and mean urinary copper excretion was 458 $\mu$g/day. Administration of 0.9 g of D-penicillamine-HCl resulted in elimination of 1.94 mg of copper per day. This provocative test is of additional diagnostic importance, since urinary copper excretion is not always markedly increased.

**Results of Treatment (Table I):**

1. Neurologic manifestations were present in eight cases and were less pronounced in three cases. One female patient had no neurologic abnormalities. In six patients (Nos. 1, 2, 6, 8, 9, 11) complete or almost complete remissions were obtained. Patients Nos. 9 and 11 showed dramatic improvement in spite of advanced disease after several years of illness. One patient had a normal pregnancy and gave birth to a healthy baby (No. 2). The other patients, however, had some residual symptoms left and all but one (No. 12), who died in the interim, regained their ability to work. One example demonstrates the recovery of manual skill by a female patient (No. 11), who had been unable to feed herself or write previously (Fig. 1).

2. Hepatic manifestations predominated in three patients (Nos. 1, 5, 6) and were less marked or absent in five cases (Nos. 7, 9-12). In 11 cases liver function tests and serial liver biopsies indicated a marked amelioration, particularly in case No. 5. This patient exhibited first progressive hepatic decompensation in the absence of neurologic disturbances.

3. Corneal Kayser-Fleischer rings disappeared completely in two patients and diminished in two others. In eight, however, they remained unchanged.

4. Significant amelioration of the patients' general condition was noted and the youngsters developed quite normally.

In general, when symptoms had been present for short periods, diagnosis was established early and treatment was instituted, symptoms disappeared quickly and permanently. In contrast, in cases with long histories and late diagnoses, residual symptoms, mainly concerning the stem ganglia, persisted in spite of treatment. Nevertheless, we agree with Scheinberg and Sternlieb[5,7,8] that treatment should be attempted for extended periods of time even in patients with advanced illness. One of our female patients (No. 10) who was sick for 12 years and completely incapacitated for several years, is able to eat and drink by herself, walks around and performs light housework now, after treatment.

Repeated measurements of urinary and serum copper during the long-term treatment gave the following results:

1. Serum copper decreased in six of seven cases. This decrease was more pronounced in patients treated for five to seven years (Table I).

2. The effect of penicillamine in promoting excretion of copper almost always decreased to such an extent

**TABLE I**

**EFFECTS OF D-PENICILLAMINE THERAPY IN PATIENTS WITH WILSON'S DISEASE**

| Patient No. | Sex | Age of onset of symptoms (years) | Age at onset of therapy (years) | Daily dose (g) | Findings before therapy** | | | Findings after therapy** | | | Copper in Serum mcg/100ml | | Copper in Urine mg/day | |
|---|---|---|---|---|---|---|---|---|---|---|---|---|---|---|
| | | | | | N | H | KF | N | H | KF | before therapy | on therapy | before therapy | on therapy |
| **Group 1a (Predominance of Parkinsonian and hepatic features)** | | | | | | | | | | | | | | |
| 1 | F | 18 | 18 | 0.9-1.35 | + | ++ | ++ | 0 | (+) | 0 | 57 | 33 | 0.67 | 2.68 |
| 2 | F | 16 | 18 | 0.6-1.35 | +++ | + | ++ | 0 | 0 | ++ | 89 | 33 | | 1.75 |
| 3 | M | 7 | 12 | 0.9-1.35 | +++ | ++ | ++ | + | (+) | (+) | 42 | 15 | 0.41 | 2.87 |
| 4 | M | 14 | 14 | 0.9 | + | ++ | + | (+) | (+) | + | 40 | 12 | 0.42 | 0.80 |
| 5 | F | 15 | 15 | 0.9 | 0 | ++++ | ++ | 0 | + | ++ | 59 | | 0.60 | 1.96 |
| 6 | M | 10 | 11 | 0.9 | (+) | +++ | ++ | 0 | + | 0 | 63 | 35 | 0.40 | 3.40 |
| **Group 1b (Pseudosclerotic type)** | | | | | | | | | | | | | | |
| 7 | F | 26 | 49 | 0.9 | +++ | (+) | ++ | + | 0 | ++ | 40 | 59 | 0.34 | 1.66 |
| 8 | M | 19 | 32 | 0.3 | +++ | + | ++ | + | ? | ++ | | | | |
| 9 | M | 22 | 27* | 0.9-1.35 | ++++ | + | ++ | (+) | 0 | (+) | 56 | 13 | 0.59 | 2.53 |
| 10 | F | 15 | 27* | 0.9 | ++++ | + | + | ++ | (+) | + | 19 | | | 0.89 |
| 11 | F | 16 | 23* | 0.9 | +++ | + | + | (+) | 0 | + | 55 | | 0.20 | 1.28 |
| 12 | F | 18 | 19 | 0.9-1.35 | +++ | (+) | + | + | 0 | + | 61 | 45 | 0.50 | 1.32 |

*Prior treatment with BAL.
**N: neurologic; H: hepatic; KF: Kayser-Fleischer rings.

TABLE II

ASYMPTOMATIC PATIENTS WITH WILSON'S DISEASE TREATED WITH D-PENICILLAMINE

| Patient No. | Sex | Age at time of diagnosis years | Age at onset of therapy years | Cerulo-plasmin* mg/100 ml | "Ravin test"** units | Copper in Serum mcg/100 ml | Copper in Urine mg/day | Copper in Liver mcg/g | Liver histology |
|---|---|---|---|---|---|---|---|---|---|
| 1 | M | 5 | 7 | <1 | 0.02 | 44 | 0.15 | 1823 | Active portal cirrhosis, ballooned cells. |
| 2 | M | 11 | 12 | 0 | 0.015 | 84 | 0.33 | 1828 | Slight portal fibrosis, fatty degeneration, ballooned cells. |
| 3 | M | 4 | 5 | 0 | 0.03 | 62 | 0.15 | 1061 | Fatty degeneration, ballooned cells. |
| 4 | M | 14 | 14 | 0 | 0.02 | 25 | 0.23 | 1130 | Fatty degeneration, ballooned cells. |
| 5 | F | 9 | 9 | 0 | 0.02 | 36 | 0.11 | 1375 | Slight portal fibrosis, fatty degeneration, ballooned cells. |
| 6 | F | 3 | 3 | 0 | 0 | 19 | 0.15 | 1460 | Normal. |

*In case No. 1 ceruloplasmin was measured quantitatively; in other cases immunelectrophoretically. **Results of Ravin test are given in Ravin-units.

that an increase in dosage was required in order to maintain a negative balance.

3. During short test periods without penicillamine urinary copper excretion was found to be diminished when compared with results obtained before the beginning of the therapy.

Group 2 consists of six clinically asymptomatic cases (siblings of known patients with Wilson's disease, aged five to 16 years now).

The diagnosis was made during the course of family examinations when the children were three to 11 years old by using the following tests:

1. Determination of serum copper and ceruloplasmin concentration (directly or by Ravin test);
2. Measurement of urinary copper excretion without and with penicillamine;
3. Liver biopsy with histologic examination and chemical determination of copper; and
4. Liver function tests.

Table II shows the data on this group and the results of treatment. No patient had any neurologic symptoms. Slight hepatomegaly was found in two patients with minor increases in serum enzyme activities. Enlargement of the spleen and hematologic abnormalities were not noted. Only in case No. 2 was a questionable beginning corneal ring found.

The biochemical findings, however, were clearly pathologic, particularly the hepatic copper concentration determined by Dr. Sternlieb.

Abnormal histologic findings were present in all liver biopsy specimens except for those of case No. 6. The

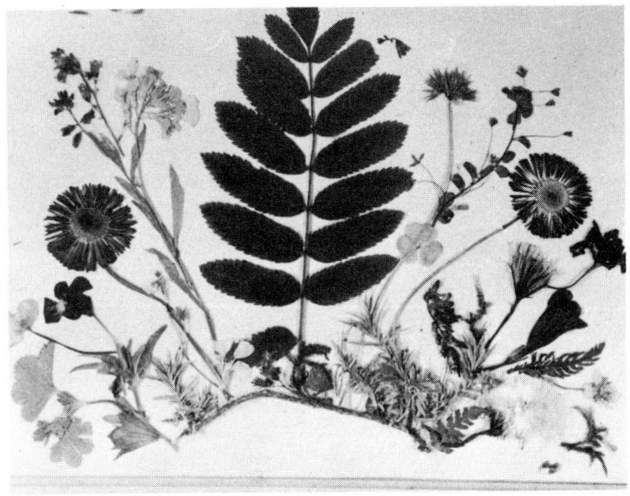

Fig. 1. Manual skill demonstrated by a recovered female patient (No. 11).

"ballooned cells," described by Anderson and Popper,[9] were detected in five cases with pathologic liver histology.

Treatment of the asymptomatic group was identical to that of group 1. Urinary copper excretion following penicillamine was not as high as in group 1, although decreases in serum and urine copper values were similar to those observed during long-term treatment. Nevertheless initial doses of 0.9 g of D-penicillamine daily could be maintained until the present.

During the two to five and one-half years of treatment, no clinical signs of Wilson's disease appeared in any of the asymptomatic patients. Corneal rings are not visible and physical development of the children

TABLE III

## Incidence of Wilson's Disease in 13 West German Families

| Family | Total number of children | Children with clinical Wilson's disease Alive | Dead | Biochemical health, siblings | Not examined |
|---|---|---|---|---|---|
| 1. Dal. | 3 | 1 | | 2 | |
| 2. Tan. | 1 | 1 | | | |
| 3. Däm. | 3 | 1 | 2 | | |
| 4. Ker. | 2 | 1 | 1 | | |
| 5. Hut. | 3 | 2 | 1 | | |
| 6. Den. | 6 | 3 | 1 | 2 | |
| 7. Pol. | 5 | 3 | | 2 | |
| 8. Schr. | 2 | 1 | 1 | | |
| 9. Bro. | 2 | 1 | 1 | | |
| 10. Ste. | 2 | 1 | 1 | | |
| 11. Krö. | 1 | 1 | | | |
| 12. Ack. | 3 | | 1 | 2 | |
| 13. Fre. | 3 | 1 | | | 2 |
| Total | 36 | 17 | 9 | 8 | 2 |
| | | 26 | | | |

continues normally. Biopsy of the liver showed marked improvement in case No. 1, some improvement in No. 5 and unchanged histologic findings in cases Nos. 2 and 4. In No. 3 liver histology seems to have worsened, possibly due to the irregularity of intake of penicillamine by the patient.

There were remarkably few side effects of treatment in our 18 patients. Only three children of one family living under poor social conditions and lacking parental care complained of gastrointestinal disturbances. In three cases serum iron decreased slightly requiring iron supplements. No disturbances of electrolyte metabolism were found. There was no need for mineral supplements.[10]

We didn't observe either allergic or nephrotic symptoms as recently described.[11,12] In one instance temporary leucopenia disappeared after discontinuing potassium sulfide. Some of our coworkers prescribe pyridoxine or nicotinic acid prophylactically although there is no uniform agreement concerning their value.

In addition, I would like to comment on some genetic aspects relating to our patients (Table III):

A family history could not be obtained in one out of the 18 cases. Therefore, an earlier patient whose siblings had undergone biochemical examination was included. In 13 families, 26 out of a total of 36 children suffered from Wilson's disease and nine of them were dead. Two children have not yet been examined. Most parents came from various regions of Germany, but some originated from a rural district where intermarriages are relatively common. Consanguinity was not found in any families for two generations.

The study of early stages of Wilson's disease demonstrates that storage of copper precedes the appearance of clinical symptoms. Copper storage therefore may be considered as the cause of the anatomical and functional lesions of the liver, in which histologic changes are found at a very early stage. In other organs (central nervous system, eyes, kidneys) copper is deposited secondarily and clinical symptoms related to these organs appear later. This is most evident with respect to the corneal ring which was not detected in any of the asymptomatic patients, although it is hardly ever absent during the advanced stages of the disease. Therefore, it cannot be regarded as an early sign of Wilson's disease.[13-15]

Additional evidence for copper-toxicity being the cause of the manifestations of Wilson's disease is the success of therapeutic "decoppering," which leads to complete recovery if organic damage is still reversible.

## *REFERENCES*


1. Walshe, J. M.: Wilson's disease. New oral therapy. *Lancet* **i:**25, 1956.
2. Wilson, S. A. K.: Progressive lenticular degeneration: a familial disease associated with cirrhosis of the liver. *Brain* **34:**295, 1911.
3. Lange, J.: Über den Klinisch asymptomatischen Morbus Wilson. *Dtsch. med. Wschr.* **87:**541, 1962.
4. Sternlieb, I. and Scheinberg, I. H.: The diagnosis of Wilson's disease in asymptomatic patients. *J. Amer. med. Ass.* **183:** 747, 1963.
5. Sternlieb, I. and Scheinberg, I. H.: Penicillamine therapy for hepatolenticular degeneration. *J. Amer. med. Ass.* **189:**748, 1964.
6. Lange, J.: Eisen, Kupfer und Eiweiss am Beispiel der Leberkrankheiten. Georg Thieme, Stuttgart, p. 53, 1958.
7. Scheinberg, I. H. and Sternlieb, I. The long-term management of hepatolenticular degeneration (Wilson's disease). *Amer. J. Med.* **29:**316, 1960.
8. Scheinberg, I. H. and Sternlieb, I.: Wilson's disease. *Ann. Rev. Med.* **16:**119, 1965.
9. Anderson, P. J. and Popper, H.: Changes in hepatic structure in Wilson's disease. *Amer. J. Path.* **36:**483, 1960.
10. Boulding, J. E.: Treatment of Wilson's disease with D-penicillamine. In *Wilson's disease: Some current concepts.* Blackwell, Oxford, p. 224, 1961.
11. Adams, D. A.; Goldman, R.; Maxwell, M. H. and Lotta, H.: Nephrotic syndrome associated with penicillamine therapy of Wilson's disease. *Amer. J. Med.* **36:**330, 1964.
12. Boudin, G. and Pépin, B.: Acidents rénaux dans deux cas de maladie de Wilson traites par la pénicillamine. *Bull. Soc. Méd. Hop. Paris* **116:**833, 1965.
13. Lange, J.: Zur Diagnostik und Therapie der hepatocerebralen Degeneration (Morbus Wilson). *Dtsch. med. Wschr.* **88:**896, 1963.
14. Lange, J.: Kupferstoffwechsel und Morbus Wilson. *Verh. dtsch. Ges. Med.* 70 Kongress p. 330, 1964.
15. Walshe, J. M. and Cumings, J. N.: *Wilson's disease. Some current concepts.* Blackwell, Oxford, 1961.

# Our Experience in the Treatment of Wilson's Disease with Penicillamine and Sodium Diethyldithiocarbamate

G. Boudin, M.D.* and B. Pépin, M.D.**

Ten patients with Wilson's disease were treated with penicillamine. One patient in whom penicillamine had to be discontinued because of the appearance of nephrotic syndrome, was treated with sodium diethyldithiocarbamate with good symptomatic response. Nephrotic syndrome was also observed in another patient treated with DL-penicillamine. While the effects of therapy on the central nervous system are clearly beneficial, long-term prognosis is limited because of the presence of liver disease.

Since our monograph of 1959[1] we have followed and treated ten cases of Wilson's disease: eight men and two women, from 14 to 42 years of age. In two cases the disease presented itself in a splanchnic form. In all cases diagnosis was confirmed by identifying a Kayser-Fleischer ring and demonstrating a deficiency of ceruloplasmin. Nine cases were treated with penicillamine alone at an average daily dose of one gram throughout the treatment. Patient eight was first treated with penicillamine,[2] then with sodium diethyldithiocarbamate (D.D.C.)[3] at a daily dose of one gram for one week out of two.

With respect to the penicillamine treatment, our experience confirms that of Walshe,[4] and Sternlieb and Scheinberg,[5] and, indeed, of most other investigators. Of our eight cases of the disease in its neurologic form treated with penicillamine, four had definitely improved, and two have been able to return to a normal way of life. One woman, over 40, resumed her post as a teacher and carried through successfully a normal pregnancy. Another of our patients underwent a serious orthopedic operation with general anesthesia. This patient's brother, however, suffering from an acute form of Wilson's disease, could not be cured. The last two patients in this series have only been treated for a few weeks.

Decrease or disappearance of the corneal ring after one to three years of treatment has been reported,[5] and was witnessed by us four times. No effect of penicillamine on osteoarticular lesions,[6] especially advanced ones, was noted. In both of our splanchnic cases we have noted that, though the hepatosplenic condition has remained unchanged, no neurologic sign has appeared after penicillamine treatment of one and two years, respectively. On the other hand, penicillamine treatment has

*Professor of Medicine, University of Paris and Clinique Médicale, Hôpital St.-Antoine, Paris.
**Professeur Agrégé (Assistant Professor), Faculty of Medicine, University of Paris and Clinique Médicale, Hôpital St.-Antoine, Paris.

## ABOUT THE SENIOR AUTHOR

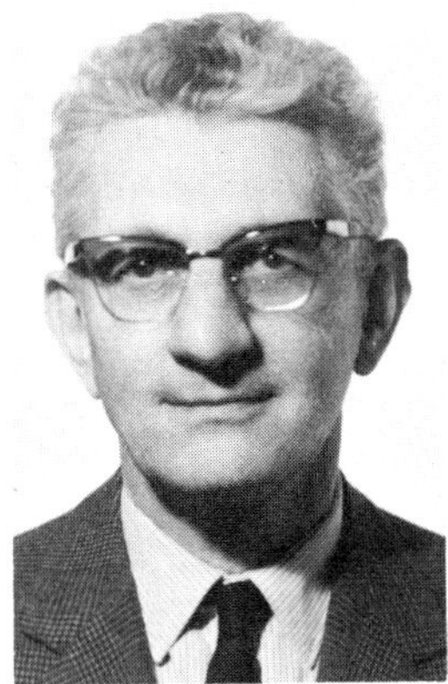

Professor Georges Boudin was born in Oyonnax (Ain) and spent most of his life in Paris. He received his training in Paris at La Salpétriere and at the Hospice de Bicêtre under Professors Alajouanine and Réne Moreau. He was Assistant Professor of Medicine in 1949. Professor Boudin has been Chief of Neurology Service at Hôpital St.-Antoine, Paris since 1954. He became Professor of General Pathology and Therapeutics at the Faculty of Medicine, University of Paris in 1960 and has been Professor of Medicine since 1963.

Besides Professor Boudin's long-standing interest in Wilson's disease (he published a book on it with Dr. Bernard Pépin in 1959) he has also studied neurologic manifestations of delirium tremens, of hypoglycemia, of syphilis of the central nervous system and the acute psychoses of epileptics.

led to renal complications in two cases: a reversible nephrotic syndrome in the first, and nephrosis and major renal insufficiency with tubular lesions, in a renal biopsy sample, in the other.[7] In both cases the nephrotic syndrome receded when penicillamine treatment was interrupted; but, in the first, death ensued because of fulminating hematemesis promoted by the corticosteroid treatment instituted against nephrosis. DL-penicillamine, a more toxic chemical for the kidneys than D-penicillamine, was used in both instances.

Our experience with D.D.C. treatment is limited to the one patient in whom we dared not resume penicillamine treatment after serious nephropathy had occurred. D.D.C. was well tolerated and effective, as our patient was able to lead a normal life through two and a half years of treatment, and even underwent a splenectomy one year ago, with splenorenal anastomosis. However, she has just died as a consequence of cirrhotic decompensation.

In conclusion, although modern therapeutics, and penicillamine in particular, have improved the prognosis in patients with Wilson's disease, this prognosis remains serious nevertheless, mainly because liver disease is far less influenced by treatment than is the central nervous system. This lays stress on the necessity henceforth to identify the disease at an early, and still asymptomatic stage, when preventive treatment may be applied.

## REFERENCES


1. Boudin, G. and Pépin, B.: Dégénérescence hépatolenticulaire. 1 vol., Masson, Paris, 1959.
2. Boudin, G.; Pépin, B. and Barraine, R.: Notre expérience du traitement de la maladie de Wilson par la pénicillamine. *Bull. Mém. Soc. Méd. Hop.,* Paris, **631:**114, 1963.
3. Boudin, G. and Pépin, B.: Essai de traitement de la maladie de Wilson par le diéthyl-dithio-carbamate de sodium. *Bull. Mém. Soc. Méd. Hop.,* Paris, **843:**116, 1965.
4. Walshe, J. M.: Treatment of Wilson's disease with penicillamine. *Lancet* **i:**188, 1960.
5. Sternlieb, I. and Scheinberg, I. H.: Penicillamine therapy for hepatolenticular degeneration. *J. Amer. med. Ass.* **748:**189, 1964.
6. Boudin, G. and Pépin, B.: Osteoarticular changes in hepatolenticular degeneration. In Walshe, J. M. and Cumings, J. N. *Wilson's Disease. Some current concepts.* Blackwell Scientific Publications. Oxford, p. 233, 1961.
7. Boudin, G. and Pépin, G.: Accidents rénaux dans deux cas de maladie de Wilson traités par la pénicillamine. *Bull. Mém. Soc. Méd. Hop.,* Paris, **833:**116, 1965.

# Treatment of Wilson's Disease

SHIBANOSUKE KATSUKI, M.D.* and MAKOTO OKUMURA, M.D.**

Three patients with Wilson's disease have been treated for three to five years with various agents, especially with BAL and penicillamine. Remarkable neurologic improvement was found in two patients. A marked decrease was noted in the hepatic copper content of one patient who failed to show neurologic improvement. Penicillamine was found to induce the most impressive cupriuresis and to be most effective in the long-term treatment of Wilson's disease.

In this report are described in detail three patients with Wilson's disease who received three to five years of treatment, and discussion of the effect of various agents, especially of BAL and penicillamine, on urinary copper excretion and clinical findings.

### Materials and Methods

The diagnosis of Wilson's disease was established by family history, neurologic examination, biochemical tests and liver biopsies. Electroencephalogram and psychometric tests were also performed. Kayser-Fleischer rings were confirmed by slit-lamp examination. Serial serum ceruloplasmin, serum copper level, and daily urinary copper excretion were determined. Urine was collected in plastic bottles. Changes in hepatic function during treatment have been followed by routine liver function tests. In two cases, liver biopsy was performed before and after the treatment for light microscopic examination and for determination of copper concentration. Copper was determined by a modified Braun-Scheffer's method[1] using sodium diethyldithiocarbamate and isoamyl alcohol. Serum ceruloplasmin level was determined by a modification of Ravin's method,[2] employing paraphenylenediamine as substrate; normal results ranged from 1.0 to 3.0 optical density units.[3] Ordinary hospital diet which contains 0.9 to 1.1 mg of copper per day (calculated from food tables) was supplied to the patients during hospitalization.

### Results

*I. (Case 14).* This female patient developed hand tremor at the age of 15 years. In January 1962, at the age of 17, she was admitted to our clinic. Examination at that time revealed Kayser-Fleischer rings, slight dysarthria, wing beating tremor in both fingers and hands and slight clumsiness in walking. Routine tests were all within normal limits. Microscopic examination of liver specimen revealed multiple copper granules in hepatic cells, but no cirrhotic changes.

Oral administration of 3.0 g EDTA daily did not result in a significant increase in urinary copper excretion.

*ABOUT THE SENIOR AUTHOR*

Dr. Shibanosuke Katsuki was born July 30, 1907 in Fukuoka Pref., Japan. He graduated from Kyushu University School of Medicine in 1930 and, after studying in Germany, became Professor of Medicine at Kumamoto University School of Medicine in 1950 and Professor of Medicine at Kyushu University School of Medicine in 1956.

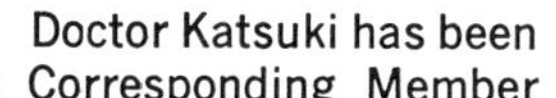

Doctor Katsuki has been a Corresponding Member of the American Neurological Association since 1960; an Honorary Corresponding Member of the American Academy of Neurology since 1966 and also since 1966 Corresponding Member of the German Neurological Society. He is presently Director and Professor of the Second Department of Internal Medicine, Faculty of Medicine, Kyushu University, Fukuoka, Japan.

*Director and Professor, Second Department of Internal Medicine, Faculty of Medicine, Kyushu University, Fukuoka, Japan.

**Senior Instructor, Second Department of Internal Medicine, Faculty of Medicine, Kyushu University, Fukuoka, Japan.

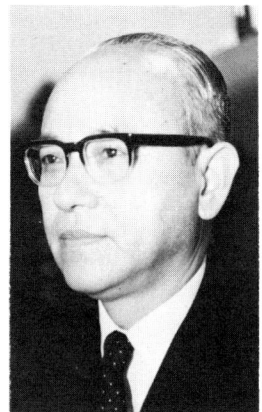

DL-penicillamine in a daily dosage of 0.4 to 1.0 g for three months induced marked cupriuresis with gradual improvement of tremors of all extremities. For seven months after her discharge in August, 1962 she continued taking 0.8 g of DL-penicillamine. She could even ride a bicycle and make a dress by herself again. However, because of difficulties in obtaining enough penicillamine in Japan at that time, another regimen had to be prescribed. On corticosteroids and antispasmodics the tremors returned in both limbs. One hundred mg of BAL (Dimercaprol) daily every other week was started in March, 1964, and was continued until January, 1966 with slight improvement of tremors. D-penicillamine was then added to BAL on alternate weeks in a daily dosage of 0.4 g. This regimen was continued until August, 1966, when she was readmitted for further examination.

At that time examination revealed much improvement in tremor and coordination (Fig. 1). Administration of 1.2 g D-penicillamine resulted in prompt and marked increase of urinary copper excretion up to 1.5 mg per 24 hours.

*II. (Case 19).* This 14-year-old female had jaundice and ascites for six months at eight years of age. At that time a diagnosis of liver cirrhosis was made. In 1962, dysarthria, salivation, difficulty in writing were noted, and she was admitted to our clinic in June, 1963. Her parents were first cousins.

Examination at that time showed hypersalivation, dysarthria, dysphasia, athetoid movement in fingers, increased muscle rigidity in both limbs and Kayser-Fleischer rings. Bromsulphalein retention was 7.4%.

Daily urinary copper excretion increased up to 1.2 and 4.4 mg following BAL and DL-penicillamine respectively. Histologic examination of her liver revealed normal structure although copper concentration was strikingly elevated (1.26 mg per g wet tissue). She remained clinically unchanged for the four months of her hospitalization. During the following eight months her symptoms progressed while no chelating agent was given. BAL was started in January, 1964, and D-penicillamine was added on alternate weeks in January, 1966. She was readmitted for further study in August 1966.

At that time neurologic findings showed no improvement, although hepatic copper content was markedly lower compared to the time of her first admission. Histologic findings did not reveal any significant changes, but large nodules on surface of liver were found by peritoneoscopy, suggesting the presence of postnecrotic cirrhosis. D-penicillamine produced marked cupriuria, although less than before.

*III. (Case 20).* This 22 year-old male student noticed tremors in his lower limbs in 1962 for which he was admitted to our clinic. Administration of DL-penicillamine induced remarkable cupriuresis with slight clinical improvement within one month. Because of difficulty in obtaining penicillamine at that time, ethinyl estradiol in

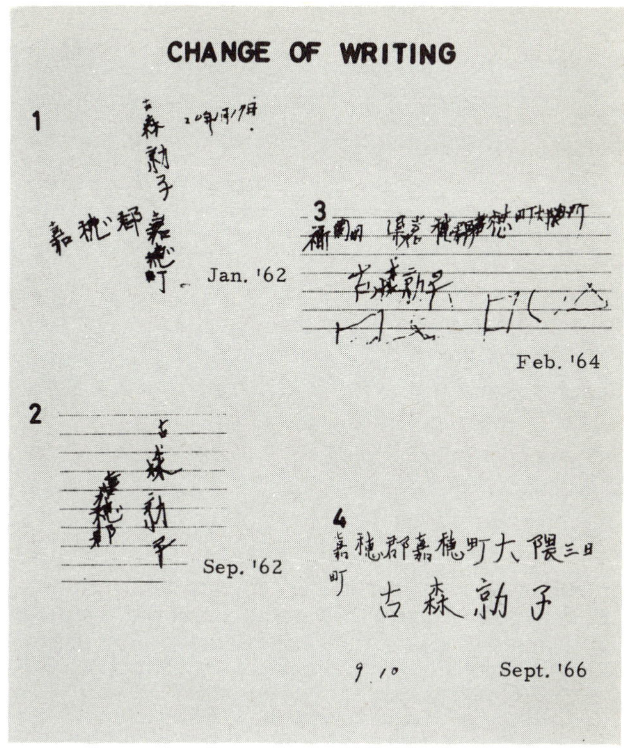


Fig. 1. Changes in handwriting during five years of treatment in Case 14.

**TABLE I**

**Effect of Various Agents on Urinary Copper Excretion**
**(mg/24 hrs.)**

| Case No. | 14 | 19 | 20 |
|---|---|---|---|
| Before Medication | 0.32 | 0.17 | 0.08 |
| During Medication (Peak) | | | |
| Betamethasone | — | 0.48 | — |
| Ethinyl estradiol | — | — | 1.07 |
| Ca-EDTA | 0.39 | — | — |
| BAL 100mg/day | 0.37 | 0.78 | 0.71 |
| 200mg/day | 0.73 | 1.27 | — |
| DL-penicillamine (1st admission) | 2.15 | 4.44 | 4.58 |
| D-penicillamine (2nd admission) | 1.86 | 2.07 | 2.19 |

a daily dosage of 0.4 to 1.0 mg was given during the following three weeks. This therapy induced a gradual increase of urinary copper excretion up to 1.07 mg per 24 hours and considerable cupriuresis persisted for several weeks after discontinuance of this drug, while serum ceruloplasmin concentration remained essentially unchanged and no neurologic improvement was observed. Following discharge, a regimen similar to that given to the two other patients was continued until his second

TABLE II

## SUMMARY OF TREATMENT RESULTS

| Case No. | 14 | | 19 | | 20 | |
|---|---|---|---|---|---|---|
| Duration of treatment (yrs.) | 5 | | 3.5 | | 3 | |
| | Before | After | Before | After | Before | After |
| Mental deterioration | + | + | + | ± | — | — |
| Dysarthria | + | ± | + | ++ | + | ± |
| Tremor | ++ | + | + | ++ | ++ | + |
| Gait disturbance | + | — | ++ | ++ | + | — |
| EEG abnormality | — | ± | ± | + | ± | ± |
| Copper Oxidase (u) | 0.14 | 0.16 | 0.09 | 0.09 | 0.01 | 0.06 |
| Serum Copper ($\mu$g/100 ml) | 113 | 62 | 52 | 54 | 29 | 37 |
| Urine Copper (mg/24 hrs.) | 0.32 | 0.06 | 0.17 | 0.08 | 0.08 | 0.05 |
| Liver Copper (mg/g w.w.) | | 0.22 | 1.26 | 0.15 | | 0.02 |
| BSP test (%, 45 min.) | 4.0 | 4.2 | 7.4 | 2.9 | 3.9 | 4.3 |

admission. At this time tremors in both limbs, clumsiness in standing and gait were all improved. Hepatic copper content was within normal limits, but peritoneoscopic and histologic findings suggested the existence of cirrhosis.

Results are summarized in Tables I and II.

Throughout the present study no untoward side effect, except transient gynecomastia during ethinyl estradiol treatment in one case, was recognized.

### Discussion

Oral administration of corticosteriods and EDTA produced neither significant increase in urinary copper excretion nor neurologic improvement. Ethinyl estradiol in the last patient induced considerable cupriuresis without beneficial effect on clinical findings. Injections of BAL promoted a moderate but steady cupriuresis in all patients, and some neurologic improvement was obtained in two cases by prolonged treatment.

The most striking cupriuretic effect and neurologic improvement were obtained by penicillamine. In the two cases (19 and 20) the initial cupriuretic effect of penicillamine was reduced to about one-half after long-term treatment. The cupriuretic effect of BAL was decreased in all three patients when courses of treatment were repeated. As explanations for the decrease in the cupriuretic effect, two possibilities have to be considered: increased tolerance to these preparations or depletion of body stores of copper.[4-6] A striking decrease in hepatic copper content was confirmed in one patient (case 19), and in one patient (case 20) hepatic copper was found to be normal after three years of treatment but in this patient the initial level had not been determined. Therefore, we prefer the assumption that the decrease in cupriuretic effect following prolonged treatment is caused by a gradual depletion of body copper stores. Yet in case 19, in spite of striking decrease in hepatic copper content her neurologic findings actually progressed during the three years of treatment. This patient probably had irreversible brain damage before the treatment had been started.

According to the observation of Tu *et al*[7] approximately one-half of the estimated dietary copper intake was absorbed in patients with Wilson's disease. To maintain favorable negative copper balance in our patients ingesting 0.9 to 1.1 mg of daily dietary copper, daily urinary copper output should be kept over 0.5 mg. Only penicillamine was considered to be satisfactory for this purpose.

### Summary

Three patients with Wilson's disease have been treated for three to five years with estrogens, corticosteroids, EDTA, BAL and penicillamine. Two patients responded favorably showing remarkable neurologic improvement. A marked decrease to one-eighth of the initial value was noted in the hepatic copper content of one patient who failed to show neurologic improvement. Penicillamine was found to induce the most impressive cupriuresis and to be most effective in the long-term treatment of Wilson's disease.

## *REFERENCES*

1. Braun, L. and Scheffer, L.: Über mikrophotometrische Bestimmung des Kupfers. *Biochem. Z.* **304**:397-403, 1940.
2. Ravin, H. A.: Rapid test for hepatolenticular degeneration. *Lancet* **i**:726-727, 1956.
3. Sasaki, S.: Clinical studies on serum ceruloplasmin. *Fukuoka Acta med.* **52**:195-227, 1961.
4. Richmond, J.; Rosenoer, V. M.; Tompsett, S. L.; Draper, I. and Simpson, J. A.: Hepato-lenticular degeneration (Wilson's disease) treated by penicillamine. *Brain* **87**:619-638, 1964.
5. Walshe, J. M.: Changing concepts of the pathogenesis of Wilson's disease. *Ann. intern. Med.* **51**:1110-1115, 1959.
6. Sternlieb, I. and Scheinberg, I. H.: Penicillamine therapy for hepatolenticular degeneration. *J. Amer. med. Ass.* **189**:748-754, 1964.
7. Tu, J. B.; Blackwell, R. Q. and Watten, R. H.: Copper balance studies during the treatment of patients with Wilson's disease. *Metabolism* **14**:653-666, 1965.